Healthcare Code Sets, Clinical Terminologies, and Classification Systems

Second Edition

Edited by Kathy Giannangelo, MA, RHIA, CCS, CPHIMS, FAHIMA

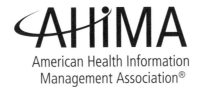

American Health Information
Management Association®

ISBN 978-1-58426-225-1
AHIMA Product No. AB201909

AHIMA Staff:
June Bronnert, RHIA, CCS, CCS-P, Reviewer
Jill S. Clark, MBA, RHIA, Reviewer

Claire Blondeau, MBA, Senior Editor
Cynthia Douglas, Developmental Editor
Katie Greenock, Editorial and Production Coordinator
Ashley Sullivan, Assistant Editor
Ken Zielske, Director of Publications

All information contained within this book, including Web sites and regulatory information, was current and valid as of the date of publication. However, Web page addresses and the information on them may change or disappear at any time and for any number of reasons. The user is encouraged to perform his or her own general Web searches to locate any site addresses listed here that are no longer valid.

AHIMA strives to recognize the value of people from every racial and ethnic background as well as all genders, age groups, and sexual orientations by building its membership and leadership resources to reflect the rich diversity of the American population. AHIMA encourages the celebration and promotion of human diversity through education, mentoring, recognition, leadership, and other programs.

American Health Information Management Association
233 North Michigan Avenue, 21st Floor
Chicago, Illinois 60601-5800

http://www.ahima.org

Contents

About the Editor and Authors

Kathy Giannangelo, MA, RHIA, CCS, CPHIMS, is a medical informaticist with Language and Computing, Inc. In this position she supports the ontology, modeling, sales, and product development activities related to the creation and implementation of natural language processing applications where clinical terminology and classification systems are utilized.

Kathy has a comprehensive background in the field of clinical terminologies and classification, with more than thirty years of experience in the health information management (HIM) field. Prior to joining L&C, she was director, practice leadership, with the American Health Information Management Association (AHIMA) in Chicago.

Kathy has served as senior nosologist for a health information services company and worked in various HIM roles, including vice president of product development, education specialist, director of medical records, quality assurance coordinator, and manager of a Centers for Disease Control and Prevention research team. Kathy has developed classification, grouping, and reimbursement systems products for healthcare providers; conducted seminars; and provided consulting assessments throughout the United States, as well as in Canada, Australia, the United Kingdom, Ireland, and Bulgaria. In addition, she has authored numerous articles and created online continuing education courses on clinical terminologies. As adjunct faculty at The College of St. Scholastica, she teaches the graduate-level course, Clinical Vocabularies and Classification Systems. In addition,

she is actively involved as a volunteer in the HIM profession at the international, national, state, and local levels.

Kathy holds a master's degree in HIM from the College of St. Scholastica.

Margaret M. Foley, PhD, RHIA, CCS, is a clinical associate professor in the HIM Department at Temple University. She has more than twenty years' experience in health information management practice. Prior to becoming a full-time educator, Margaret served as a director of medical records for a large acute care teaching hospital, a coding/reimbursement consultant and in various other administrative positions. Her research interests include birth certificate data quality, use of ICD-9-CM data, and the use of clinical terminologies in an EHR. She is also very active in various professional associations such as AHIMA and PHIMA.

Karen M. Kostick, RHIT, CCS, CCS-P, holds an associate degree in health information technology and is currently a product specialist for AHIMA.

Before joining AHIMA, Karen served as a reimbursement compliance specialist for the Department of Medicine at the University of Illinois at Chicago. Her areas of HIM specialization include acute inpatient, hospital outpatient, and physician provider coding, compliance and reimbursement methodology. Karen has also served as a clinical data analyst, coding manager, consultant, and HIM department manager.

Danielle Przychodzin, PharmD, RPh, is a clinical terminology specialist with the healthcare business of Thomson Reuters. In this role, she is involved in clinical decision support software development, management of the Thomson Reuters lexicon content, and provides expertise on the use of controlled terminologies within clinical decision support resources. In her previous role as a clinical content specialist with Thomson Reuters, she wrote drug information content for the Micromedex product and worked with interdisciplinary teams on new product development.

Prior to joining Thomson Reuters Healthcare in 2005, Danielle completed a pharmacy practice residency at Virginia Mason Medical Center in Seattle, Washington. Her current research interests are focused on the resource impacts of maintaining controlled vocabularies in clinical decision support tools.

Danielle received a BS in Molecular, Cellular and Developmental Biology from the University of Colorado in Boulder, CO, in 1994. She worked for several years as a research assistant in the areas of developmental genetics and human molecular genetics. She received a PharmD from Shenandoah University in Winchester, VA, in 2004. At present, she is enrolled in a master's program in biomedical informatics at Oregon Health and Sciences University, which she expects to complete in April 2011.

Daniel Vreeman, PT, DPT, MSc, is an assistant research professor at the Indiana University School of Medicine and a research scientist at the Regenstrief Institute, Inc. Dr. Vreeman earned a BA in biology from Cornell University and a DPT from Duke University. He completed a post-doctoral medical informatics research fellowship at the Regenstrief Institute while also earning a MS in clinical research. Dr. Vreeman's research interests are focused on improving healthcare through the use of information technology. In particular, he is interested in the role of standardized clinical vocabularies to support electronic health information exchange. He codirects the development of the international standard for laboratory and clinical observations, called LOINC, at Regenstrief. As an informatics investiga-

tor, Dr. Vreeman currently directs more than $3.5 million of extramural funding for projects related to clinical terminologies and medical informatics applications and collaborates on projects with $27 million of additional external funding. He also provides leadership and oversight to terminology services that undergird the Indiana Network for Patient Care, a regional health information exchange in central Indiana. Dr. Vreeman also teaches medical informatics at Regenstrief and Indiana University.

Judith J. Warren, PhD, RN, BC, FAAN, FACMI, is the Christine A. Hartley Centennial Professor of Nursing, the SEEDS Program Director, and coordinator of the graduate healthcare informatics specialty track at the University of Kansas School of Nursing, as well as the director of nursing informatics in the University of Kansas Center for Healthcare Informatics. Adapting electronic health record software, she developed, in partnership with Cerner Corporation, the Simulated E-hEalth Delivery System (SEEDS) to teach students how to analyze data from virtual patient case studies, simulations, and clinical experiences while developing informatics competencies. This system is now being used by fourteen other schools of nursing, one school of medicine, and one school of allied health. She is a member of the National Committee on Vital and Health Statistics (NCVHS), co-chair of its Standards Subcommittee, and member of the Executive Subcommittee, an advisory body to the Secretary of the U.S. Department of Health and Human Services on health data, statistics, and national health information policy. Dr. Warren is the past co-chair of HL7's Patient Care Technical Committee, an informatics standards development organization. She serves on the Quality Committee of the International Health Terminology Standards Development Organization (IHTSDO), which develops SNOMED CT (a leading multidisciplinary standardized terminology). Due to her knowledge of SNOMED CT, she was invited to be a member of an IHE team to develop the first profile that highlighted nursing knowledge and practice and focused on patient assessment. This team was so successful that IHE added a Nursing Subcommittee to their structure. She is a member of the organizing committee for the Nursing Terminology Summit, a member of the QSEN faculty, and consultant to TIGER. Dr. Warren is a Fellow in both the American Academy of Nursing and the American College of Medical Informatics. She has taught, published, and conducted research in nursing informatics since 1988. She is an ANCC-certified informatics nurse.

Ann Zeisset, RHIT, CCS, CCS-P is Manager of Professional Practice Resources for AHIMA. In her role, Ann provides professional expertise to AHIMA members, the media, and outside organizations on coding practice issues. She also authors and supports AHIMA online coding education, including the "Coding Basics" program, is a technical advisor for the association on ICD-9-CM and CPT coding publications, and the author of several books.

Prior to joining AHIMA in 1999, Ann served as director of Health Information/Utilization Management. Prior to this, she served in various coding roles, including coordinator of information processing, coding resource specialist, and coder. She has been an educator of coding and HIM for more than twenty years at multiple colleges. Ann has authored many coding-related articles and has presented numerous seminars and educational sessions on coding and other HIM-related topics throughout the United States, including many for Home Health professionals. Ann recently completed a one-year contract between the Foundation for Research and Education and CMS to determine potential impacts to CMS when converting from ICD-9-CM to ICD-10-CM/PCS coding systems. Ann is a frequent author and speaker on ICD-10-CM/PCS.

As a member of AHIMA, Ann has participated in various leadership positions. She has served on the Board of Directors for the Illinois Health Information Management Association, been the President of the Southern Illinois Health Information Management Association, as well as held offices and committee assignments on the regional and state level. Ann also helped organize the Coding Roundtable concept meetings designed to meet the local needs of coding professionals in Illinois and served two terms as the State of Illinois Coding Roundtable Coordinator. Ann was awarded the Distinguished Member award from SILHIMA in 2003 and the Certified Coding Specialist award in 2005.

Ann received an associate's degree in Health Information Technology from Belleville Area College in Belleville, IL, and a bachelor's degree in Organizational Leadership at Greenville College.

Acknowledgments

The authors wish to thank Ann H. Peden, MBA, RHIA, CCS, who served as external reviewer of the first edition of this text and provided excellent suggestions for its improvement. Ann is an associate professor at the University of Mississippi Medical Center.

In addition, the authors thank the following reviewers of the nursing informatics content: Claudia Bartz, PhD, RN, FAAN; Joyce Sensmeier, MS, RN, BC, CPHIMS; and Pawan Goyal, MD, MHA, PMP, CPHIMS.

Furthermore, the authors and AHIMA wish to acknowledge and thank the authors whose work they used as a base for this revision: Rita Scichilone, MHSA, RHIA, CCS, CCS-P, CHC; Mary Stanfill, RHIA, CCS, CCS-P; and especially Susan Hull, MPH, RHIA, CCS, CCS-P, who is missed by her friends, colleagues, and the HIM community.

Note to Educators

Each chapter of this book contains "Check Your Understanding" questions for discussion and/or to help the reader focus on important points within the text. The answers to these questions are provided in appendix A.

Application exercises and review quizzes also follow each chapter. The answer key for the review quizzes is contained with other resources in the instructor guide for this book. The instructor guide is available to instructors in online format from the individual book pages in the AHIMA Bookstore or through the Assembly on Education (AOE) Community of Practice (CoP). Instructors who are AHIMA members can sign up for this private community by clicking on the help icon on the CoP home page and requesting additional information on becoming an AOE CoP member. An instructor who is not an AHIMA member or a member who is not an instructor may contact the publisher at publications@ahima.org. The instructor materials are not available to students enrolled in college or university programs.

Foreword

by James J. Cimino, M.D.
Chief, Laboratory for Informatics Development
NIH Clinical Center
Senior Scientist, Lister Hill National Center for Biomedical Communication
National Library of Medicine
Adjunct Professor of Biomedical Informatics
Columbia College of Physicians and Surgeons

Healthcare today has never been more information intensive. Whether discussing improvements in quality, reduction of errors, reigning in of costs, or reaping the benefits of genomic discoveries, the underlying topic is always about information: collecting it, interpreting it, or bringing it to bear on problems. Computers, of course, can help immensely with such tasks, but in order to do so, the information has to be represented in a usable form. For most purposes, this means coding it using controlled terminologies. While healthcare informaticians have known this for decades, the rest of the healthcare community is only recently recognizing the importance of terminologies, and the need for standards.

Standards are critical, for example, for being able to collect data from disparate sites in order to merge them for population health studies. Standards also facilitate the development of systems for automated decision support, which must embody decision logic that is written in general terms (such as classes of drugs or patient conditions) but map to patient-specific information (such as particular medications or laboratory test results).

Some standards have been around for years, but were poorly attended to, while others have arisen more recently along with arguments for their acceptance. Yet, for the most part, these terminologies remained largely unknown or obscure. Developers of health information systems, collectors of data, and users of data sought out these terminologies, but often did not know where or how to get information about them. Even today, in the age of the World Wide Web, such information is hard to come by. Try, for example, to find out what the controlled terminology acronym GALEN stands for. Or see if you can find the ICD-9-CM disease table on the Department of Health and Human Services' Web site. If you somehow succeed, try to find the ICD-9-CM procedure table. Then try to figure out why it has multiple codes for the same terms (for example, 366.04 and 743.33 for nuclear cataract).

The fact is that proper use of controlled terminologies remains an obscure art, and this has been part of the reason for their slow adoption. It is still often easier for information system developers or data collection protocol designers to create their own controlled terminology, rather than trying to comprehend and deal with something that was "not invented here." This resistance persists in the face of changing national policy toward standards adoption, as articulated in the Health Insurance Portability and Accountability Act (HIPAA) and the recommendations of the National Committee for Vital and Health Statistics (NCVHS).

A national attempt to address the perfusion of standard terminologies has been the National Library of Medicine's Unified Medical Language System (UMLS), which brings together over 100 terminologies and makes them freely available. The UMLS makes many terminologies publicly accessible for the first time, but it does not explain what the terminologies should be used for or how to use them. And, in any case, understanding the UMLS itself presents additional challenges. As a result, adoption of controlled terminologies has progressed only slowly, despite 20 years of expansion in the UMLS.

The clear explanations of controlled terminologies, lacking in the UMLS, desperately needed by health professionals, health information management professionals, and health information system professionals, can be found at last in this book. Here, you can find clear definitions for terms that are all-too-often used interchangeably (and incorrectly), like "vocabulary," "terminology" and "classification." With clear definitions set forth, the book then proceeds to organize the available standards into those used for statistical and administrative functions and those used for clinical purposes.

Statistical and administrative functions have long been important motivators for coding health data, whether for reimbursement purposes or mandatory reporting. While we complain about their existence and their limitations, we should at least thank them for getting the healthcare industry on the road to computerization. The first section of the book provides detailed examinations of the history, structure, and use of each of these key terminologies in ways that could otherwise only be found in expensive, time-consuming tutorials and training classes.

Computer systems that serve administrative functions have often been adapted for clinical purposes, usually with mixed results. Consider, for example, systems that partition patient data according to visit, rather than make it available to clinicians in a longitudinal manner. As these systems have evolved to become more clinically oriented, they have developed needs for coding data at levels of detail not possible

with administrative terminologies. As a result, clinical terminologies that have lurked for decades outside of the mainstream of healthcare are finally getting appropriate attention, while others are being created *de novo* to fill gaps not covered by pre-existing terminologies. Many of these terminologies have their origins in the informatics research world and are therefore frequently described in the published, peer-reviewed literature. Nevertheless, trying to understand them from the published pieces is a bit like the blind men trying to describe the elephant. Within these pages, though, you will find eight chapters that bring together the published work on each terminology and organize them into coherent descriptions, again including history, structure and use.

Terminologies for electronic health records can be a dry subject if taken in the abstract. True understanding does not come until one examines the applications in which terminologies are used. An important bridge between standard terminologies and these applications is the set of standards used for storing and exchanging data; both of these topics are covered in respective chapters in the third section of the book.

Readers who master the first three sections will be ready to put all the pieces together. For this, they will need to understand how to access terminologies through the available terminology databases, such as the Unified Medical Language System (UMLS), and how the terminologies are actually used in healthcare applications. Both of these topics are covered in the final section.

This book covers a lot of ground. Its seven authors bring many years of experience with health data and health information systems to the table and have collected a thorough bibliography of published work that can serve as a secondary resource. Most importantly, they have brought together information that has heretofore been scattered and inaccessible to form a coherent whole. The result is a book that will be a valuable resource for anyone trying to understand the end-to-end chain of health information coding systems and their use in electronic health records: a book that is unmatched by any other current book or class.

Chapter 1

Introduction

Kathy Giannangelo, MA, RHIA, CCS, CPHIMS, FAHIMA

The coding of healthcare encounters has been one of the core functions of health information management (HIM) almost since the beginning of the profession. According to Sheehy (1991), many consider the function of identifying and organizing clinical data to be the essence of the profession. Given this observation, what better way is there to name and arrange medical content than through vocabularies, terminologies, and classifications.

The American Health Information Management Association's (AHIMA) Coding Futures Task Force studied the likely futures of HIM professionals in the domain of coding practice. The group concluded that HIM professionals must be educationally prepared to go well beyond the assignment of diagnostic and procedural codes and into broader areas of formalization that will ensure a leading position in the development of algorithmic translation, concept representation, and mapping among clinical nomenclatures and reimbursement methods (AHIMA 2000).

Today, HIM professionals deem the Health Insurance Portability and Accountability Act (HIPAA) standard code sets as the systems of significance for cataloguing diseases and procedures. These code sets include the following:

- *International Classification of Diseases, Ninth Revision, Clinical Modification* (ICD-9-CM), volumes 1–3

- Current Procedural Terminology, Fourth Edition (CPT®)

- Code on Dental Procedures and Nomenclature (CDT)

- National Drug Codes (NDCs)

- The Centers for Medicare and Medicaid Services (CMS) Healthcare Common Procedure Coding System (HCPCS)

In August 2008, a proposed rule was published to adopt ICD-10-CM and ICD-10-PCS to replace the ICD-9-CM when conducting standard transactions. A final rule published on January 16, 2009, adopted the ICD-10-CM and ICD-10-PCS code sets for all covered entities and set a compliance date of October 1, 2013. It is important to note that the compliance date must occur on October 1 in order to coincide with the effective date of annual Medicare inpatient prospective payment system (PPS) updates.

The final rule calls for adoption of ICD-10-CM to replace ICD-9-CM Volumes 1 and 2, including the official coding guidelines, for coding diseases, injuries, impairments, other health problems and their manifestations, and causes of injury, disease, impairment, or other health problems. Additionally, ICD-10-PCS replaces ICD-9-CM Volume 3, including the official coding guidelines, for the following procedures or other actions taken for diseases, injuries, and impairments on hospital inpatients reported by hospitals: prevention, diagnosis, treatment, and management. HIPAA-covered entities would be required to use these codes when diagnoses and hospital inpatient procedures need to be coded in HIPAA transactions. Because ICD-10-PCS codes are only used for inpatient hospital procedures, the ICD-10-PCS codes would not be used in outpatient transactions.

Although HIM professionals need to learn these key systems, they also need to become cognizant of and knowledgeable about many other vocabulary, terminology, and classification systems in order to prepare for the adoption of electronic health record (EHR) systems. Among others, these include:

- RxNorm

- Logical Observation Identifiers Names and Codes (LOINC®)

- Systematized Nomenclature of Medicine Clinical Terms (SNOMED CT®)

- International Classification of Functioning, Disability and Health (ICF)

In addition to broadening their perspective on vocabularies, terminologies, and classifications, HIM professionals need to understand data standards in a more global way. The Committee on Health Data Standards of the Data Council of the Department of Health and Human Services (HHS) states: "One of the biggest issues for health data today is the lack of shared data standards. The lack of shared standards increases paperwork and data collection burdens, and reduces the analytic potential of health data. Without consistent use of data standards, there is little ability to make multiple uses of or link data, which limits the usefulness of the HHS data to our public and private data customers and State partners, and vice versa. The need for shared health data standards encompasses the need for better agreement on common health data vocabularies, assurances of privacy, and other issues surrounding electronic transmission of information" (HHS Data Council 1997).

Moreover, an Institute of Medicine report titled "Patient Safety: Achieving a New Standard for Care" states: "At the most basic level, data standards are about the standardization of data elements: (1) defining what to collect, (2) deciding how to represent what is collected (by designating data types or terminologies), and (3) determining how to encode the data for transmission" (IOM 2004).

In the last several years, other organizations have been established and recently have been instrumental in data standards development and implementation. These include the Office of the National Coordinator for Health Information Technology (ONC), American Health Information Community (AHIC), Consolidated Health Informatics initiative (CHI), Healthcare Information Technology Standards Panel (HITSP), and Certification Commission for Health Care Information Technology (CCHIT). The Office of the National Coordinator for Health Information Technology (ONC) provides counsel to the Secretary of HHS and Departmental leadership for the development and nationwide implementation of an interoperable health information technology infrastructure.

AHIC began as a federal advisory body chartered to make recommendations to the Secretary of HHS on how to accelerate the development and adoption of health information technology. From inception, AHIC was conceived as an interim organization. During the transition period it was known as AHIC Successor, Inc. In 2009, the name was changed to the National eHealth Collaborative (NeHC). NeHC is an independent, sustainable public-private enterprise that brings together public, nonprofit, and private sectors into an organization for the creation and use of a secure, interoperable, nationwide health information system.

CHI was named as one of the Presidential eGov initiatives responsible for establishing a portfolio of existing clinical vocabularies and messaging standards enabling federal agencies to build interoperable federal health data systems. HITSP, a public-private partnership, is charged with the identification and harmonization of data and technical standards for healthcare. CCHIT is an organization dedicated to accelerating the adoption of interoperable health information technology throughout the U.S. healthcare system by certifying health information technology (HIT) products.

Two new official HHS advisory committees were established as a result of The American Recovery and Reinvestment Act of 2009 (HR 1). They are the Health IT Standards Committee and the Health IT

Policy Committee. The former committee will recommend technical standards, specifications, and certification criteria, and the latter committee will recommend policies for development and adoption of interoperable electronic health records and health information exchange to the National Coordinator.

This chapter provides a brief introduction to vocabularies, terminologies, and classifications and lays the foundation for the remaining chapters. Part I, Terminologies and Classifications Commonly Used for Administrative and Statistical Reporting, and Part II, Other Vocabulary, Terminology, and Classification Systems, supply further detail on the various vocabularies, terminologies, and classifications either currently in use or having the potential for use in an EHR. This material combined with that found in Part III, Data Standards for Healthcare, and Part IV, Application of Vocabularies, Terminologies, and Classification Systems, translates into a comprehensive textbook for HIM professionals. This chapter also establishes a framework for the entire textbook, whose purpose is to explain principles and applications associated with vocabulary, terminology, and classification systems for healthcare services.

Vocabulary, Terminology, and Classification Systems

Vocabulary, terminology, and classification systems are key to having the encoded data that users need to access, combine, manipulate, and share for various purposes.

Table 1.1 (see page 4) provides some reasons why vocabulary, terminology, and classification systems are needed in healthcare.

Definitions of Vocabulary, Terminology, and Classification Systems

Deciding on a definition for vocabulary, terminology, and classification is not as easy as it may sound. Although vocabulary and classification are relatively straightforward, terminology has various facets. The definitions for terminology, vocabulary, and classification are:

- A terminology is a set of terms representing a system of concepts.

- A vocabulary is a collection of words or phrases with their meanings, that is, a dictionary of those terms.

- A classification is a system that arranges or organizes like or related entities.

According to Paterno, Rynberg, and Giannangelo, what is essential in differentiating the terms is in knowing the domain in which each is employed:

- Clinical: pertains to the practice of medicine, particularly as it relates to patients.

- Reference: pertains to the terms of a field itself, such as medicine or disease; however, it is not limited to the medical field. An example in medicine of a reference would be SNOMED CT.

- Interface: refers to communication between two entities, one of which is usually an electronic system.

- Controlled: pertains to how the terms included in a vocabulary are bound or limited, such as ICD-9-CM (disease classification) and SNOMED CT (broader set of clinical terms) (Paterno, Rynberg, Giannangelo 2009).

One other related term, *ontology*, is also important to understand in the context of clinical terminologies for the EHR. An ontology in information science is a common vocabulary organized by meaning that allows for an understanding of the structure of descriptive information, which helps to facilitate interoperability.

In the HIT domain, a reference terminology is a set of concepts and relationships that provides a common consultation point for comparison and aggregation of data about the entire healthcare process. A reference terminology is a form of ontology. ICD-9-CM is not an ontology because it does not include clear definitions of terms, nor does it define relationships between terms. So, while it might be

Table 1.1.   Reasons for needing a vocabulary, terminology, or classification system

Function	Reasons for Needing a Vocabulary, Terminology, or Classification System
1. Access to complete and accurate clinical data	• Facilitates electronic data collection at the point of care • Possesses the ability to capture the detail of diagnostic studies, history and physical examinations, visit notes, ancillary department information, nursing notes, vital signs, outcomes measures, and any other clinically relevant observations about the patient • Allows many different sites and different providers the ability to send and receive medical data in an understandable and usable manner, thereby speeding care delivery and reducing duplicate testing and duplicate prescribing
2. Practitioner alerts and reminders	• Improves the quality of healthcare through the effective use of information found in other information management systems • Allows the computer to manipulate standardized data and find information relevant to individual patients for the purpose of producing automatic reminders or alerts
3. Clinical decision support systems	• Permits retrieval of relevant data, information, and knowledge for the purpose of generating patient-specific assessments or recommendations designed to aid clinicians in making clinical decisions • Provides data to consumers regarding costs and outcomes of treatment options
4. Links to medical knowledge	• Provides an organized system of data collection and retrieval, resulting in the linkage of published research with clinical care, thereby improving the quality of care through outcomes measurement
5. Research and epidemiological studies	• Allows the collection and reporting of basic health statistics • Ensures a high-quality database for accurate clinical and statistical data
6. Healthcare claims	• Provides data for use in designing payment systems and determining the correct payment for healthcare services • Identifies fraudulent or abusive practices
7. Public health	• Provides data for use in monitoring public health and risks
8. Management	• Makes available information for use in improving clinical, financial, and administrative performance

Source: MITRE Corp. Used with permission.

considered to have a defined vocabulary, ICD-9-CM does not include definitions for shared meaning. In contrast, SNOMED CT is considered an ontology because it includes both a defined vocabulary and defined relationships.

Even though there are slight differences in the definitions of terminology and vocabulary, the terms are frequently used interchangeably.

Differences among Vocabulary, Terminology, and Classification Systems

Considering the definitions, a vocabulary or a terminology provides a way to input clinical data into a record. That is, it is intended to cover a particular subject (clinical practice) and include the smallest details. The purpose of a classification is to group or categorize the details. A classification is designed to provide output and not to be used as an input device.

Table 1.2 shows some differences among vocabularies, terminologies, and classification systems based on the chosen goal and targeted user.

Data Sets and Data Interchange Standards for Healthcare

In addition to understanding the principles of nomenclature, terminology, and classification systems, HIM professionals must be educated in data set and data interchange standards. A portion of the professional definition of HIM is the statement

Table 1.2.   Differences among vocabulary, terminology, and classification systems based on the chosen goal and targeted users

	Chosen Goal	Users
Vocabulary or terminology	To facilitate electronic data collection at the point of care with terms familiar to the user	• Healthcare providers • Consumers
Vocabulary or terminology	To capture the detail of diagnostic studies, history and physical examinations, visit notes, ancillary department information, nursing notes, vital signs, outcomes measures, and any other clinically relevant observations about the patient	• Healthcare providers
Vocabulary or terminology	To allow many different sites and different providers the ability to send and receive medical data in an understandable and usable manner, thereby speeding care delivery and reducing duplicate testing and duplicate prescribing	• Healthcare providers • IS personnel
Vocabulary or terminology	To improve the quality of healthcare through the effective use of information found in other information management systems	• Healthcare providers • IS personnel
Vocabulary or terminology	To allow the computer to manipulate standardized data and find information relevant to individual patients for the purpose of producing automatic reminders or alerts	• Healthcare providers • IS personnel
Vocabulary or terminology	To permit the retrieval of relevant data, information, and knowledge for the purpose of generating patient-specific assessments or recommendations designed to aid clinicians in making clinical decisions	• Healthcare providers • IS personnel
Vocabulary or terminology	To provide an organized system of data collection and retrieval, resulting in the linkage of published research with clinical care, thereby improving the quality of care through outcomes measurement	• Data analysts • Quality management personnel • Utilization management personnel
Classification	To provide data to consumers on costs and outcomes of treatment options	• Consumers
Classification	To allow collection and reporting of basic health statistics	• Researchers • Epidemiologists
Classification	To ensure a high-quality database for accurate clinical and statistical data	• Data analysts • Researchers
Classification	To provide data that are used in designing payment systems and determining the correct payment for healthcare services	• Accounting personnel • Coding personnel • Billing personnel • Payers
Classification	To identify fraudulent or abusive practices	• Compliance personnel • Auditors
Classification	To provide data that are used in monitoring public health and risks	• Public health personnel
Classification	To make available information that can be used to improve clinical, financial, and administrative performance	• Management

that HIM professionals manage healthcare data and information resources (AHIMA 2001). To succeed in meeting this requirement, expertise in various types of data, data sets, and standards used in the exchange of data is needed. And although some data standards, such as the Uniform Hospital Discharge Data Set (UHDDS), have been in existence since the late 1960s, others have been created expressly for use in an electronic world, such as the Digital Imaging and Communications in Medicine (DICOM) standard.

Having standard vocabularies, terminologies, and classifications available means the numerous bits of data contained in the health record can be coded and shared internally and externally. But as HIM professionals know, not everyone needs exactly the same set of data. Data set standards exist for a variety of purposes. For example, the UHDDS is considered a core data set for hospital reporting. Vocabularies, terminologies, and classifications form the basis of all coded data sets and provide the data structure required for a fully interoperable EHR.

Data set standards, along with those required for the electronic exchange of data, also are evolving as the transition from paper-based records to an EHR occurs. Although HIM professionals may have heard of the acronyms *PCDS, HL7, DICOM,* or *NCPDP,* a broader understanding of these and other data sets and data interchange standards is necessary to understand how interoperability will happen.

Use of Vocabulary, Terminology, and Classification Systems in an EHR

According to the e-HIM Task Force report titled "A Vision of the e-HIM™ Future," the future state of health information is electronic, patient centered, comprehensive, longitudinal, accessible, and credible (AHIMA 2003).

In addition, the Institute of Medicine's 2003 report states that an EHR system includes the following:

- Longitudinal collection of electronic health information for and about persons, where health information is defined as information pertaining to the health of an individual or healthcare provided to an individual

- Immediate electronic access to person- and population-level information by authorized, and only authorized, users

- Provision of knowledge and decision support that enhance the quality, safety, and efficiency of patient care

- Support of efficient processes for healthcare delivery (critical building blocks of an EHR system are the EHRs maintained by providers and individuals)

The report also points out the need to clearly define a functional model of key capabilities for an EHR system. Health Level Seven (HL7), a standards-setting organization, has taken the lead in the development of an EHR functional model. In 2007, the EHR-S Functional Model Normative Standard (American National Standards Institute [ANSI]-approved) was published.

With this as the future of HIM, it is important to understand how vocabulary, terminology, and classification systems integrate into this electronic environment.

According to Amatayakul, "On a practical level for providers seeking to implement an EHR system, a controlled vocabulary would support a data structure that promotes standardization of terms. The vocabulary aids data capture, enhances database management, and helps build a data warehouse for use in executive and clinical decision support. The vocabulary also supports contributions to standard data sets, required either by law or for voluntary participation in research studies, registries, the development of clinical practice guidelines, and many other uses" (2007, 208). (In Amatayakul's book, the terms *vocabulary* and *terminology* are used as synonyms to mean a body of terms and their definitions.)

The practicality of usage of vocabularies, terminologies, and classifications within EHRs is tied to the applications that employ these systems (see figure 1.1). Thus, more than one vocabulary, terminology, and classification system is necessary to meet the needs of the applications that contain them. For example, multiple systems have been recommended as U.S. government-wide standards by the Consolidated Health Informatics eGov initiative and/or as core terminology standards by the National Committee on Vital and Health Statistics (NCVHS).

Following were the general criteria used by NCVHS to make its recommendations for the patient medical record information terminology standards:

- The extent to which the standard enables interoperability between information systems

- The ability of the standard to facilitate the comparability of data

- The aspects of the standard that support data quality, accountability, and integrity

- The degree of market acceptance of the standard

During a NCVHS Subcommittee on Standards and Security meeting in August 2002, Dr. James R.

Figure 1.1.   EHR concept overview

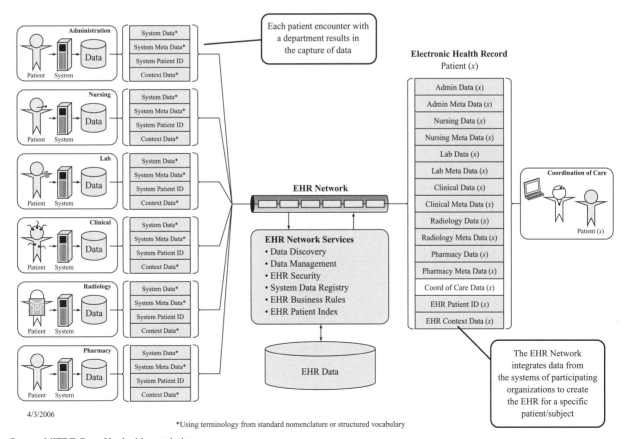

Electronic Health Record—Concept Overview

The EHR represents the integration of healthcare data from a participating collection of systems for a single patient.

4/3/2006

*Using terminology from standard nomenclature or structured vocabulary

Source: MITRE Corp. Used with permission.

Campbell presented a trilevel model showing the relationships of various vocabulary, terminology, and classification systems. He defined the layers as follows:

1. Core convergent reference terminology will deliver accurate patient records, improvement of clinical outcomes and decision support.

2. Modeled departmental, professional, and legacy terminology will provide for clinical system integration and departmental function.

3. Mapped administrative and financial classifications and codes will offer administrative and governmental reporting.

Figure 1.2 from the IOM report, *Patient Safety: Achieving a New Standard for Care,* is a modification of what Dr. Campbell presented at the NCVHS meeting.

In addition to NCVHS, the work of the Healthcare Information Technology Standards Panel (HITSP) in standards harmonization has resulted in the iden-

tification of not one but a suite of terminology standards. These standards are needed for the electronic exchange of clinical health information and as a requirement for interoperability. They use criteria for standards readiness against which to evaluate the systems before naming a standard for the use case under review. The Tier 2 Standards Readiness Criteria are:

- Suitability: The standard is named at a proper level of specificity and meets technical and business criteria of use case

- Compatibility: The standard shares common context, information exchange structures, content or data elements, security, and processes with other HITSP harmonized standards or adopted frameworks as appropriate

- Preferred standards characteristics: Approved standards, widely used, readily available, technology neutral, supporting uniformity,

Figure 1.2.   Relationships of various vocabulary, terminology, and classification systems

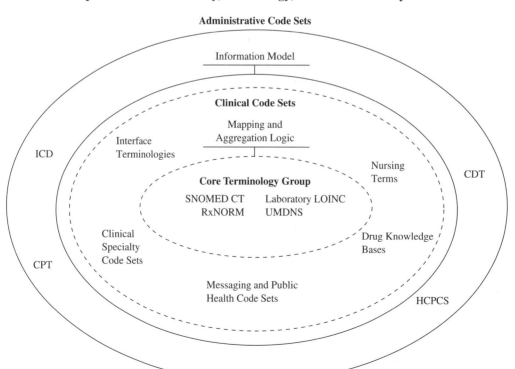

Source: Reprinted with permission from *Patient Safety: Achieving a New Standard for Care.* ©2004 by the National Academy of Sciences, courtesy of the National Academies Press, Washington, DC.

demonstrating flexibility and international usage are preferred

- Standards development organization and process: Meet selected criteria including balance, transparency, developer due process, stewardship, and others

- Total costs and ease of implementation (HITSP 2008)

With so many systems available, and some of them being quite large, a centralized location is needed in order to maintain consistent use. One such centralized database of vocabulary, terminology, and classification systems described in chapter 17 is the Unified Medical Language System® (UMLS®), a project of the National Library of Medicine. The UMLS's Metathesaurus® includes more than a hundred vocabularies, terminologies, and classifications, some in multiple languages. Many of the terminology and classification systems mentioned in this book are included in the UMLS. At an enterprise level, organizations are likely to have a terminology server which makes the encoded content usable.

As EHR systems evolve and mature, the capability of them to use standard terminologies also increases. A Gartner study in 2007 recommended organizations should consider the following depending on their EHR status (Hieb and Handler 2007):

- Implementing advanced applications: Make strong controlled medical vocabulary (CMV) capabilities a prerequisite before implementing advanced physician orders, clinical decision support, or clinical workflow functions

- Not yet purchased: Examine the current and planned CMV capabilities to ensure the EHR system will support the organization's strategic needs

- Current installation: Work with vendor to ensure the system's CMV capabilities continue to be enhanced so they will support the organization's strategic needs

Summary

Because the coding of healthcare encounters is one of the core functions of health information management, vocabulary, terminology, and classification systems have been integral to our work for a very long time. However, familiarity with what works in a paper-based environment, though necessary, is not adequate in an electronic one. Having better ways and means to understand, organize, and analyze health data will increase as the automation of health information continues. Many vocabulary, terminology, and classification systems will be necessary to meet the needs of the various electronic health record (EHR) applications.

In addition, to arrive at meaningful data comparisons, standard data representation of clinical and administrative information is necessary. Uniform data sets and standards for the electronic exchange of health record information results in the ability to send and receive medical and administrative data in an understandable and usable manner. Standard terminologies are a key element for interoperable EHRs.

Data sets are required for data capture, to enhance database management, and to help build a data warehouse for use in executive and clinical decision support. Moreover, to access, combine, manipulate, and share data for various purposes, data interchange standards are necessary. The encoded data for codified data sets needed for a number of uses and by a number of users requires more than one system. Therefore HIM professionals need to understand the differences among a vocabulary, terminology, and classification, the need for each, and how they can work together in an EHR.

References

AHIMA e-HIM Task Force. 2003. A vision of the e-HIM™ future: A report from the AHIMA e-HIM task force. Supplement to the *Journal of the American Health Information Management Association* 74(9).

Amatayakul, Margret K. 2007. *Electronic Health Records: A Practical Guide for Professionals and Organizations*, third edition. Chicago: American Health Information Management Association.

American Health Information Management Association. 2000 (January). A crystal ball for coding. *Journal of the American Health Information Management Association* 71(1).

American Health Information Management Association, 1999 and 2000 Committees on Professional Development. 2001. Health information management: Professional definition. *Journal of the American Health Information Management Association* 72(4):insert before p. 49.

Aspden, Philip, Janet M. Corrigan, Julie Wolcott, and Shari M. Erickson, editors. 2004. Patient Safety: Achieving a New Standard for Care. Report of the Committee on Data Standards for Patient Safety, Board on Health Care Services, Institute of Medicine. Washington, DC: National Academies Press.

Campbell, James R. 2002 (August 2). Letter to the chairman of the National Committee on Vital and Health Statistics (NCVHS).

Cook, Jane, Margaret Foley, Kathy Giannangelo, Marilyn Paterno, Rita Scichilone, and Kathleen Schwarz. 2009. Universal adapters: Terminology standards enable meaningful data exchange. *Journal of the American Health Information Management Association* 80(1):46–48

Department of Health and Human Services. 2008 (August 22). Proposed Rule on HIPAA Administrative Simplification: Modification to Medical Data Code Set Standards to Adopt ICD-10-CM and ICD-10-PCS. *Federal Register*. http://edocket.access.gpo.gov/2008/E8-19298.htm.

Giannangelo, Kathy. 2007. Standard Terminologies: Key Elements for Interoperable Electronic Health Records. Proceedings from the 15th Congress of the International Health Records Organizations.

Health Level Seven. 2007. Health Level Seven EHR-S Functional Model Normative Standard (ANSI-approved). http://www.hl7.org/ehr/downloads/index_2007.asp.

Healthcare Information Technology Standards Panel. 2008. http://www.hitsp.org/.

HHS Data Council. 1997. Committee on Health Data Standards. http://aspe.hhs.gov/datacncl/hdscmte.htm.

Hieb, Barry and Thomas Handler. 2007 (March 21). 2007 CPR Generation Criteria Update: Controlled Medical Vocabulary Capabilities. Stamford, CT: Gartner, Inc.

Institute of Medicine. 2004. *Patient Safety: Achieving a New Standard for Care*. Washington, DC: National Academies Press.

Institute of Medicine. 2003. Key Capabilities of an Electronic Health Record System. Letter Report of the Committee on Data Standards for Patient Safety, Board on Health Care Services, Institute of Medicine. Washington, DC: National Academies Press.

National Committee on Vital and Health Statistics. 2000 (July 6). Uniform Data Standards for Patient Medical Record Information. Report to the Secretary of the U.S. Department of Health and Human Services. National Committee on Vital and Health Statistics.

National Institutes of Health, National Center for Research Resources. 2006. Electronic Health Records Overview. The MITRE Corporation. http://www.ncrr.nih.gov/publications/informatics/EHR.pdf.

Paterno, Marilyn, Sally Rynberg, and Kathy Giannangelo. 2009. Terms for terms: A terminology guide for e-HIM professionals. *Journal of the American Health Information Management Association* 80(1):64–65, 69.

Sheehy, Kathryn H. 1991. Coding and classification systems: Implications for the profession. White paper. *Journal of the American Medical Record Association* 62:44–49.

Part I

Terminologies and Classifications Commonly Used for Administrative and Statistical Reporting

Chapter 2

International Classification of Diseases (ICD) and the U.S. Modifications

Ann Zeisset, RHIT, CCS, CCS-P

Learning Objectives

- To discuss the purpose and function of the International Classification of Diseases

- To define the uses of, and content similarities and differences among, ICD-9-CM, ICD-10, ICD-10-CM, and ICD-10-PCS

- To identify the developer, revision process, and guidelines for ICD-9-CM, ICD-10, ICD-10-CM, and ICD-10-PCS

Key Terms

Centers for Medicare and Medicaid Services (CMS)
Classification
Clinical Data Abstraction Center (CDAC)
Coding Clinic for ICD-9-CM
Cooperating Parties for ICD-9-CM
Department of Health and Human Services (HHS)
Health Insurance Portability and Accountability Act (HIPAA) of 1996
ICD-9-CM Coordination and Maintenance Committee
International Classification of Diseases, Ninth Revision, Clinical Modification (ICD-9-CM)
Morbidity
Mortality
Mortality Reference Group (MRG)
National Center for Health Statistics (NCHS)
Notice of Proposed Rulemaking (NPRM)
Prospective payment system (PPS)
Updating and Revision Committee (URC)
World Health Organization (WHO)

Introduction

This chapter discusses international classification of disease. Each classification is discussed in terms of how it was developed, its purpose, its content, its principles and guidelines, and the process for revision and updates.

International Classification of Diseases, Ninth Revision, Clinical Modification (ICD-9-CM)

The *International Classification of Diseases, Ninth Revision, Clinical Modification (ICD-9-CM)*, is a modification of the *International Classification of Diseases, Ninth Revision*, developed by the **World Health Organization** (WHO) in Geneva, Switzerland. ICD-9-CM is used in the United States to code and classify diagnoses contained in records from:

- Inpatient and outpatient hospitals
- Physician offices
- Long-term care and home health agencies
- Other healthcare encounters

In addition, ICD-9-CM (volume 3) is used to code inpatient procedures. ICD-9 has been clinically modified to meet the needs of the United States healthcare system.

Developer

WHO published the ninth revision of ICD (ICD-9), and the ICD-9-CM coding system was implemented in the United States in 1979. The Council on Clinical Classification developed ICD-9-CM under the direction of the **National Center for Health Statistics** (NCHS), which is the agency that maintains the coding system. ICD-9 was modified to meet the needs of American hospitals, and the intent of the modification was to provide a **classification** system for **morbidity** data. The clinical modification introduced a fifth-digit subclassification. The procedure classification (volume 3) is not part of the international version of ICD-9.

Purpose

Although diagnostic and procedural coding for statistics and research was the original function of the system, since 1983, ICD-9-CM also has been used to communicate information on healthcare services for the purpose of reimbursement. Today, coding for reimbursement is a vital part of healthcare operations in most types of facilities.

There are many uses of coded data, such as:

- Classifying morbidity and **mortality** information for statistical purposes
- Indexing hospital records by disease and operations
- Reporting diagnoses and procedures for reimbursement
- Storing and retrieving data
- Determining patterns of care among healthcare providers
- Analyzing payments for health services
- Performing epidemiological studies, clinical trials, and clinical research
- Measuring quality, safety, and efficacy of care
- Designing payment systems
- Setting health policy
- Monitoring resource utilization
- Implementing operational and strategic plans
- Designing healthcare delivery systems
- Improving clinical, financial, and administrative performance
- Preventing and detecting healthcare fraud and abuse
- Tracking public health and risks

Coded data are more widely used now than when the United States transitioned to ICD-9-CM in 1979. The system is outdated and needs to be replaced with a new, more robust classification system. ICD-9-CM is no longer able to respond to additional classification specificity, newly identified disease entities, and other advances. Many chapters are full, and it is estimated that the system will run out of procedure codes in appropriate, logical sections in 2009. This lack of detail in ICD-9-CM greatly restricts the data uses listed above.

Content

The official ICD-9-CM currently comprises the following three volumes:

- Volume 1, Diseases: Tabular List
- Volume 2, Diseases: Alphabetic Index
- Volume 3, Procedures: Tabular List and Alphabetic Index

The official ICD-9-CM is available only on CD-ROM from the U.S. Government Printing Office in Washington, DC. ICD-9-CM is not copyrighted, so many versions appear on the market. Although each product may offer special features, the ICD-9-CM codes themselves remain the same.

Code Composition

ICD-9-CM diagnosis codes consist of from three to five characters. The structure is three characters to the left of a decimal point and up to two additional digits to the right. All characters are numbers except for the beginning character in one of the supplementary classifications (discussed later in this chapter).

The procedure codes have at least three digits with a maximum of four digits. Two digits are placed to the left of the decimal, and one or two additional digits are placed to the right. The procedure codes are all numbers. (See table 2.1 for examples of ICD-9-CM code composition.)

Table 2.1.   Examples of ICD-9-CM code composition

ICD-9-CM Codes	Diagnoses
496	Chronic airway obstruction, not elsewhere classified
492.8	Other emphysema
491.21	Obstructive chronic bronchitis with (acute) exacerbation
ICD-9-CM Codes	**Procedures**
37.0	Pericardiocenteses
37.11	Cardiotomy

Volume 1: Tabular List

The Tabular List of Diseases and Injuries (volume 1) contains the following major subdivisions:

- Classification of Diseases and Injuries
- Supplementary Classifications (V Codes and E Codes)
- Appendices

Volume 1, Classification of Diseases and Injuries, contains chapters that classify conditions according to etiology (cause of disease) or by specific anatomical (body) system.

The Tabular List contains the following seventeen chapters:

Chapter Titles	Categories
1. Infectious and Parasitic Diseases	001–139
2. Neoplasms	140–239
3. Endocrine, Nutritional, and Metabolic Diseases, and Immunity Disorders	240–279
4. Diseases of the Blood and Blood-Forming Organs	280–289
5. Mental Disorders	290–319
6. Diseases of the Nervous System and Sense Organs	320–389

Table 2.2. ICD-9-CM subdivisions

Format	Description	Example
Sections	Sections are groups of three-digit categories that represent a single disease entity or a group of similar or closely related conditions.	ARTHROPATHIES AND RELATED DISORDERS (710–719)
Categories	Each three-digit category represents a single disease entity or a group of similar or closely related conditions.	710 Diffuse diseases of connective tissue
Subcategories	The fourth-digit subcategories provide more specificity or information regarding the etiology (cause of a disease or illness), site (location), or manifestation (display of characteristic signs, symptoms, or secondary processes of a disease or illness).	710.0 Systemic lupus erythematosus 710.1 Systemic sclerosis 710.2 Sicca syndrome
Subclassifications	The fifth-digit subclassifications provide more clinical or administrative detail.	008.61 Enteritis due to Rotavirus 410.01 Acute myocardial infarction of anterolateral wall, initial episode of care

7. Diseases of the Circulatory System   390–459

8. Diseases of the Respiratory System   460–519

9. Diseases of the Digestive System   520–579

10. Diseases of the Genitourinary System   580–629

11. Complications of Pregnancy, Childbirth, and the Puerperium   630–679

12. Diseases of the Skin and Subcutaneous Tissue   680–709

13. Diseases of the Musculoskeletal System and Connective Tissue   710–739

14. Congenital Anomalies   740–759

15. Certain Conditions Originating in the Perinatal Period   760–779

16. Symptoms, Signs, and Ill-Defined Conditions   780–799

17. Injury and Poisoning   800–999

Each chapter is divided into sections, categories, subcategories, and, when appropriate, fifth-digit subclassifications. Table 2.2 illustrates the subdivisions.

The codes in the Tabular List are arranged in numerical order in the appropriate chapters. Following is an example of a tabular entry:

603.0 Encysted hydrocele
603.1 Infected hydrocele
    Use additional code to identify organism
603.8 Other specified types of hydrocele
603.9 Hydrocele, unspecified

Fourth-digit subcategories have been expanded to the fifth-digit level to provide even greater specificity in some cases. Fifth-digit assignments and instructions may appear at the beginning of a chapter, a section, a three-digit category, or a fourth-digit category. An example of a code expanded to the fifth-digit level is 715.04, Osteoarthrosis, generalized of the hand.

Codes must be assigned to the highest level of specificity. Thus, a three-digit code cannot be assigned when a category has been subdivided and a fourth digit is available. Likewise, a four-digit subcategory cannot be assigned when a five-digit code is available.

Two supplementary classifications exist in addition to the main classification for diseases and injuries. Unlike the numeric codes in the disease classification, the supplementary classifications contain alphanumeric codes. Table 2.3 (see page 18) provides information about the ICD-9-CM supplementary classifications.

Table 2.3.   ICD-9-CM supplementary classifications

Classification	Purpose	Composition and Example
Supplementary Classification of Factors Influencing Health Status and Contact with Health Services (V01–V89)	Provided to deal with occasions when circumstances other than a disease or injury classifiable to categories 001–999 are recorded as diagnoses or problems. This may arise mainly in three ways: • Person is not currently sick, but needs health services • Person with known disease encounters healthcare for specific treatment • Person has a problem that influences health status but is not the reason for care	The codes are alphanumeric. They begin with V, followed by two numbers, a decimal, and then one or two numbers. V58.42, Aftercare following surgery for neoplasm
Supplementary Classification of External Causes of Injury and Poisoning (E800–E999)	Provided to permit classification of environmental events, circumstances, and conditions as the cause of injury, poisoning, and other adverse effects. These codes are never used in the primary position.	The codes are alphanumeric. They begin with E, followed by three numbers, a decimal, and then one number. E813.0, Motor vehicle traffic accident involving collision with other vehicle, driver

Check Your Understanding 2.1

Instructions: Complete the following exercises on a separate piece of paper.

1. The supplementary classifications of ICD-9-CM are:
    a. Alpha characters
    b. Numeric codes
    c. Alphanumeric codes
    d. None of the above

2. What is the maximum number of digits available in the diagnosis codes of ICD-9-CM?
    a. 3
    b. 4
    c. 5
    d. 6

3. What is the purpose of the Supplementary Classification of Factors Influencing Health Status and Contact with Health Services codes?
    a. When a person with a known disease encounters healthcare for a specific treatment, such as for chemotherapy or to have a cast changed
    b. When a person is not currently sick but needs health services, such as for vaccination
    c. When a problem is present that influences a person's health status but is not the reason for care, such as a history of an artificial heart valve
    d. All of the above

Volume 2: Alphabetic Index to Diseases

Volume 2 of ICD-9-CM is divided into the following three major sections:

*   The Index to Diseases and Injuries
*   The Table of Drugs and Chemicals
*   The Alphabetic Index to External Causes of Injury and Poisoning (E Codes)

Characteristics of each of the major sections are displayed in table 2.4. Figure 2.1 displays an example of the Alphabetic Index.

Conventions in ICD-9-CM

To assign diagnostic and procedural codes accurately, coding professionals must thoroughly understand the ICD-9-CM conventions. The conventions are defined in the ICD-9-CM Official Coding Guidelines for Coding and Reporting. Some of the specific conventions are discussed here.

Instructional Notations

Occasionally, instructional notations appear throughout the Tabular List to clarify information or to provide additional information. The following subsections describe the various types of instructional notes.

Figure 2.1.   Sample of the Alphabetic Index to Diseases

> **Prematurity** NEC 765.1
>   extreme 765.0
> **Premenstrual syndrome** 625.4
> **Premenstrual tension** 625.4
> **Premolarization, cuspids** 520.2
> **Premyeloma** 273.1
> **Prenatal**
>   care, normal pregnancy V22.1
>   first V22.0
>   death, cause unknown—*see* Death, fetus
>   screening—*see* Antenatal, screening
>   teeth 520.6
> **Prepartum**—*see* condition
> **Preponderance, left or right ventricular** 429.3
> **Prepuce**—*see* condition
> **PRES** (posterior reversible encephalopathy syndrome) 348.39
> **Presbycardia** 797
>   hypertensive (*see also* Hypertension, heart) 402.90
> **Presbycusis** 388.01
> **Presbyesophagus** 530.89

Includes Notes

Includes (or inclusion) notes are used throughout the Tabular List to further define or provide an example of a category or section. They usually list other common phrases used to describe the same condition.

The following includes note appears at the beginning of chapter 1:

INFECTIOUS AND PARASITIC DISEASES (001–139)

INCLUDES   diseases generally recognized as communicable or transmissible as well as a few diseases of unknown but possibly infectious origin

Excludes Notes

Excludes (or exclusion) notes are found throughout the Tabular List and are easily identified. Essentially, they should be interpreted as directions to code a particular condition listed elsewhere, usually with the code listed in the excludes note.

The following excludes note appears at the beginning of chapter 1:

INFECTIOUS AND PARASITIC DISEASES (001–139)

EXCLUDES   acute respiratory infections (460–466)
carrier or suspected carrier of infectious organism (V02.0–V02.9)
certain localized infections
influenza (487.0–487.8, 488)

Notes

Notes appear in the Tabular List and the Alphabetic Index in all three volumes of ICD-9-CM. Some notes carry an instruction to assign a fifth digit.

Mandatory Multiple Coding

Certain conditions require mandatory multiple coding. In such cases, one code describes the underlying condition (cause or etiology of the condition) and the other code identifies the manifestation(s). Mandatory multiple coding is identified in the Alphabetic Index with the second code listed in brackets. The first code identifies the underlying condition, and the second

Table 2.4.   Major sections of ICD-9-CM, volume 2

Section	Characteristics
Index to Diseases and Injuries	Includes terminology for all the codes appearing in volume 1 (Tabular List) of ICD-9-CM. The Alphabetic Index employs three levels of indentations: • Main terms • Subterms • Carryover lines
Table of Drugs and Chemicals	Reports substances to identify poisoning states and external causes of adverse effects. The table lists the poisoning code and several different E codes indicating circumstances such as assault, adverse effect, suicide attempt, accidental, or undetermined.
Alphabetic Index to External Causes of Injury and Poisoning (E Codes)	Classifies environmental events, circumstances, and other conditions as the cause of injury and other adverse effects

code identifies the manifestation or other condition that occurs as a result of the underlying condition. In such cases, both codes must be assigned and sequenced in the order listed in the Alphabetic Index.

In the Tabular List, the manifestation code acknowledges the need for multiple codes with the phrase "Code first underlying condition." The manifestation codes and the titles are listed in italic print. The codes in italic print can never be designated as the first-listed diagnoses and always require a code for the underlying condition to be listed prior to it. The mandatory multiple coding concept is illustrated in figure 2.2.

"Use Additional Code" Instruction
The instructional notation "Use additional code" is found in the Tabular List of ICD-9-CM. This notation indicates that use of an additional code may provide a more complete picture of the diagnosis or procedure. The additional code should always be assigned if the health record provides supportive documentation. If this instruction appears at the beginning of a chapter, it applies to all the codes in that chapter.

599.0   Urinary tract infection, site not specified
Use additional code to identify infectious organism, such as Escherichia coli [E. coli] (041.4)

Abbreviations
ICD-9-CM also contains abbreviations, some of which are listed here:

Figure 2.2.   Mandatory multiple coding concept

Alphabetic Index
 	
Diabetes, diabetic
   nephropathy 250.4 *[583.81]*
 	
Tabular Listing
 	
583.81   Nephritis and nephropathy, not specified as acute
            or chronic, in disease classified elsewhere
            Code first underlying diseases, as:
               amyloidosis (277.30–277.39)
               diabetes mellitus (249.4, 250.4)

- NEC (not elsewhere classifiable) is used with ill-defined terms listed in the Tabular List or with terms for which a more specific code is unavailable.

- NOS (not otherwise specified) is the equivalent of "unspecified."

Symbols and punctuation also have a role in ICD-9-CM and should be studied.

Check Your Understanding 2.2

Instructions: Complete the following exercises on a separate piece of paper.

1. Which of the following would be found in the Alphabetic Index to Diseases?
    a. Table of Drugs and Chemicals
    b. Appendices
    c. Classification of Disease and Injuries
    d. Supplementary Classifications

2. True or False. An includes note usually indicates that a condition is coded elsewhere.

3. True or False. When mandatory multiple coding is indicated, the manifestation code is listed in the index in brackets and should be listed in the second position.

ICD-9-CM Procedure Coding
Volume 3 classifies the procedure coding in ICD-9-CM and includes the Alphabetic Index and the Tabular List. Much of the same format is followed in volume 3 as in volumes 1 and 2.

Volume 3 procedure codes are used to classify hospital inpatient procedures. Hospital inpatient procedures are coded consistently when performed in the range of procedure code categories 00–86. Procedure codes outside this range may or may not be assigned based on hospital policy or whether they affect reimbursement.

The Tabular List contains seventeen chapters, and an effort was made to group similar procedures, such as operations on the endocrine system in chapter 3, categories 06–07. Because ICD-9-CM is out of room, procedure codes have been added to 00—Procedures and Interventions, Not Elsewhere

Classified. This chapter includes a mix of various types of procedures. Further, it is possible that any available codes will be utilized by unrelated procedures in the future.

Principles and Guidelines

Two departments within the **Department of Health and Human Services** (HHS), the **Centers for Medicare and Medicaid Services** (CMS) (formerly the Health Care Financing Administration [HCFA]) and NCHS, develop and maintain the ICD-9-CM Official Guidelines for Coding and Reporting. The guidelines should be used as a companion document to the official versions of ICD-9-CM.

The guidelines for coding and reporting have been developed and approved by the **Cooperating Parties for ICD-9-CM.** The Cooperating Parties are the American Hospital Association (AHA), the American Health Information Management Association (AHIMA), CMS, and NCHS. Published by HHS, the guidelines also have appeared in the *Coding Clinic* **for ICD-9-CM**, an AHA publication.

The purpose of the guidelines is to assist users in coding and reporting in situations where ICD-9-CM does not provide direction (although coding and sequencing instructions in ICD-9-CM take precedence over any guidelines). The conventions, general guidelines, and chapter-specific guidelines apply to the proper use of ICD-9-CM, regardless of the healthcare setting. A joint effort between attending physician and coder is essential to achieve complete and accurate documentation, code assignment, and diagnosis and procedure coding. The importance of consistent, complete documentation in the medical record cannot be overemphasized. Without such documentation, the application of all coding guidelines is a difficult, if not impossible, task.

It should be pointed out that the guidelines for coding and reporting are not exhaustive. The Cooperating Parties review the guidelines on an ongoing basis and develop new ones as needed. Users of ICD-9-CM should be aware that only guidelines approved by the Cooperating Parties are official. Revision of the guidelines and new guidelines are published by HHS after the Cooperating Parties have approved them. The Official Coding Guidelines currently are divided in four sections, as shown in table 2.5 (see page 22). The ICD-9-CM Official Guidelines for Coding and Reporting are available at http://www.cdc.gov/nchs/datawh/ftpserv/ftpicd9/ftpicd9.htm#guidelines.

Process for Revision and Updates

Changes and updates to ICD-9-CM are managed by the **ICD-9-CM Coordination and Maintenance (C&M) Committee,** a federal committee established in 1985 and cochaired by representatives from NCHS and CMS. ICD-9-CM undergoes biannual updates in the United States to remain current. An Official Authorized Addendum documents the changes. The official addenda for volumes 1 and 2 are available at http://www.cdc.gov/nchs/datawh/ftpserv/ftpicd9/ftpicd9.htm and for volume 3 at http://www.cms.hhs.gov/ICD9ProviderDiagnostic Codes/.

NCHS is responsible for maintaining the diagnosis classification (volumes 1 and 2); CMS is responsible for maintaining the procedure classification (volume 3). AHIMA and the AHA give advice and assistance, as do health information management (HIM) practitioners, physicians, and other users of ICD-9-CM. C&M Committee meetings are open to the public, and the discussion topics are available at http://www.cdc.gov/nchs/about/otheract/icd9/maint/maint.htm.

Check Your Understanding 2.3

Instructions: Complete the following exercises on a separate piece of paper.

1. True or False. NCHS is responsible for updating the diagnosis classification of ICD-9-CM.

2. True or False. Volume 3 of ICD-9-CM is not part of the international version of ICD-9 and is used only in the United States.

Table 2.5.   Sections of the ICD-9-CM Official Guidelines for Coding and Reporting

Section	Title	Content and Uses
I	ICD-9-CM conventions, general coding guidelines, and chapter-specific guidelines	Used by all regardless of setting Contains three parts A: ICD-9-CM conventions; B: General coding guidelines; C: Chapter-specific guidelines
II	Selection of principal diagnosis	Used by those covered by the Uniform Hospital Discharge Data Set (UHDDS) guidelines. This includes all inpatient and nonoutpatient settings (acute care, short-term, long-term care, and psychiatric hospitals; home health agencies; rehab facilities; nursing homes; and so on.). Provides information on sequencing and reporting
III	Reporting additional diagnoses	Used by those covered by the Uniform Hospital Discharge Data Set (UHDDS) guidelines. This includes all inpatient and nonoutpatient settings (acute care, short-term care, long-term care, and psychiatric hospitals; home health agencies; rehab facilities; nursing homes; and so on.). Provides information on abnormal findings, general rules, previous conditions, and uncertain diagnoses
IV	Diagnostic coding and reporting guidelines for outpatient services	Used by hospital-based outpatient services and provider-based office visits
Appendix I	Present on Admission (POA) Reporting Guidelines	

Source: NCHS, ICD-9-CM Official Guidelines for Coding and Reporting.

3. True or False. The third volume of ICD-9-CM contains the tabular and alphabetic lists of diseases.

4. Indicate disease (D) or procedure (P) for the following codes.
   - a. 496
   - b. 250.02
   - c. 51.88
   - d. 051.9
   - e. 15.3
   - f. 616.0
   - g. 00.02

International Statistical Classification of Diseases and Related Health Problems, Tenth Revision (ICD-10)

Development of the tenth revision of ICD began in 1983. Volume 1, Tabular List, was first published in 1992, followed by volume 2, Instruction Manual, in 1993, and volume 3, Alphabetic Index, in 1994. The Forty-third World Health Assembly endorsed

ICD-10 in May 1990, and the system came into use by WHO Member States in 1994. Many countries around the world have implemented ICD-10 for reporting mortality statistics, including the United States in 1999. The United States is bound by international treaty to report mortality data to WHO using ICD-10 codes.

Some of these same countries use ICD-10 to report morbidity data; others have chosen to modify ICD-10. Clinically modified systems have been implemented in both Australia (ICD-10-AM) and Canada (ICD-10 -CA). A great deal of information is available on the Internet about both of these coding systems as well as about ICD-10, ICD-10-CM, and ICD-10-PCS. A search would generate too many sources to list in this chapter, but performing such a search would be advantageous and would yield a great many topics to supplement the students' knowledge about these classification systems. One important Web site discusses ICD-10 at http:// www.who.int/classifications/icd/en/.

ICD-10 has not yet been implemented for morbidity in the United States, but a clinical modification has been developed and is discussed in detail later in this chapter.

Developer

ICD-10 is a collaborative product among WHO and ten international centers, although WHO holds the copyright. It is a statistical classification, hierarchical in structure.

ICD was developed in the early twentieth century as a way to collect data on the causes of death. As revisions were developed, it became increasingly evident that classifications needed to be considered from a broader perspective. It was recognized that the classification of sickness and injury was closely linked with the classification of causes of death.

ICD-10 provides many more categories for disease and other health-related conditions than previous revisions through its alphanumeric coding scheme. In addition, it includes chapter rearrangements, additions and revisions, and extensive changes to the mental and behavioral disorders (chapter V), the injury, poisoning, and certain other consequences of external causes (chapter XIX), and the external causes of morbidity and mortality (chapter XX). It also includes additional categories for postprocedural disorders.

Today, ICD-10 is used to record both mortality and morbidity data by many countries. The United States is the only industrialized country which has not implemented ICD-10 for morbidity reporting. Having an international coding system provides a way in which data can be collected, analyzed, interpreted, and compared.

Purpose

A classification of diseases can be defined as a "system of categories to which morbid entities are assigned according to established criteria." The purpose of ICD is to permit the systematic recording, analysis, interpretation, and comparison of mortality and morbidity data collected in different countries. The classification system then is used to translate diagnoses and diseases and other health problems from words into codes. This translation permits easy reporting, storage, retrieval, and analysis of data (ICD-10, Volume 2, Second Edition).

ICD has become the international, standard diagnostic classification for all general epidemiological and many health management purposes.

The most current version of the Tabular List of ICD-10 is available online at: http://www.who.int/classifications/apps/icd/icd10online.

Content

The content of ICD-10 is examined below in terms of the classification system's general structure, components, new features, and coding conventions.

General Structure

Although the collaborating centers discussed a different structure and evaluated other models after the ninth revision, the tenth revision maintains the long-established arrangement for morbidity and mortality statistics. This variable-axis classification places diseases, disorders, injuries, and other reasons for a patient to receive healthcare services into chapters according to what is most appropriate for general epidemiological purposes. This method influences the way diseases are grouped in ICD-10. The five ways are:

- Epidemic diseases

- Constitutional or general diseases

- Local diseases arranged by site (the body system chapters)

- Development diseases

- Injuries

Four of the five groupings are considered "special." The exception is local diseases arranged by site. The special groups bring together disorders that, for epidemiological study, make sense to be placed together rather than classified mainly by anatomical site. In other words, the conditions are assigned principally to one of the four special-group chapters, which have priority over the body system chapters.

In order to assign codes and interpret statistics properly, it is important to keep this in mind.

Structural Components

ICD-10 is divided into three volumes, consists of twenty-one chapters, and uses alphanumeric codes, described in the following subsections.

The Volumes

Volume 1, Tabular List, contains an alphanumeric listing of ICD-10 codes arranged by chapter. It also includes notes and other coding instructions. Volume 2, Instruction Manual, contains background information, instructional materials on how to use volumes 1 and 3, and rules and guidelines for mortality and morbidity coding. Volume 3, Alphabetic Index, is the alphabetical index to the diseases, disorders, injuries, and other conditions found in volume 1. Volume 1 also contains instructions on how to use the index. The Instruction Manual is available online at: http://www.who.int/classifications/icd/ICD-10_2nd_ed_volume2.pdf.

The Chapters

ICD-10 has four more chapters than the ninth revision, which contained seventeen chapters and two supplemental classifications. The tenth edition has separate chapters for diseases of the nervous system (VI), diseases of the eye and adnexa (VII), and diseases of the ear and mastoid process (VIII). Moreover, ICD-10 does not separate the codes that explain the external causes of injury and poisoning (E codes in ICD-9) and the factors influencing health status and contact with health services (V codes in ICD-9) from the core classification.

Since the ICD-10 codes begin with an alpha character, many of the chapters begin with a new letter. It is important to keep in mind that some chapters use more than one letter and some chapters share a letter. For example,

Chapter II, Neoplasms (C00–D48)

Chapter III, Diseases of the blood and blood-forming organs and certain disorders involving the immune mechanism (D50–D89)

Chapter XIX, Injury, poisoning and certain other consequences of external causes (S00–T98)

The order and content of the ICD-10 chapters has changed as well. The ICD-10 codes for diseases of the skin and subcutaneous tissue (XII) and diseases of the musculoskeletal system and connective tissue (XIII) follow the chapter on diseases of the digestive system. Next are chapters for diseases of the genitourinary system (XIV), pregnancy, childbirth, and the puerperium (XV), certain conditions originating in the perinatal period (XVI), and congenital malformations, deformations, and chromosomal abnormalities (XVII). Disorders involving the immune mechanism are included with diseases of the blood and blood-forming organs (III).

Category restructuring and code reorganization have occurred in a number of ICD-10 chapters, which has resulted in the classification of certain diseases and disorders differently from the ninth revision. For example, Streptococcal sore throat and its inclusion terms found in the infectious and parasitic disease chapter of ICD-9 are reclassified in ICD-10 to chapter X, Diseases of the Respiratory System.

The Codes

To serve a wider variety of needs for reporting mortality and healthcare data, the tenth revision has implemented a completely alphanumeric coding scheme. The first character is a letter. All the letters of the alphabet are used with the exception of the letter *U,* which has been set aside by WHO for the provisional assignment of new diseases of uncertain etiology (U00–U49) or for Bacterial agents resistant to antibiotics (U80–U89). For example, category U04 has been assigned to severe acute respiratory syndrome (SARS). When this condition is better understood, a code (or codes) will be created to classify this condition to the appropriate ICD-10 chapter.

The code letter is followed by two numbers. Each code must have the first three characters, followed by a decimal point, followed by additional characters if needed.

C19	Malignant neoplasm of rectosigmoid junction
I50.0	Congestive heart failure
S02.10	Fracture of base of skull, closed

Check Your Understanding 2.4

Instructions: Complete the following exercises on a separate piece of paper.

1. True or False. ICD-10 codes are numeric.

2. True or False. The United States uses ICD-10 for reporting mortality statistics.

3. True or False. ICD-10 is not copyrighted.

New Features

Some of the other new features of ICD-10 are:

- *Exclusion notes:* These notes have been expanded at the beginning of each chapter to clarify the hierarchy of the chapters. As explained previously, the special-group chapters have priority over the organ or system chapters. In addition, the chapters for pregnancy, childbirth, and the puerperium (XV) and certain conditions originating in the perinatal period (XVI) take precedence over the other special-group chapters.

- *Blocks:* Chapters are further subdivided into blocks of three-character categories. To explain the chapter structure, the beginning of each chapter contains a listing of blocks and, where applicable, the asterisk categories.

- *Notes:* The notes in the Tabular List apply to both mortality and morbidity use. Rules specific to one or the other are found in volume 2.

- *Drug-induced conditions:* What began with the ninth revision regarding the identification of drug-induced conditions has been expanded in the tenth revision.

- *Postprocedural disorders:* ICD-10 contains new categories placed toward the end of the body system chapters for intraoperative and postprocedural complications.

- *Complete titles:* Each ICD-10 code title is complete. In ICD-9, only a portion of the description appeared in the title, requiring users to review subcategory or category titles to gain a complete understanding of the code's meaning.

- *Etiology and manifestation:* The asterisk codes (manifestations) are found in specific three-character categories, resulting in less confusion on their appropriate use in conjunction with the dagger codes (etiology).

Conventions Used in ICD-10

Like its predecessors, ICD-10 contains conventions that must be understood and used, where necessary, in order to properly use the classification and assign accurate codes. Following is a summary of those found in the Tabular List and Alphabetic Index.

Instructional Terms and Notes

Terms or notes providing information or instructions are found either at the beginning of a chapter or a block or after a three-, four-, or five-character code. Their position is important in that the terms or notes that appear at the beginning of a chapter apply to all the categories in the chapter. The same rule applies to terms or notes found at the block or code level. Following are some examples of the various types of instructional notes and terms found in ICD-10:

- Inclusion and exclusion terms

  K31 Other diseases of stomach and duodenum

  Includes: functional disorders of stomach

  Excludes: diverticulum of duodenum (K57.0–K57.1)

  gastrointestinal haemorrhage (K92.0–K92.2)

- Includes notes and exclusion notes

  Mental and behavioral disorders (F00–F99)

      Includes: disorders of psychological development

      Excludes: symptoms, signs and abnormal clinical and laboratory findings, not elsewhere classified (R00–R99)

- Use additional code

      N34   Urethritis and urethral syndrome Use additional code (B95–B97),if desired, to identify infectious agent.

Punctuation Marks

ICD-10 uses the following punctuation marks for the purposes stated:

- Parentheses ( ) enclose supplementary words, a code contained in an excludes note, a code range for a block, or a dagger or asterisk code in the Tabular List. Parentheses are used in the Alphabetic Index to enclose nonessential modifiers, cross-referenced terms, or morphology codes.

- Square brackets [ ] are used to enclose a note or pages and direct the user elsewhere. They also are used to enclose synonyms, alternative words, and explanatory phrases.

- Colons indicate that one of the modifying terms after the main term (that is, the condition listed above the colon) is required before the code can be assigned.

- Braces { } are used to identify incomplete terms. The terms may precede or follow the brace. One or more of the terms after the brace complete or qualify the terms before the brace.

- A dash is used in both the ICD-10 index and the Tabular List. The index uses the dash to show the level of indentation. In the Tabular List, a dash preceded by a decimal point (.–) indicates an incomplete code.

  Examples:

      K63.1   Perforation of intestine (nontraumatic)

      B20   Human immunodeficiency virus [HIV] disease resulting in infectious and parasitic diseases

      C48   Malignant neoplasm of retroperitoneum and peritoneum

          Excludes: Kaposi's sarcoma (C46.1)

               Mesothelioma (C45. –)

Abbreviations

The abbreviation *NEC* stands for not elsewhere classified. A residual category, subdivision, or subclassification provides a location for "other" types of specified conditions that have not been classified elsewhere.

The abbreviation *NOS* stands for not otherwise specified. The unspecified or NOS codes are available for use when documentation of the condition identified by the provider is not specific to the defined axis.

Examples:

    Granuloma

        foreign body (in soft tissue) NEC M60.2

    R07.3 Other chest pain

        Anterior chest-wall pain NOS

Relational Terms

ICD-10 contains the following types of relational terms:

- *And:* When the term *and* is contained in code titles, it should be interpreted to mean and/or.

- *With, with mention of, associated with, in:* These terms join together conditions. The combination must be present to assign the code; however, an indication of a cause-and-effect relationship is unnecessary.

- *Without, not associated with:* These terms indicate that the two conditions should not be present together. When both conditions are present, a different code should be selected.

- *Due to, resulting in:* The cause-and-effect relationship should be clear from the documentation. In some cases, however, ICD-10 presumes a cause-and-effect relationship.

Examples:

C41.3	Malignant neoplasm of ribs, sternum and clavicle
E50.5	Vitamin A deficiency with night blindness
H33.3	Retinal breaks without detachment
J15.2	Pneumonia due to staphylococcus

Check Your Understanding 2.5

Instructions: Complete the following exercises on a separate piece of paper.

1. The chapters in ICD-10 are divided into _____ of three-character categories.

2. Which symbol directs the user elsewhere or encloses synonyms?
   a. :
   b. –
   c. { }
   d. [ ]

3. True or False. Parentheses ( ) enclose a code range for a block.

Dagger (etiology) and Asterisk (manifestation)
As in the ninth revision, a dual-classification system is available for the identification of the etiology or underlying cause and the manifestation of certain disease. In ICD-10, the dagger symbol (†) follows the code for the underlying disease, and the asterisk symbol (*) is placed after the optional code for the manifestation.

Lead Terms
The Alphabetic Index to Diseases and Nature of Injury, the Table of Neoplasms, the External Causes of Injury Index, and the Table of Drugs and Chemicals are organized in ICD-10 by lead terms describing the disease condition, other reason for an encounter with the healthcare provider, or the underlying cause or means of an injury.

Modifiers or Qualifiers
Descriptors, essential and nonessential modifiers, that further specify the lead term may be listed as subterms or in parentheses.

Cross-References
The Alphabetic Index contains the following cross-references: *see* and *see also*. The *see* cross-reference requires the coder to check another term in the index; the *see also* cross reference provides the option to review a different term in the index if the specificity is not found with the original indexed term.

Examples:
Perinephritis (*see also* Infection, kidney) N15.9
–purulent (*see also* Abscess, kidney) N15.1

Paget's disease
–with infiltrating duct carcinoma (M8541/3) *see* Neoplasm, breast, malignant

Principles and Guidelines

The guidelines for mortality and morbidity coding are located in the fourth section of volume 2, Instructional Manual. These rules have been adopted by the World Health Organization to provide guidance on selecting the underlying cause of death and main/secondary conditions analysis for morbidity data.

When reporting the underlying cause of death to WHO, the rules specified in section 4 must be applied consistently for meaningful statistics to be obtained from these data. Included are standard definitions on "underlying cause of death," "live birth," "maternal death," and many others.

As one can see from the section 4 headings listed below, a coder assigning ICD-10 codes for the underlying cause of death has many guidelines to understand and apply for appropriate reporting.

4.1   Mortality: Guidelines for certification and rules for coding

4.1.1   Causes of death

4.1.2   Underlying cause of death

4.1.3   International form of medical certificate of cause of death

4.1.4   Procedures for selection of the underlying cause of death for mortality tabulation

4.1.5   Rules for selection of the originating antecedent cause

4.1.6   Some considerations on selection rules

4.1.7   Examples of the general principle and selection rules

4.1.8   Modification of the selected cause

4.1.9   The modification rules

4.1.10   Examples of the modification rules

4.1.11   Notes for use in underlying cause mortality coding

4.1.12   Summary of linkages by code number

Process for Revision and Updates

The WHO established the **Updating and Revision Committee** (URC) in 2000 to recommend mortality and morbidity changes to ICD-10. The URC manages the update process and recommends changes to the Heads of WHO Collaborating Centres each year. Before ICD-10, updates were not made between revisions. Because health classifications provide a common language for clinicians and administra-tors and must allow for the addition of new disease processes, the need for updates was recognized. An additional group, the **Mortality Reference Group** (MRG) was established to make recommendations regarding mortality to the URC. An update cycle was established. The Tabular list is updated every three years with major changes, and annually for minor changes. The Index is updated annually with changes that do not impact the structure on the Tabular List. Each version of updates is available at: http://www.who.int/classifications/icd/icdonlineversions/en/index.html.

To better understand the updating procedure, students should review the file at http://www.who.int/classifications/committees/URC.pdf.

ICD-11

The ICD is a member of the World Health Organization's Family of International Classifications (WHO-FIC). Currently ICD is scheduled for periodic revisions and updates. A coordinated method will be used to revise ICD-10 to ICD-11. This revision will proceed in three stages. According to WHO, these stages are:

1.   Systematic review of scientific, clinical, and public health evidence relevant to classification

2.   Creation of draft ICD-11 and field-testing

3.   Development of meaningful linkages to standardized healthcare terminologies to facilitate communication, standardized data processing, and research (WHO 2007)

It is planned that content from other classifications, such as the International Classification Functioning Disability and Health (ICF), and national modifications of ICD will be included in order to improve the content and also to align the classifications. WHO anticipates that a final version of ICD-11 may be submitted to the World Health Assembly for approval by 2014.

ICD-10-CM and ICD-10-PCS

On January 16, 2009, the Department of Health and Human Services (HHS) published 45 CFR Part 162—HIPAA Administrative Simplification: Modifications to Medical Data Code Set Standards to Adopt ICD-10-CM and ICD-10-PCS, in the *Federal Register.*

In a separate final regulation, HHS adopted the updated X12 standard, Version 5010, and the National Council for Prescription Drug Programs standard, Version D.0, for electronic transactions, such as healthcare claims. Version 5010 is essential to use of the ICD-10 codes.

The final rule adopted ICD-10-CM for diagnosis coding, and ICD-10-PCS for hospital procedure coding. The new codes replace ICD-9-CM volumes 1 and 2 (for diagnosis reporting), and ICD-9-CM volume 3 (for procedure coding). They set an implementation date of October 1, 2013.

Replacement of ICD-9-CM is an absolute necessity because the code set is more than twenty years old and has become obsolete. It no longer meets the needs for accurate and complete data in this country. The terminology used in ICD-9-CM and the classification of some conditions are outdated and inconsistent with current medical knowledge. The system is rapidly running out of space and cannot accommodate many new codes to address the need for greater specificity, advances in medicine, and new diseases. In some cases, meritorious new code proposals have not been implemented simply because there is insufficient space. ICD-9-CM diagnosis codes do not pro-vide sufficient clinical detail to describe the severity or complexity of diagnoses nor does ICD-9-CM provide sufficient codes for healthcare encounters for reasons other than treatment of disease (for example, preventive medicine). ICD-9-CM is often ambiguous, lacks precision, and lacks a desired level of flexibility.

For more information on the implementation in the United States, watch the Web sites for NCHS (http://www.cdc.gov/nchs), CMS (http://www.cms.hhs.gov), and AHIMA (http://www.ahima.org/icd10).

International Classification of Diseases, Tenth Revision, Clinical Modification (ICD-10-CM)

In 1994, NCHS awarded a contract to the Center for Health Policy Studies (CHPS) to conduct a comprehensive evaluation of ICD-10 to determine whether it was a significant improvement over ICD-9-CM and should be implemented in the United States. The evaluation concluded that modifications would be necessary to make the system an improvement over ICD-9-CM, but that such modifications would be worth implementing. A technical advisory panel concluded that modifications were needed to:

*   Return to the level of specificity found in ICD-9-CM

*   Develop an improved alphabetic index

*   Modify code titles and narrative descriptions to enhance the consistency with accepted clinical practice in the United States

*   Remove codes unique to mortality coding (for example, unattended death, traumatic amputation at neck level, sudden infant death syndrome) or those designed specifically for emerging nations

*   Remove procedure descriptions included with diagnosis codes

*   Expand specificity for ambulatory and managed care encounters

- Expand to include new concepts

- Expand to include emerging diseases and more recent medical knowledge

All modifications to ICD-10 must conform to WHO conventions. WHO authorized development of the modifications of ICD-10 for use in the United States. Per the agreement with WHO, NCHS had to conform with system conventions and code structure. Moreover, any changes to code titles could not alter the meaning.

Developer

NCHS, the federal agency responsible for the use of ICD-10 in the United States, has developed a clinical modification of the classification for morbidity purposes.

ICD-10-CM represents a significant improvement over both ICD-9-CM and ICD-10. It incorporates much greater specificity and clinical detail, which will result in major improvements in the quality and usefulness of the data for all the current uses of the coding system. Moreover, information relevant to ambulatory and managed care encounters has been added.

Purpose

When **prospective payment systems** (PPSs) came into existence, the concerns for data quality, coding education, and medical record documentation received new emphasis. The consequences of inaccurate claims data in a fee-for-service environment had not been nearly as critical. Many reimbursement systems that are not based on a prospective payment methodology also require complete, accurate, and detailed coding in order to negotiate or calculate appropriate reimbursement rates, determine coverage, and establish medical necessity.

The new ICD-10-CM would be used to report diseases and conditions of patients treated in the United States healthcare system. For the coding of death certificates (mortality data), ICD-10 replaced ICD-9 as of January 1, 1999. ICD-10-CM is intended to replace ICD-9-CM, volumes 1 and 2.

Because many countries have already implemented ICD-10, continued use of ICD-9-CM causes significant difficulty in comparing international data used in public health, research and development, and the study of issues related to quality, safety, and efficacy of medical care. Even within the United States, the ability to compare mortality and morbidity data is compromised, as ICD-10 has been used in the United States for mortality statistics since 1999.

Check Your Understanding 2.7

Instructions: Complete the following exercises on a separate piece of paper.

1. True or False. Countries wishing to clinically modify ICD-10 must conform to WHO conventions.

2. True or False. A technical advisory panel concluded that a clinical modification of ICD-10 was not advantageous in the United States.

Content

The Tabular List and the Alphabetic Index have been completed but are still considered in draft form because the system has not yet been implemented. The American Health Information Management Association (AHIMA) and the American Hospital Association (AHA) conducted testing of ICD-10-CM in 2003.

Furthermore, a crosswalk between ICD-9-CM and ICD-10-CM was developed. The current draft of ICD-10-CM contains significantly more codes than exist in ICD-9-CM and offers many additional advantages.

Some of the major changes in ICD-10-CM include the following:

- The codes corresponding to ICD-9-CM V and E codes are incorporated into the main classification and are not separated into supplementary classifications as they were in ICD-9-CM.

- New diseases and conditions not uniquely identified in ICD-9-CM have been given codes.

In addition, conditions with newly discovered etiology or treatment protocols have been re-classified to a more appropriate chapter.

- Injuries are grouped by body part instead of by categories of injury.

- Excludes notes are expanded to provide guidance on the hierarchy of chapters and to clarify priority of code assignment.

- Combination codes have been created (for example, arteriosclerotic heart disease with angina).

- The concept of laterality (right–left) has been added.

- The codes for postoperative complications have been expanded and a distinction made between intraoperative complications and postprocedural disorders.

- The obstetric codes indicate which trimester the patient is in, and the codes no longer identify whether or not the patient has delivered.

- Information relevant to ambulatory and managed care encounters has been added.

- In general, the classification will allow greater specificity in code assignment.

The draft Tabular List, index, guidelines, and mappings for ICD-10-CM are available at http://www.cdc.gov/nchs/about/otheract/icd9/icd10cm.htm.

Similarities
ICD-10-CM is similar to ICD-9-CM in many ways. It is still maintained by NCHS. It has the same hierarchical structure as ICD-9-CM: all codes with the same first three characters have common traits, and each character beyond three adds greater specificity. It also has many of the same conventions and guidelines.

Moreover, ICD-10-CM has the same organization and use of notes and instructions as in ICD-9-CM. When a note appears under a three-character code, it applies to all codes within that category and instructions under a specific code apply to only that single code.

Differences
The principal changes in ICD-10-CM are in its organization and structure, code composition, and level of detail. For example, newly recognized conditions and conditions not uniquely identified in ICD-9 have been given codes, such as:

- Subsequent myocardial infarction (including site)

Conditions with a recently discovered etiology or a new treatment protocol have been reassigned to a more appropriate chapter.

Examples:
Gout: Musculoskeletal (ICD-10); endocrine (ICD-9)

Bradycardia: Symptoms (ICD-10); circulatory (ICD-9)

Sarcoidosis: Blood (ICD-10); infections (ICD-9)

Refractory anemia: Neoplasms (ICD-10); blood (ICD-9)

Structural Changes
As mentioned earlier, ICD-10-CM contains twenty-one chapters and its code composition is different from ICD-9-CM. The codes are alphanumeric with all letters used; letters *I* and *O* and numbers *1* and *0* should not be confused because the first character is always a letter.

A chapter may encompass more than one letter, and more than one chapter may share a letter. All codes in ICD-10-CM have full titles; thus, referral back to a common fourth or fifth digit is unnecessary. A sixth character has been added in some chapters for further specificity.

Code extensions have been added in the obstetrics, injury, and external cause chapters. Code extensions are letters of the alphabet and are added to the end of the code in the seventh position when applicable.

A dummy placeholder *x* is used in some codes to allow for future expansion and also to enable the use of a seventh character when the code contains fewer than seven characters.

Unlike ICD-10-PCS, in which all seven characters are utilized in all codes, ICD-10-CM codes may have as few as three characters.

The first three characters are to the left of the decimal and still represent the category. A three-character category may represent a single-disease entity (generally based on frequency or severity) or a group of closely related conditions. An example of a category is: D51, Vitamin B$_{12}$ deficiency anemia.

Most, but not all, three-character categories have been subdivided. An example of a complete three-character code is: P90, Convulsions of newborn.

Up to four characters may follow the decimal to further describe such things as etiology, anatomic site, and/or severity. However, not every code will have four characters after the decimal; the concept is the same as ICD-9-CM.

When the first three characters after the decimal are insufficient to describe the condition, an extension may appear after the three characters to the right of the decimal. Figure 2.3 shows the format of ICD-10-CM.

Organizational Changes

Following are some of the organizational changes in ICD-10-CM (some of which were mentioned in earlier sections of this chapter):

- V codes (factors influencing health status and contact with health services) and E codes (external causes of morbidity and mortality) are no longer considered supplementary; rather, they are part of the core classification.

- Sense organs have been separated from nervous system disorders, creating two new chapters for diseases of the eye and adnexa and for disorders of the ear and mastoid process.

- Injuries are grouped by body part rather than by category of injury; thus, all injuries of the head and neck are grouped together rather than all fractures or all open wounds.

- The order of some chapters has been rearranged.

- The categories for disorders of the immune system have been expanded and are placed with diseases of blood and blood-forming organs rather than with endocrine, nutritional, and metabolic diseases (as in ICD-9-CM).

- Excludes notes at the beginning of each chapter have been expanded to provide guidance on the hierarchy of chapters and to clarify priority of code assignment. For example, diseases of genitourinary system (N00–N99) (these are two of several excludes notes):

  —Excludes certain conditions originating in perinatal period
  —Excludes complications of pregnancy, childbirth, and puerperium

- After the appropriate includes and excludes notes, each chapter begins with a list of the subchapters or blocks of three-character categories. These blocks provide an overview of structure of chapter.

- Postoperative complications have been moved to procedure-specific body system chapters.

Figure 2.4 compares injury codes in ICD-10-CM with those in ICD-9-CM.

Figure 2.3.   Format of ICD-10-CM

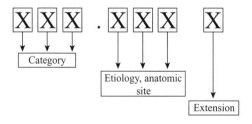

Check Your Understanding 2.8

Instructions: Complete the following exercises on a separate piece of paper.

1. True or False. The Supplementary Classification of Factors Influencing Health Status and Contact with Health Services (V codes) and the Supplementary

Classification of External Causes of Injury and Poisoning (E codes) will be supplementary classifications in ICD-10-CM.

2. True or False. There are many similarities between ICD-9-CM and ICD-10-CM.

3. True or False. Laterality can be classified in ICD-10-CM.

4. Which chapter does not use code extensions in ICD-10-CM?
   a. Injuries
   b. Neoplasms
   c. Obstetrics
   d. External causes

5. True or False. All ICD-10-CM codes are six characters in length.

6. Injuries in ICD-10-CM are grouped by

   _____.

New Features

Following are some of the new features found in ICD-10-CM:

- The creation of combination codes resolves sequencing issues (for example, pathological fractures are distinguished by underlying cause).

- With regard to laterality, the majority of affected codes are in neoplasm and injury chapters.

- The codes for postoperative complications have been expanded and a distinction made between intraoperative complications and postprocedural disorders.

Figure 2.4. Differences in injury codes, ICD-9-CM and ICD-10-CM

```
ICD-9-CM
        —Fractures (800–829)
        —Dislocations (830–839)
        —Sprains and strains (840–848)

ICD-10-CM
        —Injuries to the head (S00–S09)
        —Injuries to the neck (S10–S19)
        —Injuries to the thorax (S20–S29)
```

- Alcohol/drug abuse codes have been expanded to include information about abuse and dependence at the fourth-character level, and information about intoxication, withdrawal, mood disorders, psychotic disorders, and other specified or unspecified disorders at the fifth-character level. A sixth character further specifies manifestations.

- Injury codes enable coders to identify not only the broad category of injury (superficial injury, open wound, fracture, and so on), but also the specific injuries within the categories (abrasion, blister, contusion, external constriction, superficial foreign body, or insect bite). There is greater specification as to type and site of injury.

- There are combination codes for poisonings and external causes.

- ICD-10-CM includes other code expansions that provide greater specificity than found in ICD-9 or ICD-9-CM (for example, diabetes, epilepsy, radiation-related skin conditions, and family history)

- With regard to OB codes, fifth digits indicating episode of care have been eliminated. The last character in the code will now report the patient's trimester. Because certain OB conditions or complications occur at only one point in the obstetric period, not all codes will include all three trimesters (some codes will not include a character to describe the trimester at all).

- With regard to diabetes, controlled versus uncontrolled is not considered in the classification.

- Three chapters are significantly revised in ICD-10: chapter 5, Mental and Behavioral Disorders; chapter 19, Injury, Poisoning, and Certain Other Consequences of External Causes; and chapter 20, External Causes of Morbidity and Mortality.

- The classification of hypertension by "malignant" and "benign" has been eliminated.

- The timeframes in some codes have changed. For example, the timeframe for abortion versus fetal death in the chapter on pregnancy, childbirth, and the puerperium has been changed from twenty-two to twenty weeks.

- In the chapter on the circulatory system, the time period for acute myocardial infarction codes has changed from eight to four weeks and there are no longer subdivisions describing the initial and subsequent episodes of care.

ICD-10-CM identifies two types of excludes notes:

- Excludes 1 is a pure excludes note. It means "do not code here." The code being excluded should never appear with the code it is excluded from.

- Excludes 2 means "not included here." It is intended for use in cases where one condition may be excluded from the other, but there is a logical possibility that the patient may have both simultaneously, so both may be coded on the same record.

As stated above, some codes have extensions to the seventh character. Table 2.6 shows how some of these extensions are used. Figure 2.5 shows the level of detail in a few selected ICD-10-CM codes.

Principles and Guidelines

As mentioned earlier, a draft of the ICD-10-CM coding guidelines is currently available (version 2009). NCHS, one of the Centers for Disease Control and Prevention (CDC), an agency within HHS, developed the guidelines for coding and reporting using ICD-10-CM. The guidelines should be used as a companion document to the official government version. The guidelines for coding and reporting appear on the official government version of the ICD-10-CM and on

Table 2.6.   Use of seventh-character extensions in ICD-10-CM

Injury and External-Cause Chapters	
Seventh-Character Extension	**Definition**
A	Initial encounter
D	Subsequent encounter
S	Sequelae
Fracture Extensions	
A	Initial encounter for closed fracture
B	Initial encounter for open fracture
D	Subsequent encounter for fracture with routine healing
G	Subsequent encounter for fracture with delayed healing
K	Subsequent encounter for fracture with nonunion
S	Sequelae

Figure 2.5.   Level of detail in selected ICD-10-CM codes

Concept	Code	Description
Laterality	C50.512	Malignant neoplasm of lower-outer quadrant of left female breast
Combination Codes	K71.51	Toxic liver disease with chronic active hepatitis with ascites
Expansion of Injury Codes	S00.411A	Abrasion of right ear, initial encounter
Postoperative Complications	K91.61	Intraoperative hemorrhage and hematoma of digestive system organ or structure complicating a digestive system procedure
Expansion of diabetes mellitus codes	E11.311	Type 2 diabetes mellitus with unspecified diabetic retinopathy with macular edema
Expansion of alcohol/drug abuse codes	F10.180	Alcohol abuse with alcohol-induced anxiety disorder
Expansion of decubitus ulcer codes	L89.112	Pressure ulcer of right upper back, stage II

the NCHS Web site at http://www.cdc.gov/nchs/about/otheract/icd9/icd10cm.htm.

ICD-10-CM is in the public domain. It contains no codes for procedures; procedures are coded using the procedure classification appropriate for the encounter setting.

The conventions and guidelines apply to the proper use of ICD-10-CM for acute short-term and long-term hospital inpatient and physician office and other outpatient settings. New guidelines will be written to correspond to new codes that are added to ICD-10-CM or for types of encounters for which no guidelines exist.

There are many similarities between the guidelines in ICD-9-CM and those in ICD-10-CM. A careful review of the guidelines is imperative in order to completely understand the new coding system.

Process for Revision and Updates

The HIPAA Administrative Simplification: Modification to Medical Data Code Set Standards to Adopt ICD-10-CM and ICD-10-PCS: Proposed Rule established that an ICD-10-CM/PCS Coordination and Maintenance Committee will be formed to follow the same procedures currently used by the ICD-9-CM Coordination and Maintenance Committee to consider new codes and revisions to existing codes. Moreover, it is expected that AHA's *Coding Clinic* will continue to provide advice on coding.

Check Your Understanding 2.9

Instructions: Complete the following exercises on a separate piece of paper.

1. Fracture codes have extensions for which of the following circumstances?
   a. Initial versus subsequent encounter
   b. Routine versus delayed healing
   c. Open versus closed fracture
   d. All of the above

2. True or False. ICD-10-CM provides many combination codes for etiology/manifestation combinations.

3. True or False. In ICD-10-CM, the timeframe for an acute myocardial infarction is eight weeks.

ICD-10-Procedure Coding System (ICD-10-PCS)

Volume 3 of ICD-9-CM has been used in the United States to report inpatient procedures since 1979. Its structure has not permitted new procedures associated with rapidly changing technology to be effectively incorporated as new codes.

In 1990, the United States Health Care Financing Administration (HCFA) (now known as CMS) funded a pilot project to produce a preliminary design for a replacement for volume 3. After a review of the preliminary design, in 1995, HCFA awarded 3M Health Information Systems a three-year contract to complete development of a replacement system. The new system is the ICD-10-Procedure Coding System (ICD-10-PCS).

The index and tabular sections of ICD-10-PCS can be obtained at http://www.cms.hhs.gov/ICD10/. This site also has the ICD-10-PCS Reference Manual, forward and backward mappings between ICD-9-CM and ICD-10-PCS, and draft coding guidelines (located in the Reference Manual). Also available is a very helpful PowerPoint presentation explaining the coding system, and a document called: Development of the ICD-10 Procedure Coding System (ICD-10-PCS). Much of the detailed information provided later in this section is derived from the Development of the ICD-10 Procedure Coding System document available on the Internet.

Developer

Development of ICD-10-PCS was funded by CMS through a contract with 3M Health Information Systems. The system underwent an informal test in October 1996, which was followed by a formal test conducted by HCFA to determine whether ICD-10-PCS would be a practical replacement for ICD-9-CM procedures. Clinical Data Abstraction Centers (CDACs) were trained on the use of ICD-10-PCS and coded 5,000 records. They also compared ICD-9-CM and ICD-10-PCS codes. The CDACs found ICD-10-PCS to be an improvement over ICD-9-CM

Table 2.7.   Essential characteristics of ICD-10-PCS

Characteristics	Explanation
Completeness	There should be a unique code for all substantially different procedures.
Expandability	As new procedures are developed, the structure of ICD-10-PCS should allow them to be easily incorporated as unique codes.
Multiaxial Structure	The structure should be multiaxial, with each code character having the same meaning within a specific procedure section and across procedure sections.
Standard Terminology	There should be definitions of the terminology used. Although the meaning of specific words can vary in common usage, ICD-10-PCS should not include multiple meanings for the same term, and each term must be assigned a specific meaning.

in that it provided greater specificity in coding for use in research, statistical analysis, and administrative areas. A major strength of the system is its detailed structure, which enables users to recognize and report more precisely the procedures that were performed.

Purpose

The purpose of ICD-10-PCS was to develop a superior procedure coding system to replace volume 3 of ICD-9-CM. ICD-10-PCS has a multi-axial, seven-character, alphanumerical code structure, which provides a unique code for all substantially different procedures and allows new procedures to be easily incorporated as new codes.

Procedures in ICD-10-PCS are divided into sections that relate to the general type of procedure. The first character of the procedure code always specifies the section or type of procedure. The second through seventh characters have a standard meaning within each section but may have a different meaning across sections. In ICD-10-PCS, the term *procedure* is used to refer to the complete specification of the seven characters. All terminology in ICD-10-PCS is defined precisely, with a specific meaning attached to all terms used in the system.

Although the new coding system will likely require coders to have a greater knowledge of anatomy and physiology and complete documentation of a procedure to be available prior to coding, ICD-10-PCS appears to provide more complete and accurate descriptions of the procedures performed than does volume 3 of ICD-9-CM. All procedures on a particular body part, by a particular approach, or by

another characteristic can be easily retrieved using ICD-10-PCS data. The codes will provide very specific information about a particular procedure.

Development of ICD-10-PCS was based on four major objectives. These essential characteristics are shown in table 2.7.

Check Your Understanding 2.10

Instructions: Complete the following exercises on a separate piece of paper.

1. What are the four essential characteristics of ICD-10-PCS?
    a. _____
    b. _____
    c. _____
    d. _____

2. True or False. ICD-9-CM requires coders to have more knowledge of anatomy and physiology, but ICD-10-PCS appears to provide more complete and accurate descriptions of the procedures.

3. ICD-10-PCS was designed as a replacement for:
    a. CPT
    b. ICD-9-CM, volume 3
    c. ICD-9-CM, volumes 1, 2, and 3
    d. ICD-10

Content

ICD-10-PCS has a seven-character alphanumeric code structure. Each character has many different possible values. The digits *0–9* and the letters *A–H, J–N,* and *P–Z* are used. The letters *O* and *I* are not used in order to avoid confusion with the digits *0* and *1*. The letters and numbers are intermingled throughout the code.

Table 2.8.   Sections of ICD-10-PCS

Section	Title
0	Medical and Surgical
1	Obstetrics
2	Placement
3	Administration
4	Measurement and Monitoring
5	Extracorporeal Assistance and Performance
6	Extracorporeal Therapies
7	Osteopathic
8	Other Procedures
9	Chiropractic
B	Imaging
C	Nuclear Medicine
D	Radiation Oncology
F	Physical Rehabilitation and Diagnostic Audiology
G	Mental Health
H	Substance Abuse Treatment

Source: Centers for Medicare & Medicaid Services. 2009. ICD-10-PCS. http://www.cms.hhs.gov/ICD10.

The number of codes is extensive, with a total number estimated in the 2009 version at 72,589. There are approximately 4,000 ICD-9-CM procedure codes.

As mentioned in the preceding section, procedures are divided into sections that relate to the general type of procedure (medical and surgical, imaging, obstetrics, nuclear medicine, and so on). The first character of the procedure code always specifies the section. (See table 2.8 for the sections.)

ICD-10-PCS Manual

The ICD-10-PCS online manual is divided into parts, including:

ICD-10-PCS Tables

Index

List of Codes

The index allows codes to be located by an alphabetic look-up; however, only the first three or four characters will be identified. The index entry will

refer to a specific location in the table. Reference to the table is always required to obtain the complete code because the codes are "built" from the tables in ICD-10-PCS.

The tables in ICD-10-PCS have a completely different organization than the Tabular List in ICD-9-CM. Each page is arranged in a grid that specifies the valid combinations of character values for the code. The upper portion of the grid contains a description of the first two or three characters of the procedure code. These characters were obtained in the index. An example of one of these grids is provided in figure 2.6 (see page 38).

In addition to the online manual, ICD-10-PCS has an ICD-10-PCS Reference Manual (including the coding guidelines). These files are all available at the CMS Web site referenced above. A significant improvement was made in 2009 by adding Body Part Keys in the reference section of the online ICD-10-PCS.

Medical and Surgical Procedures

The medical and surgical procedures section is used frequently in the hospital inpatient setting, so the following demonstrates the meanings of the seven characters in this section. (See figure 2.7.) It is important to remember, however, that the characters have a slightly different meaning in each section, but that they are well defined in the coding system.

In the medical and surgical procedures section, the first character specifying the section is 0. The second character indicates the body system (for example, the endocrine system). Table 2.9 (see page 39) lists the Medical and Surgical Section (0) body systems. The tabular section provides an extensive list of the corresponding appropriate body system by body part.

Figure 2.7.   Meaning of characters for medical and surgical procedures

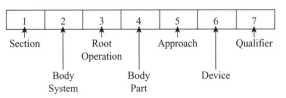

Figure 2.6.   Sample of ICD-10-PCS tabular grid

```
0: MEDICAL AND SURGICAL
D: GASTROINTESTINAL SYSTEM
B: EXCISION: Cutting out or off, without replacement, a portion of a
             body part
```

Body Part Character 4	Approach Character 5	Device Character 6	Qualifier Character 7

0 Esophagus
1 Esophagus, Upper
2 Esophagus, Middle
3 Esophagus, Lower
4 Esophagogastric Junction
6 Stomach
7 Stomach, Pylorus
8 Small Intestine
9 Duodenum
A Jejunum
B Ileum
C Ileocecal Valve
D Large Intestine
F Large Intestine, Right
G Large Intestine, Left
H Cecum
J Appendix
K Ascending Colon
L Transverse Colon
M Descending Colon
N Sigmoid Colon
P Rectum
	0 Open
	1 Open Intraluminal
	2 Open Intraluminal
	  Endoscopic
	3 Percutaneous
	4 Percutaneous
	  Endoscopic
	5 Percutaneous
	  Intraluminal
	6 Percutaneous
	  Intraluminal
	  Endoscopic
	7 Transorifice
	  Intraluminal
	8 Transorifice
	  Intraluminal
	  Endoscopic
	F Open With
	  Endoscopic
	  Assistance
		Z No Device	X Diagnostic
			Z No Qualifier

Q Anus	0 Open
	1 Open Intraluminal
	2 Open Intraluminal
	  Endoscopic
	3 Percutaneous
	4 Percutaneous
	  Endoscopic
	5 Percutaneous
	  Intraluminal
	6 Percutaneous
	  Intraluminal
	  Endoscopic
	7 Transorifice
	  Intraluminal
	8 Transorifice
	  Intraluminal
	  Endoscopic
	F Open With
	  Endoscopic
	  Assistance
	X External
		Z No Device	X Diagnostic
			Z No Qualifier

R Anal Sphincter
S Greater Omentum
T Lesser Omentum
V Mesentery
W Peritoneum
	0 Open
	3 Percutaneous
	4 Percutaneous
	  Endoscopic
	F Open With
	  Endoscopic
	  Assistance
		Z No Device	X Diagnostic
			Z No Qualifier

Source: Centers for Medicare and Medicaid Services. 2009. ICD-10-PCS. http://www.cms.hhs.gov/ICD10.

Check Your Understanding 2.11

Instructions: Complete the following exercises on a separate piece of paper.

1. True or False. ICD-10-PCS is based on a seven-character alphanumeric code. The meaning of each individual character changes according to the needs of the clinical section.

2. True or False. When assigning a code from ICD-10-PCS, the process is similar to ICD-9-CM. The term is indexed and all the characters are provided, and then the coding professional checks the code in the Tabular List.

3. In the medical and surgical section of ICD-10-PCS, what does the fifth character represent?
   a. Root operation
   b. Device
   c. Qualifier
   d. Approach

The third character indicates the root operation, which specifies the objective of the procedure (for example, con-trol). ICD-10-PCS has done an exemplary job of defining these terms. It also has included examples of each term for clarification. Table 2.10 (see page 40) provides the list of root operations with their respective definitions.

A root operation also must specify the objective of the procedure. The term *anastomosis* is not a root operation because it is a means of joining and is an integral part of another procedure such as a bypass or a resection; therefore, it can never stand alone. Incision is not a root term because it is a means of opening and is always an integral part of another procedure. Repair is only coded when none of the other operations apply and is therefore the NEC option for the root operation character. It is used when documentation and necessary information cannot be obtained from the physician indicating a more specific root operation.

The body part is specified in the fourth character and indicates the specific part of the body system on which the procedure was performed (for example, stomach).

Table 2.9.   ICD-10-PCS Medical and Surgical Section (0) body systems

Character	Title	Character	Title
0	Central Nervous Systems	H	Skin and Breast
1	Peripheral Nervous Systems	J	Subcutaneous Tissue and Fascia
2	Heart and Great Vessels	K	Muscles
3	Upper Arteries	L	Tendons
4	Lower Arteries	M	Bursae and Ligaments
5	Upper Veins	N	Head and Facial Bones
6	Lower Veins	P	Upper Bones
7	Lymphatic and Hemic System	Q	Lower Bones
8	Eye	R	Upper Joints
9	Ear, Nose, Sinus	S	Lower Joints
B	Respiratory System	T	Urinary System
C	Mouth and Throat	U	Female Reproductive System
D	Gastrointestinal System	V	Male Reproductive System
F	Hepatobiliary System and Pancreas	W	Anatomical Regions, General
G	Endocrine System	X	Anatomical Regions, Upper Extremities
		Y	Anatomical Regions, Lower Extremities

Source: Centers for Medicare and Medicaid Services. 2009. ICD-10-PCS. http://www.cms.hhs.gov/ICD10.

Table 2.10.   Root operations with their respective definitions

Operation		Definition, Explanation, Examples
Alteration	Definition	Modifying the natural anatomic structure of a body part without affecting function of the body part
	Explanation	Principal purpose is to improve appearance
	Examples	Face-lift, breast augmentation
Bypass	Definition	Altering the route of passage of the contents of a tubular body part
	Explanation	Rerouting contents around an area of a body part to another distal (downstream) area in the normal route; rerouting the contents to another different, but similar, route and body part or to an abnormal route and another dissimilar body part. It includes one or more concurrent anastomoses with or without the use of devices such as autografts, tissue substitutes, and synthetic substitutes.
	Examples	Coronary artery bypass, colostomy formation
Change	Definition	Taking out or off a device from a body part and putting back an identical or similar device in or on the same body part without cutting or puncturing the skin or a mucous membrane
	Explanation	All CHANGE procedures are coded using the approach EXTERNAL
	Examples	Urinary catheter change, gastrostomy tube change
Control	Definition	Stopping, or attempting to stop, postprocedural bleeding
	Explanation	The site of the bleeding is coded as an anatomical region and not to a specific body part.
	Examples	Control of postprostatectomy hemorrhage, control of posttonsillectomy hemorrhage
Creation	Definition	Making a new genital structure that does not take over the function of a body part
	Explanation	Used only for sex-change operations
	Examples	Creation of vagina in a male, creation of penis in a female
Destruction	Definition	Physical eradication of all or a portion of a body part by the direct use of energy, force, or a destructive agent
	Explanation	None of the body part is taken out.
	Examples	Fulguration of rectal polyp, cautery of skin lesion
Detachment	Definition	Cutting off all or a portion of the upper or lower extremities
	Explanation	The body part value is the site of the detachment, with a qualifier if applicable to further specify the level where the extremity was detached.
	Examples	Below-knee amputation, disarticulation of shoulder
Dilation	Definition	Expanding an orifice or the lumen of a tubular body part
	Explanation	The orifice can be a natural orifice or an artificially created orifice. Accomplished by stretching a tubular body part using intraluminal pressure or by cutting part of the orifice or wall of the tubular body part.
	Examples	Percutaneous transluminal angioplasty, pyloromyotomy

Table 2.10.   (Continued)

Operation	Definition, Explanation, Examples	
Division	Definition	Cutting into a body part without draining fluids and/or gases from the body part in order to separate or transect a body part
	Explanation	All or a portion of the body part is separated into two or more portions.
	Examples	Spinal cordotomy, osteotomy
Drainage	Definition	Taking or letting out fluids and/or gases from a body part
	Explanation	The qualifier DIAGNOSTIC is used to identify drainage procedures that are biopsies.
	Examples	Thoracentesis, incision and drainage
Excison	Definition	Cutting out or off, without replacement, a portion of a body part
	Explanation	The qualifier DIAGNOSTIC is used to identify excision procedures that are biopsies.
	Examples	Partial nephrectomy, liver biopsy
Extirpation	Definition	Taking or cutting out solid matter from a body part
	Explanation	The solid matter may be an abnormal byproduct of a biological function or a foreign body. The solid matter is imbedded in a body part or is in the lumen of a tubular body part. The solid matter may or may not have been previously broken into pieces. No appreciable amount of the body part is taken out.
	Examples	Thrombectomy, choledocholithotomy
Extraction	Definition	Pulling or stripping out or off all or a portion of a body part by the use of force
	Explanation	The qualifier DIAGNOSTIC is used to identify extraction procedures that are biopsies.
	Examples	Dilation and curettage, vein stripping
Fragmentation	Definition	Breaking solid matter in a body part into pieces
	Explanation	The solid matter may be an abnormal byproduct of a biological function or a foreign body. Physical force (for example, manual, ultrasonic) applied directly or indirectly through intervening body parts is used to break the solid matter into pieces. The pieces of solid matter are not taken out, but are eliminated or absorbed through normal biological functions.
	Examples	Extracorporeal shockwave lithotripsy, transurethral lithotripsy
Fusion	Definition	Joining together portions of an articular body part, rendering the articular body part immobile
	Explanation	The body part is joined together by fixation device, bone graft, or other means
	Examples	Spinal fusion, ankle arthrodesis
Insertion	Definition	Putting in a nonbiological device that monitors, assists, performs, or prevents a physiological function but does not physically take the place of a body part
	Explanation	N/A
	Examples	Insertion of radioactive implant, insertion of central venous catheter
Inspection	Definition	Visually and/or manually exploring a body part
	Explanation	Visual exploration may be performed with or without optical instrumentation. Manual exploration may be performed directly or through intervening body layers.
	Examples	Diagnostic arthroscopy, exploratory laparotomy
Map	Definition	Locating the route of passage of electrical impulses and/or locating functional areas in a body part
	Explanation	Applicable only to the cardiac conduction mechanism and the central nervous system
	Examples	Cardiac mapping, cortical mapping

(Continued on next page)

Table 2.10.   (Continued)

Operation		Definition, Explanation, Examples
Occlusion	Definition	Completely closing an orifice or the lumen of a tubular body part
	Explanation	The orifice can be a natural orifice or an artificially created orifice.
	Examples	Fallopian tube ligation, ligation of inferior vena cava
Reattachment	Definition	Putting back in or on all or a portion of a separated body part to its normal location or other suitable location
	Explanation	Vascular circulation and nervous pathways may or may not be reestablished.
	Examples	Reattachment of hand, reattachment of avulsed kidney
Release	Definition	Freeing a body part from an abnormal physical constraint by cutting or by use of force
	Explanation	Some of the restraining tissue may be taken out, but none of the body part is taken out.
	Examples	Adhesiolysis, carpal tunnel release
Removal	Definition	Taking out or off a device from a body part
	Explanation	If the device is taken out and a similar device is put in without cutting or puncturing the skin or mucous membrane, the procedure is coded to the root operation CHANGE. Otherwise, the procedure for taking out the device is coded to the root operation REMOVAL, and the procedure for putting in the new device is coded to the root operation performed.
	Examples	Drainage tube removal, cardiac pacemaker removal
Repair	Definition	Restoring, to the extent possible, a body part to its normal anatomic structure and function
	Explanation	Used only when the method to accomplish the repair is not one of the other root operations
	Examples	Herniorrhaphy, suture of laceration
Replacement	Definition	Putting in or on biological or synthetic material that physically takes the place and/or function of all or a portion of a body part
	Explanation	The biological material is nonliving or the biological material is living and from the same individual. The body part may have been previously taken out, previously replaced, or may be taken out concomitantly with the replacement procedure. If the body part has been previously replaced, a separate REMOVAL procedure is coded for taking out the device used in the previous replacement.
	Examples	Total hip replacement, bone graft, free skin graft
Reposition	Definition	Moving to its normal location or other suitable location all or a portion of a body part
	Explanation	The body part is moved to a new location from an abnormal location, or from a normal location where it is not functioning correctly. The body part may or may not be cut out or off to be moved to the new location.
	Examples	Reposition of undescended testicle, fracture reduction
Resection	Definition	Cutting out or off, without replacement, all of a body part
	Explanation	N/A
	Examples	Total nephrectomy, total lobectomy of lung
Restriction	Definition	Partially closing an orifice or the lumen of a tubular body part
	Explanation	The orifice can be a natural orifice, or an artificially created orifice.
	Examples	Esophagogastric fundoplication, cervical cerclage
Revision	Definition	Correcting, to the extent possible, a malfunctioning or displaced device
	Explanation	Revision can include correcting a malfunctioning or displaced device by taking out or putting in components of the device such as a screw or pin.
	Examples	Adjustment of pacemaker lead, adjustment of hip prosthesis

Table 2.10.   (Continued)

Operation	Definition, Explanation, Examples	
Supplement	Definition	Putting in or on biologic or synthetic material that physically reinforces and/or augments the function of a portion of a body part
	Explanation	The biological material is nonliving, or the biological material is living and from the same individual. The body part may have been previously replaced. If the body part has been previously replaced, the SUPPLEMENT procedure is performed to physically reinforce and/or augment the function of the replaced body part.
	Examples	Herniorrhaphy using mesh, free nerve graft, mitral valve ring annuloplasty, a new acetabular liner in a previous hip replacement
Transfer	Definition	Moving, without taking out, all or a portion of a body part to another location to take over the function of all or a portion of a body part
	Explanation	The body part transferred remains connected to its vascular and nervous supply.
	Examples	Tendon transfer, skin pedicle flap transfer
Transplantation	Definition	Putting in or on all or a portion of a living body part taken from another individual or animal to physically take the place and/or function of all or a portion of a similar body part
	Explanation	The native body part may or may not be taken out, and the transplanted body part may take over all or a portion of its function.
	Examples	Kidney transplant, heart transplant

Source: Centers for Medicare and Medicaid Services. 2009. ICD-10-PCS. http://www.cms.hhs.gov/ICD10.

The fifth character indicates the approach or the technique of the procedure. Table 2.11 (see page 44) provides the surgical approaches.

The device is specified in the sixth character and is only used to specify devices that remain after the procedure is completed. If no device is applicable, the letter *Z* is used.

There are four general types of devices:

- Biological or synthetic material that takes the place of all or a portion of a body part (skin grafts and joint prosthesis)

- Biological or synthetic material that assists or prevents a physiological function (IUD)

- Therapeutic material that is not absorbed by, eliminated by, or incorporated into a body part (radioactive implant)

- Mechanical or electronic appliances used to assist, monitor, take the place of, or prevent a physiological function (cardiac pacemaker, orthopedic pins).

The seventh character is for the qualifier. The qualifier has a unique meaning for individual procedures. It could be used to identify the second site included in a bypass or to identify that a biopsy is a diagnostic procedure.

Principles and Guidelines

Several general principles were followed in the development of ICD-10-PCS. (See table 2.12 on page 45.) Further, ICD-10-PCS draft coding guidelines developed for ICD-10-PCS are available at http://www.cms.hhs.gov/ICD10/.

Process for Revision and Updates

CMS/3M has updated ICD-10-PCS each year since it was published. The HIPAA Administrative Simplification: Modification to Medical Data Code Set Standards to Adopt ICD-10-CM and ICD-10-PCS; Proposed Rule established that an ICD-10-CM/PCS Coordination and Maintenance Committee will be formed to follow the same procedures currently used by the **ICD-9-CM Coordination and Maintenance**

Table 2.11.   Surgical approaches

Approach Value	Approach Definition
Open	Cutting through the skin or mucous membrane and any other body layers necessary to expose the site of the procedure
Percutaneous	Entry, by puncture or minor incision, of instrumentation through the skin or mucous membrane and/or any other body layers necessary to reach the site of the procedure
Percutaneous Endoscopic	Entry, by puncture or minor incision, of instrumentation through the skin or mucous membrane and/or any other body layers necessary to reach and visualize the site of the procedure
Via Natural or Artificial Opening	Entry of instrumentation through a natural or artificial external opening to reach the site of the procedure
Via Natural or Artificial Opening, Endoscopic	Entry of instrumentation through a natural or artificial external opening to reach and visualize the site of the procedure
Open with Percutaneous Endoscopic Assistance	Cutting through the skin or mucous membrane and any other body layers necessary to expose the site of the procedure, and entry, by puncture or minor incision, of instrumentation through the skin or mucous membrane and any other body layers necessary to aid in the performance of the procedure
External	Procedures performed directly on the skin or mucous membrane and procedures performed indirectly by the application of external force through the skin or mucous membrane

Committee to consider new codes and revisions to existing codes. This was reiterated in the Final Rule as the process going forward.

Check Your Understanding 2.12

Instructions: Complete the following exercises on a separate piece of paper.

1. What is the root operation for bypass, one coronary artery to left internal mammary artery in ICD-10-PCS?

2. What root operation would be used to describe the following in ICD-10-PCS?
   a. Kidney transplant
   b. Appendectomy
   c. Diagnostic bronchoscopy
   d. Lithotripsy, bladder stone

3. True or False. A device in ICD-10-PCS applies only to devices that remain after the procedure is completed.

Summary

The uses being made of coded data go well beyond the purposes for which coding systems were designed or even contemplated in the 1970s. ICD was used primarily in the hospital inpatient setting for indexing purposes at the time ICD-9-CM was implemented. Used in many more healthcare settings, ICD-9-CM became a key component of several American healthcare reimbursement systems. Many reimbursement systems that are not based on a prospective payment methodology also require complete, accurate, and detailed coding in order to negotiate or calculate appropriate reimbursement rates, determine coverage, and establish medical necessity. However, ICD-9-CM is now seen as being woefully inadequate for meeting the needs of noninpatient hospital settings or serving the many other purposes for which ICD data are currently used.

The ICD system was originally intended to collect mortality data from governments worldwide. Accordingly, ICD-10 was first used for the coding of national mortality data. The United States began using ICD-10 to code and classify mortality data from death certificates in January 1999. The World Health Organization published ICD-10 in its hard-copy version in 1992 (Tabular List), 1993 (Instruction Manual), and 1994 (Alphabetical Index). Several countries currently use ICD-10 for morbidity classification, but others have clinically modified ICD-10

Table 2.12.   General principles followed in the development of ICD-10-PCS

Guideline	Explanation
Diagnostic information is not included in procedure description	The disease or disorder is not specified in procedures.
Not otherwise specified (NOS) options restricted	Many NOS options are provided in ICD-9-CM, but these options are restricted in ICD-10-PCS. A minimal level of specificity is required for components in the procedure.
Limited use of "not elsewhere classified" (NEC) option	ICD-9-CM will often provide an NEC option. All possible components of a procedure are specified in ICD-10-PCS. Thus, in general, there is no need for an NEC option, although ICD-10-PCS does use this in very limited situations when necessary. For example, because new devices are being developed, there is an NEC option for devices until the new device can be explicitly added to the coding system.
Level of specificity	Based on combinations of the seven alphanumeric characters, all possible procedures were defined. A code was created for any procedure that could be performed.

for that purpose. WHO has authorized development of modifications of ICD-10 under specific requirements.

Based on ICD-10, ICD-10-CM was created to classify diagnoses and reasons for visits in all healthcare settings. ICD-10 is used in the United States solely as a mortality classification for the coding of death certificates. A morbidity classification contains substantially more detail than is required in a mortality classification.

ICD-10-CM is intended to replace volumes 1 and 2 of ICD-9-CM; ICD-10-PCS has been developed to replace volume 3 of ICD-9-CM. ICD-10-PCS has evolved during its development based on extensive input from many segments of the healthcare industry. The multiaxial structure of the system combined with its detailed definition of all terminology will permit a precise specification of procedures for use in statistical analysis and administrative areas. Moreover, it will enhance the ability of health information coders to determine accurate procedure codes with minimal effort.

References

AHIMA. 2008. http://www.ahima.org/ICD10.

AHIMA. 2008. Introduction to ICD-10 mortality. Online training course. http://campus.ahima.org/campus/course_info/ICD10MORT/ICD10M_info.html.

AHA. 2008. Central Office on ICD-9-CM. http://www.ahacentraloffice.org.

Bowman, Sue. 2008. Why ICD-10 is worth the trouble. *Journal of the American Health Information Management Association* 79(3):24–29.

Centers for Medicare and Medicaid Services. 2008. ICD-10-PCS. http://www.cms.hhs.gov/ICD10/.

Centers for Medicare and Medicaid Services. 2008. http://www.cms.hhs.gov.

Federal Register. Vol. 73. No. 164. Friday, August 22, 2008. http://www.access.gpo.gov/su_docs/fedreg/a080822c.html.

Giannangelo, Kathy. 2004. The regulatory journey to destination 10: Understanding the process for adoption of ICD-10-CM and ICD-10-PCS. AHIMA Web Extra. http://library.ahima.org/xpedio/groups/public/documents/ahima/bok1_023199.hcsp?dDocName=bok1_023199.

Johns, Merida L. 2007. *Health Information Management Technology.* Chicago: American Health Information Management Association.

National Center for Health Statistics. 2008. http://www.cdc.gov/nchs.

National Center for Health Statistics. 2008. *About the International Classification of Diseases, Tenth Revision, Clinical Modification (ICD-10-CM).* http://www.cdc.gov/nchs/about/otheract/icd9/abticd10.htm.

National Center for Health Statistics. 2008. *ICD-9-CM Official Guidelines for Coding and Reporting.* http://www.cdc.gov/nchs/datawh/ftpserv/ftpicd9/ftpicd9.htm#guidelines.

National Center for Health Statistics. 2008. ICD-10-CM and guidelines (draft). http://www.cdc.gov/nchs/about/otheract/icd9/icd10cm.htm.

Schraffenberger, Lou Ann. 2008. *Basic ICD-9-CM Coding.* Chicago: American Health Information Management Association.

Official Authorized Addendum. http://www.cdc.gov/nchs/datawh/ftpserv/ftpicd9/ftpicd9.htm or http://www.cms.hhs.gov/ICD9ProviderDiagnosticCodes/.

U.S. Department of Health and Human Services. 2008. *International Classification of Diseases, 9th Revision, Clinical Modification.* Washington, DC: U.S. Government Printing Office.

World Health Organization. 2007. Production of ICD-11: The overall revision process. http://www.who.int/classifications/icd/ICDRevision.pdf.

World Health Organization. 2008. ICD Revision Process: towards ICD-11. http://www.who.int/classifications/network/ICD_11Rejkjavik.pdf.

World Health Organization. 2008. History of the development of the ICD. http://www.who.int/classifications/icd/en/HistoryOfICD.pdf.

World Health Organization. 2008. The WHO Updating & Revision Committee. http://www.who.int/classifications/committees/URC.pdf.

World Health Organization. 2008. Description of the International Statistical Classification of Diseases and Related Health Problems Instructional Manual. http://www.who.int/classifications/icd/ICD-10_2nd_ed_volume2.pdf.

World Health Organization. 2007. *International Statistical Classification of Diseases and Related Health Problems, Tenth Revision.* Geneva: World Health Organization.

World Health Organization. 2008. http://www.who.int/classifications/icd/en/.

World Health Organization. 2008. ICD Online Versions. http://www.who.int/classifications/icd/icdonlineversions/en/index.html.

World Health Organization. 2008. Current online version (2007). http://www.who.int/classifications/apps/icd/icd10online/.

Application Exercises

1. Go to the Web site for ICD-10-PCS http://www.cms.hhs.gov/ICD10/. Review the Introduction to ICD-10-PCS. Do a detailed analysis of the meanings of each of the seven characters and turn in a report to your instructor.

2. Create a table showing the similarities and differences among ICD-9-CM, ICD-10, ICD-10-CM, and ICD-10-PCS.

3. Go to the AHIMA Web site on ICD-10 (http://www.ahima.org/ICD10), AHIMA Communities of Practice and/or the Body of Knowledge to research the most current information on the status and expected implementation dates of ICD-10-CM and ICD-10-PCS in the United States. Summarize your findings in a report to the class.

Review Quiz

1. Which classification system is currently in use in the United States to provide diagnostic and procedural coding for many purposes, including reimbursement?
   a. ICD-9
   b. ICD-9-CM
   c. ICD-10
   d. ICD-10-CM

2. True or False. ICD-9-CM is published in four volumes.

3. True or False. V codes and E codes are referred to as supplementary classifications in ICD-9-CM.

4. Which section(s) of the ICD-9-CM Official Guidelines for Coding and Reporting are followed for the coding of hospital inpatients?
   a. Section I
   b. Section I, II
   c. Section I, II, III, IV
   d. Section I, II, III

5. True or False. Home health agencies do not have any specific ICD-9-CM Official Coding Guidelines.

6. Using table 2.8, identify the first character that would be assigned to the following procedures for ICD-10-PCS.
   a. Gait training
   b. Cholecystectomy
   c. Computerized tomography, spine
   d. Cranioplasty

7. What is the root operation for tendon transfer in ICD-10-PCS?

8. True or False. A unique meaning for individual procedures in ICD-10-PCS is a qualifier. The following procedure would have a qualifier reported: hysteroscopy with biopsy.

9. What is contained in the volume 3 of ICD-10?
   a. Tabular List
   b. Alphabetic Index
   c. Instruction Manual
   d. Coding Guidelines

10. Includes and excludes notes are used in:
    a. ICD-9-CM
    b. ICD-9-CM and ICD-10-CM
    c. ICD-9-CM, ICD-10-CM, and ICD-10
    d. ICD-10 and ICD-10-CM

11. What does (.–) mean in ICD-10?
    _____

12. ICD-11 will be submitted to the _____ for approval.
    a. World Health Assembly
    b. National Center for Health Statistics
    c. World Health Organization
    d. National Committee on Vital and Health Statistics

13. Why does ICD-9-CM need to be replaced?
    a. It contains outdated terminology.
    b. There is no room to expand.
    c. The codes do not provide sufficient clinical detail.
    d. All of the above

14. True or False. If you were coding in ICD-10-CM and had a patient with traumatic arthritis due to an old fracture, you would assign extension J.

15. True or False. ICD-10-CM provides a greater level of detail and more specificity than ICD-10.

Chapter 3

Current Procedural Terminology (CPT®)

Ann Zeisset, RHIT, CCS, CCS-P

Learning Objectives

- To review the development and purpose of CPT

- To identify and describe the types of CPT codes

- To discuss component parts of CPT

- To review the process for updating CPT codes

Key Terms

CPT Editorial Panel
Counseling
Evaluation and management (E/M) codes
Modifier
Separate procedure
Semicolon
Surgical package

Introduction

This chapter discusses the American Medical Association's (AMA) Current Procedural Terminology (CPT), a comprehensive terminology describing diagnostic and therapeutic procedures and medical and surgical services. The chapter focuses on the content of CPT, the process for updating the terminology, and principles of its application.

Developer

The AMA developed CPT to describe medical services and procedures performed by physicians and other healthcare providers. As a procedural terminology, CPT contains no diagnosis codes. One of the most widely used terminologies in healthcare, CPT was first introduced in 1966 and has subsequently been published in four editions. In 1983, the Centers for Medicare and Medicaid Services (CMS) adopted CPT as the standard for physician and hospital outpatient service coding. With implementation of the Health Insurance Portability and Accountability Act (HIPAA) code sets standards, CPT in combination with the Healthcare Common Procedure Coding System (HCPCS) became the only acceptable system for reporting services in these settings. These services include, but are not limited to:

- Physician services
- Physical and occupational therapy services
- Radiologic procedures
- Clinical laboratory tests
- Other medical diagnostic procedures
- Hearing and vision services
- Transportation services including ambulance

In addition, CPT codes are reported with ICD-9-CM diagnostic codes to obtain reimbursement for outpatient services in physician offices, hospital outpatient and freestanding ambulatory surgery centers, and other outpatient settings.

Purpose

The CPT system is published annually with January 1 as the effective date for the use of the updated CPT codes. The one exception to this rule is that CPT category III and vaccine product codes are released twice per year, with release dates of January 1 and July 1 and effective dates for use six months later. Further CPT category II codes released changes are meant to be applied prospectively from the effective date. The purpose of CPT is "to provide a uniform language that will accurately describe medical, surgical, and diagnostic services, and will thereby provide an effective means for reliable nationwide communication among physicians, patients, and third parties" (AMA 2009). CPT is used to report physician services, many nonphysician services, and surgical services performed in hospital outpatient departments and ambulatory surgery centers. Although it was originally developed as a way to report physician services as accurately as possible for reimbursement, CPT now is also used for healthcare trending and planning, benchmarking, and measurement of quality of care.

Check Your Understanding 3.1

Instructions: Complete the following exercises on a separate piece of paper.

1. True or False. The AMA developed CPT primarily to describe medical services and procedures performed by physicians and other healthcare providers.

2. Which clinical setting below does *not* submit CPT codes for reimbursement?
   a. Physician offices
   b. Hospital inpatient services
   c. Hospital outpatient services
   d. Ambulatory surgery centers

Content

CPT is composed of three types of codes: category I, category II, and category III.

Category I Codes

Category I codes are five-digit numeric codes. For a procedure to receive a category I CPT code, it first must be:

- Performed by many healthcare professionals across the country and a distinct service

- Approved by the Food and Drug Administration (FDA) or with approval imminent within a given CPT cycle

- Of proven clinical efficacy

- Not a fragmentation of another procedure or reportable by current CPT codes

- Not a means to report extraordinary circumstances of another CPT code (AMA 2008)

Thus, new technologies or procedures of unproven efficacy would not receive CPT codes. An example of a category I code is: 27830, Closed treatment of proximal tibiofibular joint dislocation; without anesthesia.

Category II Codes

Introduced in 2004, category II codes are five-character alphanumeric codes with an *F* in the fifth position. These codes are supplemental tracking codes that can be used for performance measurement. They are reported in addition to standard **evaluation and management (E/M) codes**, not in place of them.

Category II codes are intended to facilitate data collection on quality of care by coding certain services that support performance measurements and have been agreed on as contributing to good patient care. The use of category II codes is completely optional. They are used only in conjunction with category I codes and cannot be reported alone. An example of a category II code is 3014F, Screening mammography results documented and reviewed.

Category III Codes

Introduced in 2002, category III codes are five-character temporary alphanumeric codes with a *T* in the fifth position. These codes are used to describe emerging technologies that do not yet qualify for regular CPT codes. Category III codes will be ar-

chived after five years unless there is a demonstrated need for their continued existence. Some category III codes may become category I codes when the procedure satisfies the criteria for inclusion as a category I code outlined above. Medicare, Medicaid, and many private insurance companies accept category III codes for reimbursement purposes.

Category III status does not imply clinical efficacy, safety, or applicability to clinical practice. The category III codes do not conform to the usual requirements for category I codes. Where a category III code exists, it must be used in place of an unlisted category I CPT code. An example of a category III code is 0052T, Replacement or repair of thoracic unit of a total replacement heart system (artificial heart).

Category III codes may or may not eventually become category I codes. In any event, category III codes will be archived five years after publication or revision in the CPT code book, unless there is demonstrated need that the temporary status is still needed. If a category III code is archived after five years, and it has not been given a category I status, the unlisted category I code would then be assigned.

Both category II and category III codes are assigned in simple numerical and chronological order and do not reflect the organization of the rest of the CPT book.

CPT is part of a larger coding system called the Healthcare Common Procedure Coding System (HCPCS), which contains both CPT codes and HCPCS National Codes. HCPCS codes are required for reporting physician services and hospital outpatient services. (See chapter 4.)

Check Your Understanding 3.2

Instructions: Complete the following exercises on a separate piece of paper.

1. CPT category I codes are used to describe:
    a. New technology procedures
    b. Procedures that are widely performed
    c. Procedures that Medicare recognizes as covered entities
    d. All of the above

2. Which of the following statements about category II codes is *not* true?
   a. Category II codes are alphanumeric.
   b. Category II codes are used in conjunction with category I codes.
   c. Category II codes describe emerging technologies.
   d. Category II codes were introduced into CPT in 2004.

3. CPT codes are part of a larger system known as:
   a. Healthcare Common Procedure Coding System (HCPCS)
   b. ICD-9-CM
   c. Uniform Hospital Discharge Data Set (UHDDS)
   d. Unified Medical Language System (UMLS)

Organization of CPT

As noted above, CPT is organized into three categories of codes. The codes in the main section (category I codes) are intended to describe procedures and services performed by physicians and other healthcare professionals. The main section of CPT is divided into the following sections:

- Evaluation and management
- Anesthesiology
- Surgery
- Radiology
- Pathology and Laboratory
- Medicine

In addition to these six sections, there is an introduction, an index, and thirteen appendices. The appendices are as follows:

- Appendix A, Modifiers
- Appendix B, Summary of Additions, Deletions, and Revisions
- Appendix C, Clinical Examples
- Appendix D, Summary of CPT Add-on Codes
- Appendix E, Summary of CPT Codes Exempt from Modifier 51

- Appendix F, Summary of CPT Codes Exempt from Modifier 63
- Appendix G, Summary of CPT Codes that Include Moderate (Conscious) Sedation
- Appendix H, Alphabetic Index of Performance Measures by Clinical Condition or Topic
- Appendix I, Genetic Testing Code Modifiers
- Appendix J, Electrodiagnostic Medicine Listing of Sensory, Motor, and Mixed Nerves
- Appendix K, Product Pending FDA Approval
- Appendix L, Vascular Families
- Appendix M, Summary of Crosswalked Deleted CPT Codes

Each of the main CPT sections is further subdivided into subsections.

Evaluation and Management

Evaluation and management (E/M) codes are designed to report physician work as performed in different clinical settings. With a few exceptions, E/M codes are based on the practitioner's documentation of history, physical examination, and medical decision making. The subsections within the E/M section are as follows:

- Office or other outpatient services
  —New patient
  —Established patient
- Hospital observation services
  —Observation care discharge services
  —Initial observation care
    New or established patient
- Hospital inpatient services
  —Initial hospital care
    New or established patient

- —Subsequent hospital care

    Observation or inpatient care services

    Hospital discharge services

- Consultations

    —Office or other outpatient consultations

    New or established patient

    —Inpatient consultations

    New or established patient

- Emergency department services

    New or established patient

    —Other emergency services

- Critical care services

- Nursing facility services

    —Initial nursing facility care

    New or established patient

    —Subsequent nursing facility care

    —Nursing facility discharge services

    —Other nursing facility services

- Domiciliary, rest home (for example, boarding home), or custodial care services

    —New patient

    —Established patient

- Domiciliary, rest home (for example, assisted living facility), or home care plan oversight services

- Home services

    —New patient

    —Established patient

- Prolonged services

    —Prolonged physician service with direct patient contact

- —Prolonged physician service without direct patient contact

- —Physician standby services

- Case management services

    —Anticoagulant management

    —Medical team conferences

    Direct contact with patient and/or family

    Without direct contact with patient and/or family

- Care plan oversight services

- Preventive medicine services

    New patient

    Established patient

    —Counseling risk factor reduction and behavior change intervention

    New or established patient

    Other preventive medicine services

- Non-face-to-face physician services

    —Telephone services

    —Online medical evaluation

- Special E/M services

    —Basic life and/or disability evaluation services

    —Work related or medical disability evaluation services

- Newborn care services

    —Delivery/birthing room attendance and resuscitation services

- Inpatient neonatal intensive care services and pediatric and neonatal critical care services

    —Pediatric critical care patient transport

    —Inpatient neonatal and pediatric critical care

—Initial and continuing intensive care services

- Other evaluation and management services

Anesthesia

The anesthesia section is used to report the administration of anesthesia for designated surgical services, including general, regional, supplemented local, or other supportive services. The anesthesia code reported includes the pre- and postprocedure anesthesia visit, the anesthesia care during the procedure, the administration of fluids and/or blood, and the usual monitoring services, such as EKG, temperature, blood pressure, oximetry, capnography, and mass spectrometry). The leading *0* in each code number is reported. The subsections of the anesthesia section are as follows:

- Head
- Neck
- Thorax (chest wall and shoulder girdle)
- Intrathoracic
- Spine and spinal cord
- Upper abdomen
- Lower abdomen
- Perineum
- Pelvis (except hip)
- Upper leg (except knee)
- Knee and popliteal area
- Lower leg (below knee, includes ankle and foot)
- Shoulder and axilla
- Upper arm and elbow
- Forearm, wrist, and hand
- Radiological procedures
- Burn excisions or debridement
- Obstetric
- Other procedures

Surgery

The surgery section is by far the largest in CPT. It is divided into subsections based on body system. Within each subsection, the next level of subdivision is body part, then type of procedure, and finally body parts within procedures. Examples of subsections include the following:

- General
- Integumentary system
- Musculoskeletal system
- Respiratory system
- Cardiovascular system
- Hemic and lymphatic systems
- Mediastinum and diaphragm
- Digestive system
- Urinary system
- Male genital system
- Reproductive system procedures
- Intersex surgery
- Female genital system
- Maternity care and delivery
- Endocrine system
- Nervous system
- Eye and ocular adnexa
- Auditory system
- Operating microscope

Radiology

Within the radiology section, subsections are based on type of diagnostic or therapeutic procedure and then by body part. The subsections are as follows:

- Diagnostic radiology (includes diagnostic imaging, computed tomography, magnetic resonance imaging, magnetic resonance angiography)

- Diagnostic ultrasound
- Radiologic guidance
- Breast, mammography
- Bone/joint studies
- Radiation oncology
- Nuclear medicine

Pathology and Laboratory

Within the pathology and laboratory section, subsections are based on type of diagnostic procedure performed. Subsections include the following:

- Organ or disease-oriented panels
- Drug testing
- Therapeutic drug assays
- Evocative/suppression testing
- Consultations (clinical pathology)
- Urinalysis
- Chemistry
- Hematology and coagulation
- Immunology
- Transfusion medicine
- Microbiology
- Anatomic pathology
- Cytopathology
- Cytogenetic studies
- Surgical pathology
- In vivo (e.g., transcutaneous) laboratory procedures
- Other procedures
- Reproductive medicine procedures

Medicine

The medicine section of CPT contains a variety of codes that describe procedures that are not appropri-ate for reporting elsewhere within CPT. The subsections of the medicine section are as follows:

- Immune globulins
- Immunization administration for vaccines/toxoids
- Vaccines/toxoids
- Psychiatry
- Biofeedback
- Dialysis
- Gastroenterology
- Ophthalmology
- Special otorhinolaryngologic services
- Cardiovascular
- Noninvasive vascular diagnostic studies
- Pulmonary
- Allergy and clinical immunology
- Endocrinology
- Neurology and neuromuscular procedures
- Medical genetics and genetic counseling services
- Central nervous system assessments/tests
- Health and behavior assessment/intervention
- Hydration, therapeutic, prophylactic, diagnostic injections and infusions, and chemotherapy and other highly complex drug or highly complex biologic agent administration
- Photodynamic therapy
- Special dermatological procedures
- Physical medicine and rehabilitation
- Medical nutrition therapy
- Acupuncture
- Osteopathic manipulative treatment

- Chiropractic manipulative treatment

- Education and training for patient self-management

- Non-face-to-face nonphysician services

- Special services, procedures, and reports

- Qualifying circumstances for anesthesia

- Moderate (conscious) sedation

- Other services and procedures

- Home health procedures/services

- Medication therapy management services

The subsections are further divided into subcategories, then headings, and finally procedures/services. For example, procedure 24600, Treatment of closed elbow dislocation; without anesthesia, is located within the surgery section, musculoskeletal subsection, humerus (upper arm) and elbow subcategory, fracture and/or dislocation heading. Within procedure groupings, the progression is usually from either proximal to distal or least to most complex.

Inclusion of a procedure code within a particular subsection of CPT does not restrict its use to practitioners within that specialty; any practitioner can use any code. For example, both emergency department physicians and orthopedic surgeons treat fractures and both can use the fracture treatment codes within the musculoskeletal subsection of CPT.

CPT has an Alphabetic Index and a Tabular List. The index contains an alphabetic listing of entries that may include:

- Procedure, service, or examination (for example, appendectomy, physical therapy, electrocardiography)

- Organ or anatomic site (for example, humerus, liver)

- Diagnosis or condition (for example, aortic stenosis, fracture)

- Synonym (for example, Seminin, followed by a note to see Antigen, prostate specific)

- Eponym (for example, Silver procedure, Shelf procedure)

- Abbreviation (for example, EEG, ERCP)

Following each entry is a single CPT code, several CPT codes separated by commas, a series of CPT codes, or a combination of CPT codes. The Alphabetic Index serves as a guide to the Tabular List; it is not recommended to assign a code from the index alone. Each of the suggested codes must be reviewed in its entirety, and the code that most accurately describes the procedure performed should be assigned.

To illustrate, following are the listings in the index for pancreas:

Anastomosis		
	With intestines	48520–48540, 48548
Anesthesia		00794
Biopsy		48100
	Needle Biopsy	48102
Cyst		
	Anastomosis	48520–48540
	Repair	48500
Debridement		
	Peripancreatic tissue	48105
Excision		
	Ampulla of Vater	48148
	Duct	48148
	Partial	48140–48146, 48150, 48154, 48160
	Peripancreatic tissue	48105
	Total	48155–48160
Lesion		
	Excision	48120
Needle biopsy		48102
Placement		
	Drainage	48000–48001
Pseudocyst		
	Drainage	

Open	48510
Percutaneous	48511
Removal	
Calculi (Stone)	48020
Removal Transplanted	
Allograft	48556
Repair	
Cyst	48500
Resection	48105
Suture	48545
Transplantation	48160, 48550, 48554–48556
Allograft Preparation	48550–48552
Islet Cell	0141T, 0142T, 0143T
Unlisted Services and Procedures	48999
X-ray with Contrast	74300–74305
Injection Procedure	48400

Check Your Understanding 3.3

Instructions: Complete the following exercises on a separate piece of paper.

1. True or False. Evaluation and management codes are generally assigned on the basis of documentation of history, physical examination, and medical decision making.

2. A complete list of CPT modifiers and their definitions is included in which appendix of CPT?
   a. A
   b. B
   c. C
   d. D

3. Which of the following is *not* a subsection of the radiology section of CPT?
   a. Nuclear medicine
   b. Magnetic resonance imaging
   c. Diagnostic ultrasound
   d. Radiation oncology

4. The Alphabetic Index of CPT includes which of the following types of listings?
   a. Procedures
   b. Diagnoses
   c. Abbreviations
   d. All of the above

Principles and Guidelines

The AMA develops guidelines for CPT use. The guidelines may appear in the form of coding notes in several places, including:

- At the beginning of a section. Notes at the beginning of a section apply to all codes within the section and may include information such as:

  —Integral components of a service

  —Definitions of terms/codes

  —Directions to assign additional codes

- At the beginning of a subsection

- Before or following a specific code

In addition, the AMA publishes *CPT Assistant*, a monthly magazine that provides official coding advice, and the annual *Insider's View*, a review, with extensive clinical rationales, of the new and revised codes for each year. Only the AMA can develop official guidelines for CPT coding, although CMS also issues guidelines that relate to the use of CPT for reimbursement purposes.

Guidelines for Reporting E/M Codes

E/M codes are used primarily to describe cognitive physician services. As noted, they are assigned based on documentation of history, physical examination, and medical decision making, with a few exceptions.

History

CPT defines the history as follows:

- Chief complaint, usually in the patient's own words, is a concise statement of the symptom, problem, condition, diagnosis, or other factor that is the reason for the encounter.

- History of present illness, which in turn is defined in terms of:

  —Location (for example, pain in the right lower quadrant of the abdomen)

—Quality (for example, pain)

—Severity (for example, pain rated 7 on a scale of 10, or severe pain)

—Timing (for example, pain lasting for up to an hour)

—Context (for example, pain occurring when lying down)

—Modifying factors (for example, pain improved with aspirin, rest, and so on)

—Associated signs and symptoms (for example, pain accompanied by nausea and vomiting)

- Review of systems is an inventory of body systems obtained through a series of questions designed to elicit signs and/or symptoms. The systems as defined by the AMA are:

—Constitutional (for example, fever, weight loss)

—Eyes (for example, blurred vision, double vision)

—Ears, nose, mouth, and throat (for example, diminished hearing, throat pain)

—Cardiovascular (for example, chest pain, palpitations)

—Respiratory (for example, shortness of breath, difficulty breathing)

—Gastrointestinal (for example, abdominal pain, diarrhea)

—Genitourinary (for example, difficulty voiding, pain on urination)

—Musculoskeletal (for example, joint pain, stiffness upon awakening)

—Integumentary (for example, skin rash, breast pain)

—Neurological (for example, loss of sensation, dizziness)

—Psychiatric (for example, feelings of helplessness and hopelessness)

—Endocrine (for example, heat or cold intolerance)

—Hematologic/lymphatic (for example, easy bruising, swollen glands)

—Allergic/immunologic (for example, history of allergies)

- Past history is a review of the patient's past illnesses, treatments, and injuries, including:

—Prior major illnesses or injuries

—Prior operations

—Prior hospitalizations

—Current medications

—Allergies (for example, drugs, foods)

—Age-appropriate immunization status

—Age-appropriate feeding/dietary status

- Social history is a review of past and current activities and interactions, including:

—Marital status and/or living arrangements

—Current employment and past occupational history

—Use of drugs, alcohol, and tobacco

—Educational level/literacy

—Sexual history and habits

—Other relevant social factors

- Family history is a review of medical events in the patient's family, including:

—Parents' and siblings' morbidity and mortality, especially as related to the presenting concerns or risk of morbidity

—Family history of congenital defects

—Family history of hereditary conditions

Physical Examination

For purposes of CPT, the AMA recognizes the following body areas:

- Head, including face ("head normocephalic, face symmetrical")

- Neck ("range of motion of the neck normal," "no thyroid masses palpable")

- Chest, including breasts and axilla ("chest symmetrical, lungs clear")

- Abdomen ("abdomen flat, no masses palpable")

- Genitalia, groin, and buttocks ("genitalia without masses, groin without palpable nodes")

- Back ("back straight with normal range of motion")

- Each extremity ("right upper extremity in a cast, remainder of extremities without loss of range of motion")

The physical examination also may be defined in terms of organ systems. The following organ systems are recognized:

- Eyes ("pupils equal, react to light and accommodation")

- Ears, nose, mouth, and throat ("ear canals clean, nose without congestion")

- Cardiovascular ("heart sounds normal without murmurs, rubs, or gallops")

- Respiratory ("breath sounds clear to auscultation and percussion")

- Gastrointestinal ("abdomen is flat and soft, without tenderness or masses")

- Genitourinary ("no tenderness of the genitalia")

- Musculoskeletal ("range of motion of all joints within normal limits")

- Skin ("no rashes or areas of discoloration")

- Neurologic ("normal sensation to pinprick and light touch in all dermatomes tested")

- Psychiatric ("alert and oriented to time, place, person, and station")

- Hematologic/lymphatic/immunologic ("no bruising, glandular enlargement")

Medical Decision Making

Medical decision making is the most cognitive of the three criteria for assigning E/M codes and the most difficult to quantify. CPT recognizes the following levels of medical decision making:

- Straightforward

  —Minimal number of diagnoses or management options

  —Minimal or no data to be reviewed

  —Minimal risk of complications, morbidity, mortality

- Low complexity

  —Limited number of diagnoses or management options

  —Limited amount or complexity of data to be reviewed

  —Low risk of complications, morbidity, mortality

- Moderate complexity

  —Multiple diagnoses or management options

  —Moderate amount or complexity of data to be reviewed

  —Moderate risk of complications, morbidity, mortality

- High complexity

  —Extensive diagnoses or management options

  —Extensive amount or complexity of data to be reviewed

—High risk of complications, morbidity, mortality

The Principle of Counseling

Counseling is defined as being a discussion of one or more of the following topics:

- Diagnostic results, impressions, and/or recommended diagnostic studies

- Prognosis

- Risks and benefits of management

- Instruction for management

- Importance of compliance

- Risk factor reduction

- Patient and family education

If counseling or coordination of care makes up more than 50 percent of a patient encounter, time is a key factor in determining the level of service, rather than the nature of the presenting problem. When counseling is a major part of a patient visit, documentation is very important. The visit note should include the topic of the counseling, the number of minutes spent counseling, and the plan for follow-up.

Guidelines for Coding Critical Care Codes

Although critical care codes are a type of E/M code, they are not defined by documentation of history, physical examination, and medical decision making. Rather, critical care codes are defined by time, the nature of the problem, and the nature of the treatment.

Critical care services should be reported in conjunction with a critical illness or injury, which is defined as an illness or injury that acutely impairs one or more vital organ systems such that there is a high probability of imminent or life-threatening deterioration in the patient's condition (CPT 2008). CPT goes on to state that critical care service involves decision making of high complexity to assess, ma-

nipulate, and support vital organ system failure and/or to prevent further life-threatening deterioration of the patient's condition. According to CPT, examples of vital organ system failure include, but are not limited to, central nervous system failure, circulatory failure, shock, and renal, hepatic, metabolic, and/or respiratory failure.

Guidelines for Reporting Surgery Codes

The surgery section has a number of unique guidelines. An example is the principle of surgical package.

The Principle of the Surgical Package

Within the surgery section of CPT, the principle of the **surgical package** (also referred to as the global surgical package) applies. This concept is based on a single, readily identifiable procedure that may contain a number of services. Per CPT guidelines, the following services are always included in each operation:

- Local infiltration, metacarpal/metatarsal/digital block, or topical anesthesia

- Subsequent to the decision for surgery, one related E/M encounter on the date immediately prior to, or on the date of, the procedure

- Immediate postoperative care, including dictating operative notes, talking with family and other physicians

- Writing orders

- Evaluating the patient in the postanesthesia recovery room

- Typical postoperative follow-up care (CPT 2008)

Another, slightly different definition for surgical package, as defined by the Medicare program, is as follows:

- Preoperative visits, beginning with the day before a surgery for major procedures and the day of surgery for minor procedures

- Intraoperative services that are normally a usual and necessary part of a surgical procedure

- Postsurgical complications that do not require additional trips to the operating room

- Postoperative visits (follow-up visits) during the postoperative period of the surgery that are related to recovery from the surgery

- Postoperative pain management provided by the surgeon

- Supplies, except those identified as exclusions

- Miscellaneous services including items such as dressing changes; local incisional care; removal of operative pack, and removal of cutaneous sutures, staples, line wires, tubes, drains, casts, and splints; insertion, irrigation, and removal of urinary catheters, routine peripheral intravenous lines, nasogastric and rectal tubes; and changes or removal of tracheostomy tubes (CMS 2008)

Guidelines for Reporting Separate Procedures

In CPT, a **separate procedure** is commonly part of another, more complex procedure. The guidelines for reporting separate procedures generally apply when one procedure designated as a separate procedure is performed with another procedure rather than with an E/M service. If the separate procedure is an integral part of the other procedure, it is not reported separately. However, when a separate procedure is performed independently or is otherwise unrelated to another procedure performed during the same session, it may be reported separately with a modifier attached.

Guidelines for Reporting Unlisted Procedure Codes

Unlisted procedure codes appear throughout the CPT system. These codes, many of which end in xxx99,

are used to report procedures for which a category I code, a category III code, or a HCPCS code does not exist. When any of the above do exist, they must be used instead of the unlisted procedure code.

When an unlisted procedure code is reported for reimbursement purposes, the payer will likely require additional documentation. For a surgical procedure, an operative report is always required, and additional information also may be requested.

Guidelines for Using Modifiers

CPT codes can be customized by the use of one or more **modifiers,** which are listed in appendix A of the CPT manual each year. Modifiers are two-digit extensions added to a CPT code to indicate that a particular event modified the service or procedure without changing its basic definition. Modifiers may be used in the following circumstances (this list is not all inclusive):

- A service/procedure has both a professional and a technical component.

- A service/procedure was performed at more than one anatomic site, or by more than one physician.

- A service/procedure has been reduced or expanded in scope.

- A service/procedure was performed bilaterally.

- An unusual event occurred during the service/procedure.

- Only part of a service was done.

- An adjunctive service was done.

- A service or procedure was provided more than once.

Like the rest of CPT, CPT modifiers may change in meaning or be deleted through the update process. Most CPT modifiers may be used with physician services, but only select ones can be reported with hospital outpatient services. Within physician services, some modifiers can be used only with E/M codes, others only with surgical codes, and others with all codes. Appendix A in CPT indicates which of these modifiers may be used in each circumstance.

In addition to the CPT modifiers, there are HCPCS Level II modifiers. (See chapter 4.) HCPCS modifiers also may be used with CPT codes. However, relatively few HCPCS Level II modifiers have been approved for hospital outpatient department use.

Guidelines for Using the Semicolon

The **semicolon** has a special meaning in CPT. In order to make the page format less cluttered, common information is not repeated. Within a code set, an initial code may contain a procedure description, a semicolon, and additional information. The information to the left of the semicolon applies to that code and all the codes indented under it; the information to the right of the semicolon changes. For example:

36800   Insertion of cannula for hemodialysis, other
        purpose (separate procedure); vein to vein
36810   arteriovenous, external (Scribner type)
36815   arteriovenous, external revision, or closure

The complete description for code 36810 is Insertion of cannula for hemodialysis, other purpose (separate procedure); arteriovenous, external (Scribner type), and the complete description for code 36815 is Insertion of cannula for hemodialysis, other purpose (separate procedure); arteriovenous, external revision, or closure.

Check Your Understanding 3.4

Instructions: Complete the following exercises on a separate piece of paper.

1. Which of the following is *not* a requirement for inclusion of a code in CPT?
   a. Many healthcare professionals across the country must perform the procedure.
   b. The procedure must be FDA approved or with approval imminent within a given CPT cycle.
   c. Medicare must cover the procedure.
   d. The procedure must be of proven clinical efficacy.

2. True or False. Category II codes describe emerging technologies.

3. Which set of E/M codes below is not assigned based on documentation of history, physical examination, and medical decision making?
   a. Inpatient consultations
   b. Office visits
   c. Critical care services
   d. Hospital observation services

4. Which circumstance below cannot be reflected with a CPT modifier?
   a. A service/procedure that has both a professional and a technical component
   b. A service/procedure that has been reduced or expanded in scope
   c. A service/procedure that does not yet have a specific CPT code
   d. A patient that has a bilateral procedure performed

Process for Revision and Updates

Category I codes are updated annually. A **CPT Editorial Panel** develops them with the assistance of the CPT Advisory Committee. The Editorial Panel is composed of seventeen members. Of that number, eleven are physicians from various medical specialty societies, with one position reserved for a member with expertise in performance measurement. Further, one physician is nominated from each of the following organizations: Blue Cross and Blue Shield Association, America's Health Insurance Plans, the American Hospital Association, and Centers for Medicare and Medicaid Services (CMS). The other two positions are reserved for two members of the CPT Health Care Professionals Advisory Committee. In addition, advisors also support the work of the CPT Editorial Panel.

Category II codes are updated three times a year. The Performance Measures Advisory Group (PMAG) reviews their content. The PMAG is an advisory body to the CPT Editorial Panel and is composed of representatives from the AMA, Agency for Healthcare Research and Quality (AHRQ), CMS, The Joint Commission, the National Committee for Quality Assurance (NCQA), and the Physician Consortium for Performance Improvement, with solicited input from various specialty societies and other agencies.

Because they are intended to report emerging technologies and must respond quickly to changes in treatment methods, category III codes are updated semiannually on the AMA/CPT Web site. The most current version of category III codes can be downloaded from the AMA Web site at http://www.ama-assn.org/ama/pub/category/3885.html.

Anyone can request a change to CPT, including the addition of new codes (in any category), the deletion of old codes, and changes in code description. The change form may be downloaded from the AMA Web site under CPT/applying for codes at http://www.ama-assn.org/ama/pub/category/3112.html. The AMA Web site discusses the process for updating CPT in detail at http://www.ama-assn.org/ama/pub/category/3882.html.

Recommendations from the AMA CPT-5 Project Executive Project Advisory Group resulted in the creation of category II and III codes.

Summary

The American Medical Association developed CPT as a procedural terminology to describe medical services and procedures performed by physicians and other healthcare providers. CPT is used to report physician services, many nonphysician services, and surgical services performed in hospital outpatient departments and ambulatory surgery centers. Although it was originally developed as a way to report physician services for reimbursement as accurately as possible, CPT now is used for healthcare trending and planning, benchmarking, and measurement of quality of care as well.

References

American Medical Association. 1992–2008. *CPT Assistant.* Chicago: American Medical Association.

American Medical Association. 2008. *CPT Changes 2008: An Insider's View*. Chicago: American Medical Association.

American Medical Association. 2009. *Current Procedural Terminology (CPT),* fourth edition. Chicago: American Medical Association.

Centers for Medicare and Medicaid Services. 2008. Internet-Only Manuals (IOMs) Medicare Claims Processing Manual, Chapter 12-Physicians/Nonphysician Practitioners. http://www.cms.hhs.gov/manuals/downloads/clm104c12.pdf.

Additional Resources

http://www.ama-assn.org/ama/pub/category/3885.html. This link is to the portion of the AMA Web site on category III CPT codes.

http://www.ama-assn.org/ama/noindex/category/17467.html. This link is to the portion of the AMA Web site on category II CPT codes.

http://www.ama-assn.org/ama/pub/category/3113.html. This is the CPT home page on the AMA Web site.

Application Exercise

Visit the AMA Web site at http://www.ama-assn.org/ama/pub/category/3882.html to review the process for requesting a new CPT code. A new procedure has been developed at your university teaching hospital: an endoscopic total hip replacement (femoral head only). Complete forms to request a new CPT code. The forms can be downloaded from http://www.ama-assn.org/ama1/pub/upload/mm/362/catiandiiiform.doc. You can request either a category I or III code for your procedure. (Note: Do not actually submit your code request to the AMA.)

Review Quiz

1. True or False. Only members of the American Medical Association can request changes to CPT.

2. "A concise statement of the symptom, problem, condition, diagnosis, or other factor that is the reason for the encounter" defines the:
    a. History of present illness
    b. Chief complaint
    c. Review of systems
    d. Primary diagnosis

3. Which of the following services is not included in CPT surgical package guidelines?
    a. Subsequent to the decision for surgery, one related E/M encounter on the date immediately prior to, or on the date of, the procedure
    b. Immediate postoperative care, including dictating operative notes, talking with family and other physicians
    c. Writing orders
    d. E/M service for postoperative care related to a complication.

4. Which of the following statements about category II codes is false?
   a. They are mandatory.
   b. They are updated biannually by the AMA.
   c. They are alphanumeric codes.
   d. They cannot be reported alone.

5. True or False. If a category III code exists to describe a procedure, an unlisted category I code may not be reported.

6. Which of the following is not a section in CPT?
   a. Surgery
   b. Evaluation and management
   c. Radiology
   d. Miscellaneous

7. Which of the following services is not included in an anesthesia code?
   a. The pre- and postanesthesia visit
   b. Central venous catheter placement
   c. Administration of fluids and/or blood
   d. Monitoring of EKG, temperature, and blood pressure

8. True or False. It is appropriate to report separately a procedure that is not an integral part of another procedure.

9. Which of the following bodies can issue official CPT coding guidelines?
   a. The American Hospital Association and the American Medical Association
   b. The American Medical Association
   c. The Centers for Medicare and Medicaid Services, the American Hospital Association, and the American Medical Association
   d. The Centers for Medicare and Medicaid Services and the American Medical Association

10. Which of the following is not a level of medical decision making?
    a. Straightforward
    b. Low complexity
    c. Moderate complexity
    d. Extensive complexity

11. Critical care services must satisfy three criteria. They are:
    a. History, physical examination, and medical decision making
    b. The nature of the problem, the nature of the treatment, and time
    c. Medical decision making, time, and physician specialty
    d. Location of the patient, specialty of the physician, and time

12. Which of the following is not considered part of counseling for CPT purposes?
    a. Diagnostic results and impressions
    b. Prognosis
    c. Interactive psychotherapy
    d. Risk factor reduction

13. The numbering system of category III codes reflects:
    a. The simple numerical sequence in which they were added
    b. The overall organization of category I codes
    c. The type of technology being reported
    d. The physician specialty to which they apply

14. True or False. CPT contains no terminologies or codes that address osteopathic or chiropractic manipulative services.

15. Marital status and/or living arrangements, current employment and past occupational history, and educational level/literacy are all part of the:
    a. Past history
    b. Social history
    c. Review of systems
    d. Family history

Chapter 4

Healthcare Common Procedure Coding System (HCPCS)

Kathy Giannangelo, MA, RHIA, CCS, CPHIMS, FAHIMA

Learning Objectives

- To discuss the history of the development of Healthcare Common Procedure Coding System (HCPCS)

- To explain the use and structure of HCPCS

- To identify and describe the levels of HCPCS

Key Terms

American Medical Association (AMA)
Carriers
Current Dental Terminology (CDT)
Dental codes
Descriptor
Durable medical equipment (DME)
Fiscal intermediary (FI)
HCPCS level I
HCPCS level II
Healthcare Common Procedure Coding System (HCPCS)
Medicare Administrative Contractors (MACs)
Miscellaneous codes
Permanent national codes
Temporary national codes

Introduction

The **Healthcare Common Procedure Coding System** (HCPCS) is a standardized system for healthcare providers and medical suppliers to report professional services, procedures, and supplies. HCPCS is required for reimbursement of ambulatory services provided in healthcare settings. This includes not only physician reimbursement, but also an expanding array of ambulatory services. HCPCS is published by the Centers for Medicare and Medicaid Services (CMS).

Since 1983, regardless of the deletion and addition of codes, CMS has maintained the intention of HCPCS, which is to meet the operational needs of the Medicare/Medicaid reimbursement programs. HCPCS is used not only for reimbursement, but also for benchmarking, trending, planning, and measurement of quality of care. This chapter examines the history and current practice of HCPCS.

Developer

Introduced in 1983, HCPCS, formerly called the HCFA Common Procedure Coding System, was developed to standardize the coding systems used to process Medicare and Medicaid claims. This system also was developed to promote uniform reporting and statistical data collection of medical procedures, supplies, products, and services. The name of the system was changed in 2001 when the agency that administers the Medicare and Medicaid programs changed its name from the Health Care Financing Administration to the Centers for Medicare and Medicaid Services (CMS).

In 1985, the federal government required physicians to use HCPCS codes to report services provided to Medicare patients, and, in October 1986, CMS required physicians to use HCPCS codes to report services provided to Medicaid patients. Section 9343(g) of the Omnibus Reconciliation Act of 1986 required hospitals (effective July 1, 1987) to report ambulatory surgery services, radiology, and other diagnostic services using HCPCS codes (HCFA 2000).

Purpose

HCPCS (usually pronounced "hick picks") is a collection of codes and descriptors used to represent healthcare procedures, supplies, products, and services. HCFA (now CMS) found out during the 1980s that it was necessary to develop the HCPCS system because not all supplies, procedures, and services could be coded using the Current Procedural Terminology (CPT) system. (See chapter 3.) The primary purpose of the HCPCS coding system is to meet the operational needs of Medicare and Medicaid reimbursement programs.

Check Your Understanding 4.1

Instructions: Complete the following exercises on a separate piece of paper.

1. What is the purpose of HCPCS?

2. What organization was responsible for developing HCPCS?

3. True or False. HCPCS codes describe physician and nonphysician services.

Composition

HCPCS is divided into two principal subsystems: level I and level II.

HCPCS Level I

HCPCS level I comprises the CPT coding system, a system maintained and published by the **American Medical Association** (AMA). Level I codes include five character codes and two-digit modifiers. Developed in 1966, CPT is a uniform coding system consisting of descriptive terms and identifying codes that are used primarily to identify medical services and procedures furnished by physicians and other healthcare professionals. Physicians and other healthcare professionals use CPT to identify services and procedures for which they bill public or private health insurance programs. The AMA makes decisions regarding the addition, deletion, or modification of CPT codes. The CPT codes in level I of HCPCS do not include codes needed to report medical items or services that are regularly billed by suppliers other than physicians.

The CPT coding system, or HCPCS level I, is discussed in detail in chapter 3.

HCPCS Level II

Development and use of **HCPCS level II** began in the 1980s. Level II codes are referred to as alphanumeric codes because they consist of a single alphabetical letter followed by four numeric digits. Also called national codes, level II codes are maintained by CMS. Level II of HCPCS is a standardized coding system that is used primarily to identify products, supplies, and services not included in the CPT codes. The system describes classifications of like products that are medical in nature by category for the purpose of efficient claims processing. Although level II codes are used for billing purposes, decisions regarding the addition, deletion, or modification of HCPCS are made independent of the process for making determinations regarding coverage and payment.

Principles and Guidelines for HCPCS Level II

HCPCS is not a methodology or system for making coverage or payment determinations. Each payer makes determinations on coverage and payment outside this coding process. Moreover, the existence of a code does not, in itself, determine coverage or noncoverage for an item or service. Rather, HCPCS ensures uniform reporting on claims forms of items or services that are medical in nature. Public and private insurance programs need such a standardized coding system to ensure the uniform reporting of services on claims forms by providers and suppliers and for meaningful data collection.

The descriptors of the codes identify like items or services rather than specific products or brand/trade names.

Types of HCPCS Level II Codes

There are several types of HCPCS level II codes depending on their purpose and who is responsible for establishing and maintaining them.

Permanent National Codes
Maintained by the CMS HCPCS Workgroup, **permanent national codes** provide a standardized coding system that is managed jointly by private and public insurers. The Workgroup includes representatives from Medicare, Medicaid, and the Pricing, Data Analysis, and Coding (PDAC) contractor. Members are responsible for reviewing requests for additions, deletions, and revisions to the codes and formulating preliminary coding recommendations for presentation to the public for comment. Coding decisions are coordinated with public and private insurers. During the public meetings, CMS also presents initial recommendations regarding payment methodology. Subsequently, the Workgroup convenes to prepare their final coding recommendations. However, CMS is the final decision-making authority concerning requests for permanent HCPCS level II codes. Permanent codes are updated annually on January 1.

Dental Codes
Published by the American Dental Association (ADA), the **Current Dental Terminology** (CDT) lists the **dental codes** used for billing dental procedures and supplies. These codes are a separate category of national codes and are included in HCPCS level II. Decisions regarding any changes of CDT are made by the ADA, not the CMS HCPCS Workgroup.

The Department of Health and Human Services (HHS) has an agreement with the ADA to include CDT as a set of HCPCS level II codes for use in billing for dental services. CDT is discussed in detail in chapter 6.

Miscellaneous Codes
Miscellaneous codes are used when a supplier submits a bill for an item or service for which no existing national code adequately describes the item or service being billed. These codes include miscellaneous, or not otherwise classified, codes and allow suppliers to begin billing immediately for a service

or item as soon as the Food and Drug Administration (FDA) permits the service or item to be marketed, even though no distinct code describes it.

Miscellaneous codes can be used during the period of time a request for a new code is being considered under the HCPCS review process. Utilization of miscellaneous codes also helps to avoid the inefficiency of assigning distinct codes for items or services that are rarely furnished or for which few claims are expected.

When using a miscellaneous code, submit documentation to the payer who will receive the claim. For **durable medical equipment**, prosthetics, orthotics, and supplies (DMEPOS), the PDAC contractor should be contacted about coding questions. A number of factors are taken into consideration by the PDAC when making a determination on whether or not a miscellaneous code should be used.

Temporary National Codes

Members of the CMS HCPCS Workgroup develop **temporary national codes**, which are independent of the permanent national codes. Temporary national codes give insurers the flexibility to establish codes that are needed before the next annual update for permanent national codes or until consensus can be reached on a permanent national code. Temporary codes do not have an expiration date. However, if a permanent code is created to replace a temporary one, then the temporary code is deleted and a cross-reference is established to the new permanent code

Temporary codes may be changed on a quarterly basis. Typically, they are implemented within 90 days, which is the time needed to prepare and issue implementation instructions and assistance to suppliers and to enter the new code into CMS's and the contractors' computer systems and initiate user education.

The types of temporary codes are as follows:

- C codes are used exclusively for the hospital outpatient prospective payment system purposes. Only Medicare claims submitted by hospital outpatient departments may contain these codes.

- G codes are used to identify professional healthcare procedures and services where normally one would expect to use a CPT code but currently no CPT code exists.

- H codes are used by Medicaid agencies when State law mandates separate codes for reporting mental health services such as alcohol and drug treatment services.

- K codes are for use by the durable medical equipment (DME) **Medicare Administrative Contactors** (MACs) when existing permanent national codes do not include the codes needed to implement a DME MAC medical review policy.

- Q codes are used to identify services that would be not be given a CPT code, such as drugs and other types of medical services that are not identified by national level II codes, but for which codes are needed for claims-processing purposes.

- S codes are used by private insurers to report drugs, services, and supplies for which there are no national codes, but for which codes are needed by the private sector to implement policies, programs, or claims processing.

- T codes are designated for use by state Medicaid agencies to establish codes for items for which there are no permanent national codes and for which codes are necessary to administer the Medicaid program. (T codes are not used by Medicare but can be used by private insurers.)

Check Your Understanding 4.2

Instructions: Complete the following exercises on a separate piece of paper.

1. Describe HCPCS levels I and II.

2. What are temporary codes? How are they used?

3. What are permanent national codes? How are they used?

4. What are miscellaneous codes? How are they used?

HCPCS level II national codes represent more than 4,000 separate categories of like items or services that encompass millions of products from different manufacturers. When submitting a claim, providers and suppliers are required to use one of these codes to identify the items they are billing. The **descriptors** assigned to codes represent the official definition of the items and services that can be billed using those codes; they do not refer to specific products. The reason the descriptors do not refer to specific products is to avoid the appearance of endorsement of particular products through HCPCS.

Index

The index for level II codes is alphanumeric and is listed alphabetically. The service or supply name is followed by the code. The index for HCPCS level II codes may be found at http://www.cms.hhs.gov/HCPCSReleaseCodeSets/ANHCPCS/list.asp.

Services and Products in HCPCS Level II

The following sections describe the codes that represent services and products in HCPCS level II.

A Codes: Transportation Services, including Ambulance

This code range includes ground and air ambulance, nonemergency transportation (taxi, bus, automobile, wheelchair van), and ancillary transportation-related fees. Examples include A0225, Ambulance service, neonatal transport, base rate, emergency transport, one way, and A0390, advanced life support (ALS) mileage (per mile).

A Codes: Medical and Surgical Supplies

This code range covers a range of medical, surgical, and other supplies and accessories related to durable medical equipment (DME). DME-related supplies, accessories, maintenance, and repair required to ensure the proper functioning of DME is generally covered by Medicare under the prosthetic devices provision. Examples include A4206, Syringe with needle, sterile 1 cc, each; A4330, Perineal fecal collection pouch with adhesive, each; and a series of codes (A5500–A5513) for diabetic footwear. Special dressings

(A6000–A6551) also are included in this area as are supplies of some radiopharmaceutical imaging agents (A9500–A9700). Other imaging agents are included in the C codes (temporary outpatient PPS) section of HCPCS.

B Codes: Enteral and Parenteral Therapy

The B codes are for supplies, formulae, nutritional solutions, and infusion pumps. Examples of each include B4034, Enteral feeding supply kit; syringe fed, per day; B4150, Enteral formula, nutritionally complete with intact nutrients, includes proteins, fats, carbohydrates, vitamins and minerals, may include fiber, administered through an enteral feeding tube, 100 calories = 1 unit; B4168, Parenteral nutrition solution; amino acid, 3.5%, 500 ml = 1 unit, home mix; and B9002, Enteral nutrition infusion pump, with alarm.

C Codes: Outpatient PPS (Temporary)

The C codes are used to report drugs, biologicals, and devices eligible for transitional pass-through payments for hospitals and for items classified in new-technology ambulatory payment classifications (APCs) under the outpatient prospective payment system (OPPS). Included in this section are codes for devices such as infusion pump, non-programmable, temporary (implantable) (C2626), procedures such as magnetic resonance angiography (MRA) of the chest without and with contrast (C8911), brachytherapy source, palladium 103, per source (C1720), and some drugs, such as galsulfase (C9224).

D Codes: Dental Procedures

The D (dental) codes are a separate category of national codes. The CDT code set is copyrighted by the ADA.

E Codes: Durable Medical Equipment

E codes include DME such as canes (E0105, Cane, quad or three-prong, includes canes of all materials, adjustable or fixed, with tips), crutches (E0117, Crutch underarm, articulating, spring assisted, each), walkers (E0130, Walker, rigid [pickup] adjustable or fixed height), and commodes (E0163, Commode chair, mobile or stationary, with fixed arms). Also included in this section are:

- Decubitus care equipment (E0176, Air pressure pad or cushion, nonpositioning)

- Bath and toilet aids (E0241, Bathtub wall rail, each)

- Hospital beds (E0295, Hospital bed, semi-electric [head and foot adjustment], without side rails, with mattress)

- Oxygen and related respiratory equipment (E0461, Volume control ventilator, without pressure support mode, may include pressure control mode, used with noninvasive interface [for example, mask])

- Monitoring equipment (E0607, Home blood glucose monitor and E0619, Apnea monitor, with recording feature)

- Safety equipment (E0700, Safety equipment [for example, belt, harness or vest])

Neurostimulators are included here, as are infusion supplies (E0776, IV pole), traction (E0860, Traction equipment, over door, cervical), wheelchair accessories (E0968, Commode seat, wheelchair), and wheelchairs (E1140, Wheelchair; detachable arms, desk or full-length, swing-away, detachable footrests). Artificial kidney machines also are included in this section (E1594 Cycler dialysis machine for peritoneal dialysis), as are other devices such as power wheelchairs and accessories.

G Codes: Procedures/Professional Services (Temporary)

G codes are used to identify professional healthcare procedures and services that would otherwise be coded in CPT, but either no CPT codes exist or the HCPCS code provides a level of detail required by CMS. Examples include such diverse services as observation services in hospitals (G0263, Direct admission of patient with diagnosis of congestive heart failure, chest pain, or asthma for observation services that meet all criteria for G0244) and positron

emission tomography (PET) scanning (G0252, PET imaging, full and partial-ring PET scanners only, for initial diagnosis of breast cancer and/or surgical planning for breast cancer).

Additionally, there are codes for end-stage renal disease (ESRD) services that do not fall within the composite rate (G0326, ESRD related services for home dialysis [less than full month], per day, for patients between 12 and 19 years of age) and codes for complex radiation therapy using robotic linear accelerators (G0339–G0340).

H Codes: Alcohol and Drug Abuse Treatment Services

H codes are used by those Medicaid agencies mandated by state law to establish separate codes for identifying mental health services that include alcohol and drug treatment services. Included in this section are codes to report detoxification (H0014, Alcohol and/or drug services; ambulatory detoxification), medication administration (H0033, Oral medication administration, direct observation), prenatal care (H1000, Prenatal care, at-risk assessment), and various therapies (H2032, Activity therapy, per 15 minutes; H2019, Therapeutic behavioral services, per 15 minutes; and H2024, Supported employment, per diem).

J Codes: Drugs Administered Other Than by Oral Method

J codes include drugs that ordinarily cannot be self-administered, such as drugs administered by other than oral means (J0120–J3590), chemotherapy drugs (J8999–J9999), immunosuppressive drugs, and inhalation solutions (J7602–J7799).

The Table of Drugs can be found at http://www.cms.hhs.gov/HCPCSReleaseCodeSets/ANHCPCS/list.asp.

K Codes (Temporary Codes)

K codes were established for use by the DME MACs. These codes are developed when current permanent national codes for supplies and certain product categories do not include the codes needed to implement a DME MAC medical review policy.

There are K codes for wheelchairs and wheelchair accessories that are not listed in the E code section (K0019, Arm pad, each), spinal orthotics that are not included in the L code section (K0114, Back support system for use with wheelchair, with inner frame, prefabricated), and various miscellaneous codes (K0602, Replacement battery for external infusion pump owned by patient, silver oxide, 1.5 volt, each). Because they are temporary, codes in this section are added and deleted regularly.

L Codes: Orthotic Procedures and Devices

L codes include orthotic and prosthetic procedures and devices as well as scoliosis equipment, orthopedic shoes, and prosthetic implants. Codes in the orthotics section are extremely specific.

Example:

L0490, TLSO (thoracolumbosacral orthosis), sagittal-coronal control, one-piece rigid plastic shell with overlapping reinforced anterior, with multiple straps and closures, posterior extends from sacrococcygeal junction and terminates at or before the T9 vertebra, anterior extends from the symphysis pubis to xiphoid, anterior opening, restricts gross trunk motion in sagittal and coronal planes, prefabricated, includes fitting and adjustment

In addition to spinal orthoses, there are codes for extremity orthoses (L1971, ankle-foot orthosis [AFO], plastic or other material with ankle joint, prefabricated, includes fitting and adjustment), for orthopedic shoes (L3219, Orthopedic footwear, men's shoe, oxford, each), and for repair of orthotic devices (L4205, Repair of orthotic device, labor component, per 15 minutes).

L Codes: Prosthetic Procedures

The procedures in this section are considered "base" or basic procedures and may be modified by listing terms/procedures or special materials from the "additions" sections and adding them to the base procedure. Although termed *procedures*, these codes are not surgical procedures but, rather, codes for fabrication of prostheses. Included are codes for prostheses for knee disarticulation (L5150, Knee disarticulation [or through knee], molded socket, external knee joints, shin, SACH foot), additions and replacements to prostheses (L5704, Custom-shaped protective cover, below knee), breast prostheses (L8020, Breast prosthesis, mastectomy form), and elastic support garments. Also included in this section are codes for prosthetic implants such as implantable breast prostheses (L8600, Implantable breast prosthesis, silicone or equal), artificial larynx (L8500), and some joint replacements (L8641, Metatarsal joint implant).

M Codes: Medical Services

M codes include office services, cellular therapy, prolotherapy, intragastric hypothermia, intravenous (IV) chelation therapy, and fabric wrapping of an abdominal aneurysm. These services do not qualify for CPT codes because they are either not of proven efficacy or considered obsolete modalities.

P Codes: Pathology and Laboratory Services

The P codes include chemistry, toxicology, and microbiology tests, screening Papanicolaou procedures, and various blood products. Included in this section are codes for laboratory procedures now considered to be obsolete (for example, P2033, Thymol turbidity, blood), blood products (P9038, Red blood cells, irradiated, each unit), and codes for travel allowances to collect specimens (P9604, Travel allowance one way in connection with medically necessary laboratory specimen collection drawn from homebound or nursing homebound patient; prorated trip charge).

Q Codes (Temporary)

Because they are temporary, the Q codes can change rapidly. Among the codes in this section as of this writing are code Q0136, Injection, epoetin alpha (for non-ESRD use), per 1000 units; codes for oral antiemetics given in conjunction with chemotherapy; codes for new technology intraocular lenses; more radiopharmaceutical codes; and codes for casting and splinting supplies.

R Codes: Diagnostic Radiology Services

R codes are used for the transportation of portable x-ray and/or EKG equipment.

S Codes: Temporary National Codes (Non-Medicare)

Private insurers use S codes to report drugs, services, and supplies for which there are no national codes, but for which codes are needed by the private sector to implement policies, programs, or claims processing. The Medicaid program also uses these codes. However, they are not payable by Medicare.

National T Codes (Temporary)

T codes are designed for use by state Medicaid agencies for items for which there are no permanent national codes, but for which codes are necessary to administer the Medicaid program. Medicare does not use T codes, but private insurers may do so.

V Codes: Vision Services

V codes include vision-related supplies, including spectacles, lenses, contact lenses, prostheses, intraocular lenses, and miscellaneous lenses. The codes in this section are very specific as to type of lens.

V Codes: Hearing Services

V codes describe hearing test and related supplies and equipment, speech-language pathology screenings, and the repair of augmentative communication systems. Also included are dispensing fees for hearing aids.

HCPCS Modifiers

HCPCS level I modifiers are developed by the AMA and, as mentioned earlier, are described in detail in chapter 3. HCPCS level II modifiers are developed by CMS and are used with codes to explain various circumstances of procedures and/or services. Modifiers also are used to enhance a code narrative in order to describe the circumstances of each procedure or service and how it applies to an individual patient. In some situations, insurers instruct suppliers to add a modifier in order to provide additional information regarding the service or item identified by the HCPCS code.

Level II HCPCS modifiers are either alphanumeric or two letters in the range A1–VP. Examples of level II modifiers include:

LT   Left side
RT   Right side

E1   Upper left, eyelid
E2   Lower left, eyelid
F1   Left hand, second digit
F2   Left hand, third digit
LC   Left circumflex coronary artery
LD   Left anterior descending coronary artery
RC   Right coronary artery

National modifiers may be used with both levels of HCPCS codes. It is recommended that the CMS Web site (http://www.cms.hhs.gov/HCPCSRelease CodeSets/02_HCPCS_Quarterly_Update.asp# TopOfPage) be checked regularly for modifiers that may change or be added throughout the year. In accordance with HIPAA rules, CMS requires all providers to report HCPCS modifiers valid at the time a service is performed.

Check Your Understanding 4.3

Instructions: Complete the following exercises on a separate piece of paper.

1. Indicate the HCPCS II section title for each of the following:
    a. D codes
    b. E codes
    c. M codes
    d. V codes

2. True or False. Modifiers can be used with both levels of HCPCS codes.

Process for Revision and Updates

Maintenance and distribution of HCPCS level II codes is the responsibility of CMS. Under the Medicare Modernization Act, the methodology for revising codes was updated in 2004 in an effort to permit more public input into the process. The updates include:

*   *Expansion of the public meetings:* Public meetings relate to all public requests for HCPCS codes for products, supplies, and services. Notice of Public Meetings for All New Public Request for Revisions to the HCPCS Coding and Payment Determinations appears in the Feder-

al Register at: http://www.gpoaccess.gov/nara/ index.html. Agenda items for the meetings are published in advance, including descriptions of the coding requests, the requestor, and the name of the product or service. This information may be found at http://www.cms.hhs .gov/MedHCPCSGenInfo/08_HCPCSPublic Meetings.asp#TopOfPage. This information provides an opportunity for the public to become aware of coding changes under consideration and of opportunities for public input into decision making.

- *Implementation of a reconsideration process:* CMS is looking into implementing an appeals process whereby denied applicants will be allowed to appeal the decision and be given the opportunity to have their application reconsidered during the same coding cycle.

- *Publication of notice of decisions:* All preliminary decisions are published on the CMS Web site prior to public meetings to facilitate effective public discussion and comment.

Applicants are notified, in writing, of the final decision on their application by mid-November, and all modifications to the HCPCS codes are incorporated into the HCPCS level II annual update. The update is published on the official HCPCS Web site, http://www.cms.hhs.gov/hcpcsreleasecodesets/ ANHCPCS/list.asp#TopOfPage, by mid November.

Any supplier or manufacturer can request an HCPCS code. (See figure 4.1 for the HCPCS decision tree for external requests to add or revise codes.) The application can be downloaded, with instructions, from the CMS Web site at http://www.cms .hhs.gov/MedHCPCSGenInfo/01a_Application_ Form_and_Instructions.asp#TopOfPage. In order to be considered, the application must be submitted by early January of the year prior to the implementation year. Thus, to receive a 2010 HCPCS code, the application must be submitted by January 5, 2009.

Among the items of data required on the application are the following:

- The FDA status of the device or drug, as appropriate

- A description of what the device, drug, or service does

- Whether or not the item is durable

- The usual medical purpose of the item

- Similar items

- Any payment history for the item

- Why there is no appropriate existing code for the item

- Settings in which the item is used

Three types of coding modifications to HCPCS can be requested:

- *That a code be added:* When no distinct code describes a product, one may be requested. If a request for a new code is approved, addition of a new HCPCS code does not necessarily mean that Medicare will cover the item. Whether an item identified by a new code is covered is determined by the Medicare law, regulations, and medical review policies and not by assignment of a code.

- *That the language used to describe an existing code be changed:* When there is an existing code, a recommendation to modify it can be made when an interested party believes that the descriptor for the code needs to be modified to provide a better description of the category of products represented by the code.

- *That an existing code be deleted:* When an existing code becomes obsolete or is duplicative of another code, a request can be made to delete the code.

The review process is conducted against the following criteria to determine whether there is a demonstrated need for a new or modified code or the need to remove a code:

Figure 4.1.   HCPCS decision tree for external requests to add or revise codes

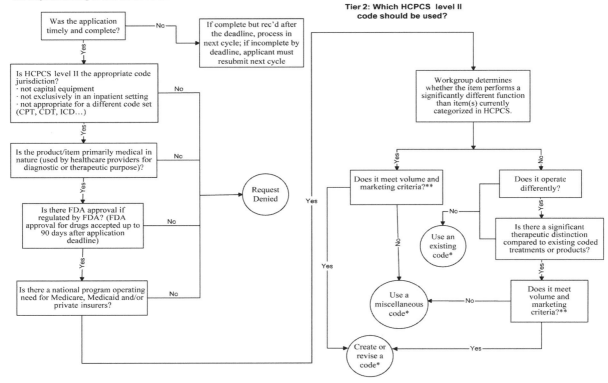

*Subject to national program operating need
**For drugs, volume and marketing criteria are waived, and "yes" is assumed for the purpose of following the decision tree

- When an existing code adequately describes the item in a coding request, no new or modified code is established. An existing code adequately describes an item in a coding request when it describes products either with functions similar to the item in the coding request or without significant therapeutic distinctions.

- When an existing code describes products that are almost the same in function with only minor distinctions from the item in the coding request, the item in the coding request may be grouped with that code and the code descriptor modified to reflect the distinctions.

- A code is not established for an item that is used only in the inpatient setting or for an item that is not diagnostic or therapeutic in nature.

- A new or modified code is not established for an item unless the FDA allows the item to be marketed.

- There must be sufficient claims activity or volume, as evidenced by three months of marketing activity, so that the addition of a new or modified code enhances the efficiency of the system and justifies the administrative burden of adding or modifying a code.

- The determination to remove a code is based on whether it is obsolete (for example, products no longer are used or other more specific codes have been added) or duplicative and no longer useful (for example, new codes better describe items identified by existing codes). The HCPCS Workgroup uses the criteria mentioned above in developing its recommendations; it does not include cost as a factor.

HCPCS and Medicare Requirements

In accordance with the Social Security Act, federal laws governing Medicare require CMS to contract with entities to process and pay Medicare claims and associated services. **Fiscal intermediaries** (FIs) and **carriers** process these claims for Medicare. FIs contract with CMS to serve as the financial agent between providers and the federal government in the local administration of Medicare Part A claims. Carriers contract with CMS to serve as the financial agent that works with providers and the federal government to locally administer Medicare Part B claims.

The Medicare Prescription Drug, Improvement and Modernization Act of 2003 (MMA) enables the CMS to make significant changes to the Medicare fee-for-service program's administrative structure. Through implementation of Medicare Contracting Reform (or section 911 of the MMA), CMS is in the process of replacing the claims payment contractors with the new contract entities called **Medicare Administrative Contractors** (MACs). CMS has 6 years—between 2005 and 2011—to complete the transition of Medicare fee-for-service (FFS) claims-processing activities from the FIs and carriers to the MACs.

The CMS regulation published on August 17, 2000 (45 CFR 162.10002) to implement the HIPAA requirement for standardized coding systems established the HCPCS level II codes as the standardized coding system for describing and identifying substances, equipment, supplies, or other items used in healthcare services that are not identified by the HCPCS level I, CPT codes. Public and private insurers were required to be in compliance with the August 2000 regulation by October 1, 2002.

Summary

Introduced in 1983 by the Health Care Financing Administration (now the Centers for Medicare and Medicaid Services [CMS]), HCPCS is divided into two levels of codes. This classification system is referred to as level I and level II of HCPCS. Level I codes are CPT codes. Level II codes are used for equipment, supplies, and services not covered by CPT, and include modifiers that can be used with both levels of codes. Level III codes were eliminated to comply with the Health Insurance Portability and Accountability Act of 1996.

Pronounced "hick picks," HCPCS is primarily used by physicians and healthcare providers to report the services and procedures they deliver. This system ensures uniform reporting on claims forms of items or services that are medical in nature.

References

American Dental Association. 1996. *Current Dental Terminology (CDT-2)*. Chicago: American Dental Association.

American Medical Association. 2008. http://www.ama-assn.org.

Centers for Medicare and Medicaid Services. 2008. http://www.cms.hhs.gov/home/medicare.asp.

Centers for Medicare and Medicaid Services. 2008. Transactions and Code Sets Regulations. http://www.cms.hhs.gov/TransactionCodeSetsStands/02_TransactionsandCodeSetsRegulations.asp#TopOfPage.

Health Care Financing Administration. 2000. Program Memorandum Intermediaries. Transmittal A-00-09. http://www.cms.hhs.gov/transmittals/downloads/A000960.PDF.

Grider, Debra. 2004. *Coding with Modifiers: A Guide to Correct CPT and HCPCS Level II Modifier Usage*. Chicago: American Medical Association.

Smith, Gail. 2008. *Basic CPT/HCPCS Coding*. Chicago: American Health Information Management Association.

Willard, Dianne. 1998. HCFA requires use of modifiers for hospital outpatient services. *Journal of the American Health Information Management Association* 69(6):75–78.

Application Exercise

Visit the HCPCS Web site at http://www.cms.hhs .gov/MedHCPCSGenInfo/08_HCPCSPublicMeetings .asp#TopOfPage. Click on the link for the list of codes under consideration for the next update. Select one or two codes for which you would like to develop comments. Write up your comments and submit them to your instructor.

Review Quiz

1. True or False. HCPCS was developed by CMS to report physician and nonphysician services.

2. HCPCS was first implemented in the United States to meet the operational needs of Medicare and Medicaid in which year?
   a. 1990
   b. 1988
   c. 1983
   d. 1973

3. True or False. HCPCS includes three levels of codes.

4. The first level of HCPCS consists of:
   a. CPT codes
   b. CDT codes
   c. NCD codes
   d. DSM IV codes

5. HCPCS level II codes are also known as:

   a. Focus codes
   b. Mandatory codes
   c. National codes
   d. Final codes

6. What organization(s) is responsible for maintenance and distribution of HCPCS level II codes?
   a. The Joint Commission
   b. AHA, AMA
   c. AMA, ANA
   d. CMS

7. True or False. HCPCS level II codes were named as one of the standardized code sets under HIPAA.

8. Level I and permanent level II HCPCS codes are updated:
   a. Quarterly
   b. Semiannually
   c. Annually
   d. Monthly

9. Which of the following is not a type of HCPCS level II temporary code?
   a. G codes
   b. Q codes
   c. T codes
   d. E codes

10. Decisions regarding the modification, deletion, or addition of HCPCS dental codes are made by:
    a. AMA
    b. NDC
    c. ADA
    d. CMS

Chapter 5

National Drug Codes (NDCs)

Danielle Przychodzin, PharmD, RPh

Learning Objectives

- To discuss the history, development, and use of National Drug Codes (NDCs)

- To identify and describe the components of NDCs

- To present the information available in the *NDC Directory*

- To review the process for updating NDCs

- To relate current principals and guidelines for using NDCs

Key Terms

Catalog name

Centers for Medicare and Medicaid Services (CMS)

Department of Health and Human Services (HHS)

Drug Listing Act 1972

Food and Drug Administration (FDA)

Food, Drug and Cosmetic Act (FDCA)

Labeler

National Drug Code (NDC)

National Drug Code (NDC) Directory

Package code

Product code

Product trade name

Introduction

National Drug Codes (NDCs) serve as product identifiers for human drugs and biologics. The NDC system was originally established as an essential part of an out-of-hospital drug reimbursement program under Medicare and has since found wider application. The NDC system is the Health Insurance Portability and Accountability Act (HIPAA) standard medical data code set for reporting drugs and biologics for retail pharmacy transactions. NDC numbers are included in the part D data, which is collected by the **Centers for Medicare and Medicaid Services** (CMS) from transactions between pharmacies and Medicare part D sponsors. As of 2008, the NDC, in combination with the Healthcare Common Procedure Coding System (HCPCS) code, is required on Medicaid reimbursement forms for use in processing manufacturer drug rebates for physician-administered drugs.

This chapter discusses why the NDC system was developed and by what agency. It also describes the components of the codes as they are listed in the *NDC Directory*.

Developer and Purpose

The National Drug Code (NDC) system was designed to serve as a universal product identifier for frequently-prescribed drugs. The NDC system was compiled into a directory that was published annually from 1969 to 1972. Some segments of the healthcare industry considered the directories essential for third-party reimbursement programs. However, due to the voluntary nature of the system, it did not meet the needs of the federal Food and Drug Administration (FDA) for a complete inventory of all commercially distributed drug products.

In 1972, the **Food, Drug and Cosmetic Act** (FDCA) was amended to make submission of information on all commercially marketed drugs mandatory. Under its new name, the **Drug Listing Act of 1972** dictated expansion of the NDC system to include human over-the-counter (OTC) drugs and veterinary drugs. (The registration of blood or blood components currently is not required, although this topic is under discussion.) The impact of the Drug Listing Act made it necessary to suspend publication of the *NDC Directory* until its provisions could be implemented and all submitted data could be processed. Between 1973 and 1976, only one directory, the 1976 directory, was published, and it was limited to human prescription drugs and selected OTC drugs that physicians often prescribe, including insulin. The next directory was published in 1980, which was followed by two more in 1982 and 1985.

The current edition of the *NDC Directory* is available in book form, as data files for download, and free online at http://www.fda.gov/cder/ndc/database/default.htm. The *NDC Directory* includes prescription drugs and selected OTC and homeopathic products. All domestic and foreign firms (manufacturers, repackagers, and labelers) marketing drug products in the United States must obtain a labeler code and register their products in the *NDC Directory*.

Owned by the FDA and distributed by the **Department of Health and Human Services** (HHS), the directory lists more than 123,000 prescription drugs. The Center for Drug Evaluation and Research within the FDA oversees the *NDC Directory*. It is important to note that the listing of a firm or product in the *NDC Directory* does *not* equate to FDA approval, imply the product is a "drug" as defined by federal law, or mean the product is eligible for reimbursement (FDA 2008b).

The National Drug Code system is utilized extensively for billing and reimbursement purposes, but it also plays a significant role in protecting public health. The FDA uses the *NDC Directory* to verify drug imports, monitor adverse drug events, manage drug recalls, and evaluate the drug impacts of natural disasters or terrorist threats. The *NDC Directory* is also used to identify the ingredients of marketed drugs and as a resource for the inspection of drug facilities.

Check Your Understanding 5.1

Instructions: Complete the following exercises on a separate piece of paper.

1. What is the purpose of NDCs?

2. True or False. NDCs were originally established as part of a drug reimbursement program under Medicare.

3. What impact did the Drug Listing Act have on NDCs?

4. True or False. The current *NDC Directory* is limited to prescription drugs and selected OTC and homeopathic products.

5. True or False. A drug product must be FDA-approved before it is listed in the *NDC Directory*.

Content

Each drug product listed under Section 510 of the Food, Drug and Cosmetic Act (FDCA) is assigned a unique ten-digit, three-segment number. The NDC is composed of three parts representing the labeler/vendor code, product code, and trade package code.

A **labeler** is any firm that manufactures, repacks, or distributes a drug product. The FDA assigns a code to each labeler, which is the first part of the three-part NDC (see table 5.1). For labeler codes 1 through 9999, the first part of the NDC code is four digits; for labeler codes 10,000 through 99,999, the first part of the NDC code is five digits.

The second part of the NDC is the **product code**. The product code is assigned by the firm and identifies a specific strength, dosage form, and formulation for a particular firm (see table 5.2).

The **package code** is also assigned by the firm. It identifies package size and comprises the third part of the NDC (see table 5.3).

NDCs have one of the following configurations: 4-4-2, 5-3-2, or 5-4-1.

For consistency with the HIPAA standard, other government agencies may display the NDC in an eleven-digit format using leading zeros. For example, the Centers for Medicare and Medicaid Services (CMS) displays the labeler code as five digits with leading zeros if needed; the product code as four digits with leading zeros if needed; and the package size as two characters with leading zeros if needed. If a labeler code begins with a digit other than zero, it is a 5 digit format. To avoid confusion between the 5-3-2 and 5-4-1 formats, the FDA stores complete NDCs with an asterisk "*" placeholder (instead of a leading zero) for product and package codes (see table 5.4).

Check Your Understanding 5.2

Instructions: Complete the following exercises on a separate piece of paper.

1. True or False. NDCs are assigned to all drugs under the Food, Drug, and Cosmetic Act

2. Describe the components of NDCs.

3. List the components of the NDC that are assigned by the firm.

4. Visit the *NDC Directory* at http://www.fda.gov/cder/ndc/database/. Review the search and query features. Then go to Search by Firm Name and type in EISAI INC. List your findings.

Table 5.1.   Example of labeler codes

Labeler Code	Firm Name
0069	PFIZER LABORATORIES DIV PFIZER INC.
68546	TEVA NEUROSCIENCE INC.

Table 5.2.   Example of labeler and product codes

Labeler Code	Product Code	Firm Name	Trade Name	Strength
0069	5510	PFIZER LABORATORIES DIV PFIZER INC.	ZYRTEC TABLETS	10MG
0069	5530	PFIZER LABORATORIES DIV PFIZER INC.	ZYRTEC SYRUP	1MG/ML
0069	5500	PFIZER LABORATORIES DIV PFIZER INC.	ZYRTEC TABLETS	5MG

Table 5.3.   Example of labeler, product, and package codes

Labeler Code	Product Code	Package Code	Firm Name	Trade Name	Strength	Packsize
0069	5510	66	PFIZER LABORATORIES DIV PFIZER INC.	ZYRTEC TABLETS	10MG	100
0069	5510	96	PFIZER LABORATORIES DIV PFIZER INC.	ZYRTEC TABLETS	10MG	3
0069	5510	62	PFIZER LABORATORIES DIV PFIZER INC.	ZYRTEC TABLETS	10MG	14
0069	5510	79	PFIZER LABORATORIES DIV PFIZER INC.	ZYRTEC TABLETS	10MG	1 × 30

Table 5.4.   Example of complete NDC, labeler, product, and package codes

Complete NDC	Labeler Code	Product Code	Package Code	Firm Name	Trade Name	Strength	Packsize
00069-5510-66	0069	5510	66	PFIZER LABORATORIES DIV PFIZER INC.	ZYRTEC TABLETS	10MG	100
17856-0731-*2	17856	0731	2	ATLANTIC BIOLOGICALS CORPORATION	ZYRTEC TABLETS	10MG	100
66105-*675-10	66105	675	10	AQ PHARMACEUTICALS INC.	ZYRTEC TABLETS	10MG	100

Note the leading zero added to the 4-digit labeler code (first row) to meet the 5-4-2 requirement.

The NDC Directory

The *NDC Directory* is available in a limited print version, as data files for integration (ACSII), or online at the FDA Web site (http://www.fda.gov/cder/ndc/database). The *NDC Directory* contains the information discussed in the following section.

NDC Directory Content

The content of the *NDC Directory* includes such information as the product trade name or catalog name, dosage form, active ingredients, strength and unit, package size and type, and FDA-approved application number for each product.

Product Trade Name or Catalog Name

The product trade names or catalog names used in the directory are generally those supplied by the label-

ers (firms) as required under the FDCA. All product names appearing in this directory are limited to a maximum of 100 characters. Minor editorial changes have been made in instances where information normally included with the name appears elsewhere in the product description. For example, the dosage form may be deleted when it is furnished as part of the product name or the strength may be removed from the product name when it also appears in other data fields.

When a number is an integral part of the product name, normal computer sort procedures will place the numeric character before the first alphabetic character. Therefore, a product with a numeric character in the first position of the name (for example, lst AID CREAM) will be found at the beginning of the alphabetic list. Product names that include special characters such as a dash (-), a slash (/), or a space normally appear before all alphabetic characters. Thus, "A-A-A SOLUTION" precedes "AAA SOLUTION." The designations

United States Pharmacopoeia (USP) or *National Formulary (NF)* also may be deleted from product names. Occasionally, however, the terms *not NF* and *not USP* have been left as part of the name.

Symbols indicating trademarked or registered products also had to be omitted because of computer input capabilities. These deletions are not intended in any way to deprive the labeler of the protection afforded under patent, trademark, registration, or copyright laws or regulations.

Dosage Form

In the print directory, the dosage form is a ten-character abbreviation. Multiple dosage forms are concatenated, or linked together. The online directory provides dosage forms and routes of administration as alphabetic terms with 240- and 60- character limits, respectively. The directory's electronic data files provide the complete lists of alphabetic terms with dosage form and route of administration codes (3 digits each) for linking the data tables together. The directory also provides a table of abbreviations for both dosage form and routes of administration.

Active Ingredient(s)

In the print directory, each product's active ingredients are listed alphabetically. A maximum of two active ingredients per product is listed. A product that contains more than two active ingredients is indicated with the abbreviation *etc.* on the third line. The online directory also provides the product's active ingredients alphabetically; however, the online version is not limited to two active ingredients per product. The directory's electronic data files provide a product's active ingredients via two separate files (FORMULAT.TXT and LISTINGS.TXT) that are linked to form the complete data set.

Strength

Strength is indicated after the active ingredient. For products that have equivalent ingredients, the strength expressed is that of the equivalent. For some combination products, the strength is that which is commonly recognized for that formulation. The product itself also has a strength/unit. For products with a single active ingredient, it is the strength of that active ingredient. For multiple active ingredient products, the strength is either "COMBO" or a concatenation of the multiple strengths. (See table 5.5.)

Unit

Unit refers to a unit of measure corresponding to strength. This nonmandatory field contains the unit code for a single entity product, such as milligram (MG), ampule, or trace. The directory provides a table of abbreviations for units and their definitions.

Package Size and Type

Package size and type appear in the directory as reported by the labeler or firm.

FDA-Approved Application Number

The New Drug Application (NDA) or the Abbreviated New Drug Application (ANDA) number indicates the product has been approved by the FDA for marketing. A designation of *Other* in the application number field means the product has not been approved for both safety and efficacy under an NDA or ANDA, may be subject to the Drug Efficacy Study Implementation (DESI), and/or the FDA may still be awaiting data for approval. (DESI applies to drugs approved between 1938 and 1962, when only safety was assessed.)

Table 5.5.   Example of a product with multiple strengths

Labeler Code	Firm Name	Trade Name	Strength
00069	PFIZER LABORATORIES	ZYRTEC TABLETS	5MG
00069	PFIZER LABORATORIES	ZYRTEC TABLETS	10MG

Organization of the Print NDC Directory

The *NDC Directory* is divided into sections

- Alphabetical Index by Product Trade Name
- Numeric Index of Products by National Drug Code
- Alphabetic Index by Firm Name

The first two sections contain drug product information and the last section contains drug establishment information.

Alphabetical Index by Product Trade Name

The first line in the Alphabetic Index by Product Trade Name lists the product trade name or catalog name. Two products that have the same trade name are listed in numerical order. The second line contains the labeler's short name. The third line includes the drug class code(s) followed by line four with the new drug application number (for example, NDA/ANDA). The line(s) following the NDA indicate the active ingredient(s) listed alphabetically, with the strength and unit specified next to each ingredient. The labeler code and product code, separated by dashes, are on the next line along with the dosage form and route(s) of administration. The last line(s) of this section consists of the NDC number, including package code, and the trade package size and type for the product. This line is repeated for each package size available for that particular product.

Numeric Index of Products by National Drug Code

The Numeric Index of Products by National Drug Code is arranged numerically by labeler code, and within the labeler code, numerically by product code. The first line contains the labeler code and the short name of the labeler. Subsequent lines list each product for that labeler. Each of these lines contains the NDC labeler and product code as well as the trade name or catalog name.

Alphabetic Index by Firm Name

The Alphabetic Index by Firm Name contains the names and addresses of establishments whose products appear in the directory. The first line contains the short name of the firm in alphabetical order and the NDC labeler code. Subsequent lines contain the firm address.

Organization of the Online NDC Directory

The online *NDC Directory* offers free access to the information above via a search/query page. The query page provides searching functionality based upon Proprietary Name, Active Ingredient, Application Number, NDC Number, or Firm Name. Content within the site is hyperlinked to facilitate navigation between related content.

Organization of the NCD Directory ASCII Data Files

NDC Directory data files are available as free downloads from the FDA Web site for system integration via ASCII import. The 11 files contain both product information and firm information that can be linked together for use in electronic databases. For more information, including file names and descriptions, visit http://www.fda.gov/cder/ndc/index.htm.

Principles and Guidelines

Although the February 2003, Final Rule on Health Insurance Reform: Modifications to Electronic Data Transaction Standards and Code Sets repeals adoption of the NDC system for institutional and professional claims, it does state that the NDC system remains the HIPAA standard medical data code set for reporting drugs and biologics for retail pharmacy transactions.

The final rule does not identify a standard medical data code set for reporting drugs and biologics in nonretail pharmacy transactions. However, absence of a code set does not preclude the use of NDCs. A health plan could require a provider to use either of the applicable code sets, NDC or HCPCS, permitted by the implementation guides. In other words, covered entities could continue to report drugs and biologics as they prefer and agree on with their trading partners, using either the NDC or HCPCS code set.

The Deficit Reduction Act (DRA) of 2005 requires all state Medicaid agencies to collect rebates from drug manufacturers for covered physician-administered (or physician-provided) drugs. Physician-administered drugs include any outpatient drug which is administered (or provided) to a patient with a reimbursement claim from a provider instead of a pharmacy. According to the DRA, covered drugs are not restricted to injectable drugs but include any physician-administered drug regardless of the method of administration. The types of practice sites required to collect National Drug Codes on reimbursement claim forms include, but are not limited to, physician offices, clinics and outpatient hospital departments. Medicaid claims will continue to be priced based upon the HCPCS code, with the NDC and corresponding units being used for manufacturer rebate processing. Medicare primary claims will also require NDCs with HCPCS codes. As of January 2008, federal financial participation is dependant upon a State Medicaid agency's compliance with the DRA. Additional information regarding this change can be found at http://www.cms.hhs.gov/ContractorLearningResources/downloads/JA5835.pdf. A crosswalk listing of NDCs assigned to individual HCPCS codes is updated monthly and available online from Noridian at http://www.dmepdac.com/crosswalk/index.html. Further guidance on the implementation and compliance requirements for the DRA may be obtained from individual state Medicaid Web sites.

Without a single, standard medical code set for reporting all drugs and biologics in nonretail pharmacy transactions, implementation guidelines vary. Some health plans use a combination of the code sets to determine reimbursement for outpatient institutional, physician, and pharmaceutical (chemotherapy and some injectable) services. Further guidance on the use of NDC codes must be obtained from the individual health plan.

Process for Revision and Updates

The FDA updates the *NDC Directory* quarterly within five working days after the end of March, June, September, and December. Weekly updates are available via the Internet at http://www.fda.gov/cder/. Instructions for submitting changes to the FDA can be found online at http://www.fda.gov/cder/drls/default.htm.

After the initial listing, foreign and domestic firms marketing products in the United States are required to update their drug-listing information twice yearly (at the end of June and December). However, changes in formulation, labeling, packaging, manufacturing site, and so on must be reported as soon as they occur.

Summary

The National Drug Code (NDC) system is a set of medical codes maintained and approved by the **Food and Drug Administration**. NDCs are unique numbers assigned to all drugs and biologics. The Secretary of the Department of Health and Human Services adopted this code set as the standard for reporting drugs and biologics on standard retail pharmacy transactions. National Drug Codes are required for Medicaid reimbursement of physician-administered drugs under the Deficit Reduction Act of 2005. In addition, many healthcare plans use a combination of NDC and HCPCS drug codes to determine reimbursement for outpatient institutional, physician, and pharmaceutical (chemotherapy and some injectable) services.

References

Brouch, Kathy. 2003 (March). Standard medical data code set. *CodeWrite*. American Health Information Management Association.

Centers for Medicare and Medicaid Services. 2008. http://www.cms.hhs.gov/.

Department of Health and Human Services. 2003 (February 20). Final Rule on Health Insurance Reform: Modifications to Electronic Data Transaction Standards and Code Sets. *Federal Register*. http://www.aspe.hhs.gov/admnsimp/FINAL/FR03-8381.pdf.

Department of Health and Human Services. 2005. Frequently Asked Questions about HIPAA Code Sets. http://www.aspe.hhs.gov/admnsimp/faqcode.htm.

Department of Health and Human Services. 2008 (April 17). Medicare Shared Systems Modifications Necessary to Accept and Crossover to Medicaid National Drug Codes (NDC) and Corresponding Quantities Submitted on CMS-1500 Paper Claims. MLN Matters Article. http://www.cms.hhs.gov/MLNMattersArticles/downloads/MM5835.pdf.

Department of Health and Human Services. 2008 (May 28). Final Rule on Medicare Program; Medicare Part D claims Data. *Federal Register*. http://frwebgate5.access.gpo.gov/cgi-bin/PDFgate.cgi?WAISdocID=675049112791+0+2+0&WAISaction=retrieve.

National Drug Code Directory. 2008. http://www.fda.gov/cder/ndc/database/.

National Drug Code query site. 2008. http://www.fda.gov/cder/ndc/database/docs/queryndctn.htm.

NDC/HCPCS Crosswalk. 2008. http://www.dmepdac.com/crosswalk/index.html.

U.S. Food and Drug Administration Center for Drug Evaluation and Research. 2008a. Drug Registration and Listing System. http://www.fda.gov/cder/handbook/druglist.htm.

U.S. Food and Drug Administration Center for Drug Evaluation and Research. 2008b. The National Drug Code Directory. http://www.fda.gov/cder/ndc/.

U.S. Food and Drug Administration Center for Drug Evaluation and Research. 2008c. http://www.fda.gov/cder/ndc/index.htm.

Workgroup for Electronic Data Interchange. 2001. NDC codes: A white paper giving a general overview and possible solutions associated with NDCS replacing HCPCS drug codes for institutional and professional billing. Strategic National Implementation Process, Translations Sub Work Group of the Workgroup for Electronic Data Interchange. http://www.wedi.org/snip/public/articles/ndc.pdf.

Workgroup for Electronic Data Interchange. 2005. http://www.wedi.org/snip/public/articles/ndc.pdf.

Additional Information

Requests for more specific drug product information may be submitted in writing to FDA's Freedom of Information staff at:

Food and Drug Administration
Freedom of Information Office, HFI-35
5600 Fishers Lane
Rockville, MD 20857
Telephone: (301)827-6500 FAX: (301)443-1726

Application Exercise

NDC codes are published in the Physician Desk Reference (PDR). Go to the library or obtain a copy a PDR. Then write a report describing how the NDCs are listed.

Review Quiz

1. Product names used in the *NDC Directory* are usually supplied by:
    a. Retail pharmacies
    b. AMA
    c. AHA
    d. Firms (labelers)

2. Labeler codes may be composed of
    a. 3 digits, 4 digits
    b. 4 digits, 4 digits
    c. 4 digits, 5 digits
    d. None of the above

3. What organization was responsible for development of the National Drug Codes?
    a. AHA
    b. The Joint Commission
    c. FDA
    d   None of the above

4. True or False. The Drug Listing Act had an impact on National Drug Codes.

5. True or False. NDCs are assigned to all drugs under the Drug, Food and Cosmetic Act.

6. The Deficit Reduction Act of 2005 requires State Medicaid agencies to provide which codes for reimbursement of physician-administered drugs?
    a. ICD-9-CM and NDC
    b. ICD-9-CM and NCPDP
    c. HCPCS and NDC
    d. HCPCS and ICD-9-CM

Chapter 6

Current Dental Terminology (CDT)

Karen Kostick, RHIT, CCS, CCS-P

Objectives

- To learn about the development and purpose of dental procedural terminology

- To identify the responsible party for developing and updating the Code

- To become familiar with information contained in the Code

- To describe the components of a CDT code

- To review the process for updating the Code

Key Terms

American Dental Association (ADA)
Code Revision Committee (CRC)
Council on Dental Benefit Programs
Current Dental Terminology (CDT)

Introduction

The dental procedure code set called the Code on Dental Procedures and Nomenclature is generally referred to as the "Code" and published as **Current Dental Terminology** (CDT). This code set is recognized as the standard dental procedural code reference for dentists practicing in academic, clinical, and administrative settings. This chapter reviews the Code on Dental Procedures and Nomenclature with discussions of its development, history, purpose, principles, and maintenance.

Developer

The Code was developed and is published by the **American Dental Association** (ADA). The ADA was founded in 1859 and provides advocacy, research, and professional development to the dentistry profession throughout the United States.

The Code was first published in the *Journal of the American Dental Association* (JADA) in 1969. JADA published six iterations until the seventh version, which became effective on January 1, 1991. This version was published in a separate educational manual titled Current Dental Terminology, 1st edition (CDT-1).

Development of CDT-1 began in 1986 when the **Council on Dental Benefit Programs** decided to develop an educational manual that would include a standard set of codes describing dental procedures. It was thought that such a manual would enable dentists to document and report the care rendered to their patients and also provide dental office practices with valuable instructive resources on how to report and process insurance claims. The manual was developed with support from dentists, dental office practice staff, and the healthcare insurance industry.

The latest edition of the Code is published in the manual titled *CDT 2009/2010* and is in effect January 1, 2009 through December 31, 2010.

In 1999, the ADA and the Centers for Medicare and Medicaid Services (CMS) entered into a license agreement for the electronic and print use of CDT. Although CDT is included in the CMS Healthcare Common Procedural Coding System (HCPCS) level II code set, only the ADA makes decisions on CDT code modification. Indeed, the ADA owns all property rights, title, and interest in CDT.

Purpose

According to the ADA, "The continuing belief is that publication of the *Code in the Current Dental Terminology (CDT) manual* encourages use of this terminology to document procedures, and to communicate accurate information on procedures and services to agencies involved in adjudicating dental claims" (ADA 2008b, i). CDT is recognized as the official code set to be used in reporting medical services and procedures performed by dental professionals under the Health Insurance Portability and Accountability Act (HIPAA) Electronic Transactions and Code Set Standards.

Content

The preface to the CDT manual provides a history of the Code and instructions on how to use the manual. The manual is divided into sections, which are discussed in the following subsections.

Section 1: Code on Dental Procedures and Nomenclature (Code)

This section includes twelve dental service categories. Each category contains the applicable five-character alphanumeric codes. The service categories and code series are as follows:

Service Category	Code Series
I. Diagnostic	D0100–D0999
II. Preventive	D1000–D1999
III. Restorative	D2000–D2999
IV. Endodontics	D3000–D3999
V. Periodontics	D4000–D4999
VI. Prosthodontics, removable	D5000–D5899
VII. Maxillofacial Prosthetics	D5900–D5999
VIII. Implant Services	D6000–D6199

IX.	Prosthodontics, fixed	D6200–D6999
X.	Oral and Maxillofacial Surgery	D7000–D7999
XI.	Orthodontics	D8000–D8999
XII.	Adjunctive General Services	D9000–D9999

Section 2: Changes to the Code

Section 2 provides a detailed overview of the revisions to procedure code nomenclatures and descriptors changed from the previous version of the Code.

Section 3: Tooth Numbering and the Oral Cavity

Section 3 includes information on two major systems used by the ADA for tooth numbering. The Universal/National System is the common system used in the United States, and the International Standards Organization System is most frequently used outside the United States.

Section 4: ADA Dental Claim Form Completion Instructions

Section 4 provides a sample ADA dental claim form with comprehensive instructions on how to complete it. The ADA dental paper claim form is consistent with the HIPAA standard electronic claim transaction data content. Updates on completing the ADA dental claim form are posted on the ADA's Web site.

The CDT manual notes a third-party payer reimbursement policy may differ from how a dentist submits a claim for payment. For example, the manual notes the presence of a dental code does not necessarily mean that the procedure or service being reported on the claim form is covered by the patient's dental insurance benefit plan.

Section 5: Questions and Answers on the Code and ADA Claim Form

The questions and answers in section 5 are published to assist users in understanding and determining accurate procedural code assignment. The questions are organized by the twelve dental service categories and a final group on claim form issues. Additional questions and answers are made available on the ADA Web site at http://www.ada.org/prof/resources/topics/cdt/faq.asp.

Section 6: Glossary

Section 6 includes an alphabetical clinical term listing of dental conditions and procedures. Insurance and reimbursement terms as they relate to dental practice management also are included.

Section 7: Numeric Index to the Code

Section 7 is categorized into the twelve service categories found in section 1. Procedure codes are listed for each service category, along with page numbers to locate the code in section 1 and any change to a CDT code (revision, addition, deletion) from the last version of the Code. If a question and answer in section 5 exists for one of the codes, the page where this information is found is also listed.

Section 8: Alphabetical Index to the Code

Section 8 includes an alphabetical listing of dental terms, along with the assigned codes and applicable page numbers to view further information on the nomenclature and description, any changes, questions and answers, and glossary information for the listed code.

Users of the Code are invited to submit comments on the manual's technical content and format to the ADA's Council on Dental Benefit Programs. The **Code Revision Committee** is responsible for the update of the Code. Guidelines, evaluation criteria, and instructions on how to submit comments and changes to the Code itself are provided in the manual and on the ADA Web site.

Check Your Understanding 6.1

Instructions: Complete the following exercises on a separate piece of paper.

1. What is the dental procedure code set often referred to as?

2. Who is the developer of current dental terminology?

3. CDT 1 was published and implemented for use in:
    a. 1986
    b. 1991
    c. 2000
    d. None of the above

4. Who contributed to the development of the CDT manual?
    a. Dentists
    b. Healthcare insurance industry
    c. Dental practice management staff
    d. All of the above

5. True or False. The Centers for Medicare and Medicaid Services (CMS) owns the property rights, title, and interest in CDT.

Principles and Guidelines

This section looks at guidelines that apply to sections 1 and 8 of the CDT manual.

Section 1: Code on Dental Procedures and Nomenclature

Dental service and procedure codes are organized first by the twelve procedure categories and then by procedural subcategories followed by code number and nomenclature. Narrative descriptors are optional and may be added to subcategories or to a dental procedure code.

An individual dental procedure code includes at least the first two of the following three components:

1. *A dental procedure code* is a five-character alphanumeric code that begins with the letter D and is followed by four numerals. Each code identifies a specific dental procedure.

2. A *nomenclature* is a concise written definition of a dental procedure code.

3. A *descriptor* is an optional written narrative that provides additional information on the intended use of a dental procedure code.

Changes in the current version of the Code are identified by two symbols. A bullet symbol (•) identifies a new procedure code, and a triangle symbol (▲) identifies a revision to a code nomenclature, code descriptor, or both. The change symbols are included before the appropriate code number, nomenclature, and descriptor. Invalid dental codes for the current version of the Code are deleted and no longer present.

For certain procedure codes, when the nomenclature of a code includes a "by report" notation, the CDT manual instructs a dental procedure narrative description be reported with the claim submission.

Examples of such codes include unspecified dental procedures and those with nomenclature specifically indicating the need to report additional information. Unspecified codes are available for all the categories except for the preventive section. The dental treatment narrative description then can be used for claim-processing purposes by third-party payers.

The ADA instructs a licensee that a code nomenclature may be abbreviated only when printed on billing forms that have space limitations and advises that code descriptors cannot be modified by a licensee.

Tables 6.1 (see page 96) and 6.2 (see page 97), taken from the CDT manual, illustrate the organization and guidelines contained in the Code and provide a review of Code categories and subcategories.

Section 8: Alphabetical Index to the Code

The Alphabetical Index lists dental terms in alphabetical order. The dental code and the appropriate page number(s) follow each dental term in the index. The page number(s) that follows the listing designates where to locate pertinent code information in one or more sections of the manual. In some instances, a dental term is further specified by the inclusion of additional information for appropriate code assignment. Some of the medical terms refer users to see another dental term in the index. Finally, the index notes "No separate code" for certain dental terms, which instructs the user not to assign a CDT code.

Table 6.3 (see page 99), taken from the CPT manual, illustrates examples from the CDT manual index.

Table 6.1.   Section 1 code on dental procedures and nomenclature

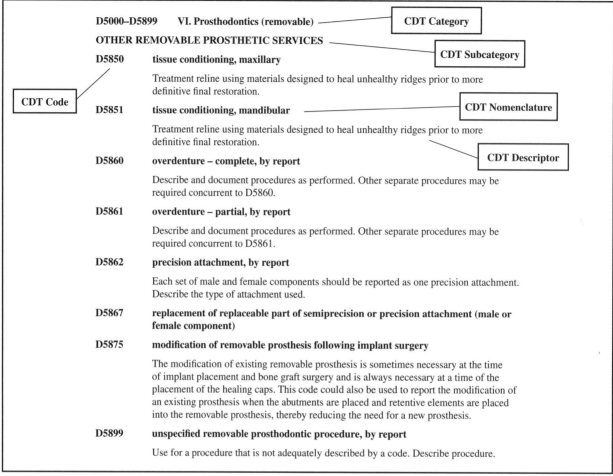

Source: CDT Code Manual. 2008.

Check Your Understanding 6.2

Instructions: Complete the following exercises on a separate piece of paper.

1. What are the required components of a CDT code?

2. True or False. A dental procedure code consists of a five-character alphanumeric code.

3. Dental codes are first organized by:
    a. Procedural categories
    b. Subcategories
    c. Sections
    d   Code number and nomenclature

4. Which of the following CDT code categories include apexification/recalcification procedures?
    a. D0100–D0999
    b. D1000–D1999
    c. D2100–D2999
    d. D3000–D3999

5. Describe the types of dental procedures and reporting guideline when the nomenclature of a code includes "by report."

Table 6.2.   Code categories and subcategories

Category of Service	Code Series	Subcategories
1. Diagnostic	D0100–D0999	Clinical oral evaluations Radiographs/diagnostic imaging (including interpretation) Tests and examinations Oral pathology laboratory
2. Preventive	D1000–D1999	Dental prophylaxis Topical fluoride treatment (office procedure) Other preventive services Space maintenance (passive appliances)
3. Restorative	D2000–D2999	Amalgam restorations (including polishing) Resin-based composite restorations—direct Gold foil restorations Inlay/onlay restorations Crowns—single restorations only Other restorative services
4. Endodontics	D3000–D3999	Pulp capping Pulpotomy Endodontic therapy on primary teeth Endodontic therapy (including treatment plan, clinical procedures, and follow-up care) Endodontic retreatment Apexification/recalcification procedures Apicoectomy/periradicular services Other endodontic procedures
5. Periodontics	D4000–D4999	Surgical services (including usual postoperative care) Nonsurgical periodontal service Other periodontal services
6. Prosthodontics (removable)	D5000–D5899	Complete dentures (including routine postdelivery care) Partial dentures (including routine postdelivery care) Adjustments to dentures Repairs to complete dentures Repairs to partial dentures Denture rebase procedures Denture reline procedures Interim prosthesis Other removable prosthetic services
7. Maxillofacial prosthetics	D5900–D5999	
8. Implant services	D6000–D6199	Presurgical services Surgical services Implant-supported prosthetics Other implant services
9. Prosthodontics, fixed	D6200–D6999	Fixed partial denture pontics Fixed partial denture retainers—inlays/onlays Fixed partial denture retainers—crowns Other fixed partial denture services

(*Continued on next page*)

Table 6.2.   (Continued)

Category of Service	Code Series	Subcategories
10. Oral and maxillofacial surgery	D7000–D7999	Extractions (includes local anesthesia, suturing, if needed, and routine postoperative care)
		Surgical extractions (includes local anesthesia, suturing, if needed, and routine postoperative care)
		Other surgical procedures
		Alveoloplasty—surgical preparation of ridge
		Vestibuloplasty
		Surgical excision of soft tissue lesions
		Surgical excision of intra-osseous lesions
		Excision of bone tissue
		Surgical incision
		Treatment of fractures—simple
		Treatment of fractures—compound
		Reduction of dislocation and management of other temporomandibular joint dysfunctions
		Repair of traumatic wounds
		Complicated suturing (reconstruction requiring delicate handling of tissues and wide undermining for meticulous closure)
		Other repair procedures
11. Orthodontics	D8000–D8999	Limited orthodontic treatment
		Interceptive orthodontic treatment
		Comprehensive orthodontic treatment
		Minor treatment to control harmful habits
		Other orthodontic services
12. Adjunctive general services	D9000–D9999	Unclassified treatment
		Anesthesia
		Professional consultation
		Professional visits
		Drugs
		Miscellaneous services

Source: CDT Code Manual. 2008.

Process for Revision and Updates

Revisions to the Code are effective and published biannually at the beginning of odd-numbered years. In 2001, the **Code Revision Committee** (CRC) was established to maintain the Code. The CRC represents the ADA, America's Health Insurance Plans, the Blue Cross/Blue Shield Association, CMS, Delta Dental Plans Association (DDPA), National Association of Dental Plans, and National Purchaser of Dental Benefits. The Code voting membership includes one representative from each payer sector and six representatives from the ADA Council on Dental Benefit Programs. The addition of representatives from the ADA's Council on Dental Benefit Programs provides an equal voting balance between the payer sector and the dental community.

The ADA manages and provides staff to coordinate the technical review and revision process. Members of the dental profession, third-party payers, or other users of the CDT manual may submit a code change request at any time. The ADA provides detailed instructions, guidelines, evaluation criteria, and three versions of code change request forms: an addition form, a revision form, and a deletion form. Requests for category and subcategory service changes also have their own

Table 6.3.   Examples from the Alphabetical Index to CDT codes

Term	Code(s)	Page Reference by CDT Manual Section			
		1 Code	2 Changes	5 Q&As	6 Glossary
Acid etch; part of resin procedure	No separate code				183
Coronoidectomy	D7991	65			
Debridement • endodontic • periodontal, full mouth	D3221 D4355	1928		153 141,155	
Whitening (see bleaching)				174, 175	189

Source: CDT Code Manual. 2008.

forms. Each change request requires the submitter to complete the appropriate form and then return it to the ADA Council on Dental Benefit Programs Division.

Change requests received by October 1 of an odd-numbered year are reviewed by the CRC for inclusion in the next version of the Code. For example, change requests received from October 1, 2008, through October 1, 2009, will be considered to the Code version effective January 1, 2011.

The CRC review process includes biannual open meetings held in odd-numbered years and an annual meeting in even-numbered years. Requested code changes are evaluated and voted on by the CRC during this time. CRC teleconference calls, as well as individual review of each code change request, also are performed prior to the scheduled meetings.

Table 6.4 provides criteria for use when submitting a version of the code change request form. These evaluation criteria also are used by the CRC for each change request as noted on the ADA Web site at http://www.ada.org/prof/resources/topics/cdt/change_guidelines.asp or http://www.ada.org/prof/resources/topics/cdt/change_evaluation.asp.

The goal for incorporating new codes is to reflect clinical dentistry advancement and to include revisions that can be recognized and adopted by all users of the Code. Each updated edition includes a summary section of CDT code additions and revisions.

If necessary, the ADA provides an errata sheet after printing the CDT manual. Additional information on the Code revision and update process can be found by visiting http://www.ada.org/prof/resources/topics/cdt/change.asp.

Table 6.4.   Guidelines for submitting change requests to the Code*

A suggested addition to the Code should represent a distinct dental procedure that: • Is part of current dental practice • Is performed as a separate procedure • Is not now included in the Code
A suggested revision to the Code should address omissions or ambiguities within a current procedure code's nomenclature or descriptor.
A suggested deletion from the Code should address a procedure that is no longer considered current or acceptable dental practice.
Frequency of occurrence should be considered when submitting a request, as the Code is not intended to accommodate procedures that are delivered on an infrequent basis.
ADA "Acceptance" or "Approval" programs should not be the sole basis on which a procedure code is added.
Additions, deletions, or changes to the Code may be considered to allow for compliance with state and federal rules and regulations relating to dental treatment.
Previously submitted, but not accepted, change requests must be accompanied by new information in order to be reconsidered.

*Any requests that do not meet these guidelines are not likely to receive favorable consideration during the evaluation process.

Source: *Dental Professionals* Topics A–Z: Code on Dental Procedures and Nomenclature. 2008. http://www.ada.org/prof/resources/topics/cdt/change_guidelines.asp. Courtesy of the American Dental Association (ADA).

Check Your Understanding 6.3

Instructions: Complete the following exercises on a separate piece of paper.

1. True or False. Revisions to the Code are effective and published biannually at the beginning of even-numbered years.

2. Who represents the Code's voting membership?

3. True or False. Each updated edition of the Code includes a summary section of CDT code additions and revisions.

4. Who manages and provides staff to coordinate the Code's technical review and revision process?
   a. Centers for Medicare and Medicaid Services (CMS)
   b. American Dental Association (ADA)
   c. Delta Dental Plans Association (DDPA)
   d. None of the above

5. True or False. The Code Revision Committee represents the ADA, America's Health Insurance Plans, and the Centers for Medicare and Medicaid Services.

Summary

The Code on Dental Procedures and Nomenclature's CDT for procedures and services is a procedural terminology developed by the American Dental Association (ADA). It is designed as a reference manual for the dentistry profession, practice management staff, and third-party payers. The Code provide a standardized code set to document procedures and to report information on procedures and services to agencies involved with the administration of dental benefit plans. The CDT codes are recognized as a national standard set for reporting dental procedures and services under the Health Insurance Portability and Accountability Act of 1996 (HIPAA). The ADA holds the copyright for the Code, and the Code may be purchased in an electronic or paper copy format.

References

American Dental Association. 2008a. A-Z Topics, Code on Dental Procedures and Nomenclature. http://www.ada.org/prof/resources/topics/cdt/faq.asp.

American Dental Association. 2008b. Current *Dental Terminology (CDT-2009/2010)*. Chicago: American Dental Association.

Acknowledgment

Frank Pokorny
Manager, Dental Codes Standards and
    Administration
Council on Dental Benefit Programs
American Dental Association

Application Exercise

1. Review the ADA request and review process for the development of new CDT codes. Familiarize yourself with the responsibilities of the Code Revision Committee, meeting activities, submitter request forms, review process, and time line. Use the following URLs to complete this project: http://www.ada.org/prof/resources/topics/cdt/committee.asp, http://www.ada.org/prof/resources/topics/cdt/timeline.asp, and http://www.ada.org/prof/resources/topics/cdt/change_request.asp.

2. Describe the current Code Revision Committee timeline for review and action on requests to revise the Code.

3. Describe the guidelines that are intended to assist the submitter of a change request.

4. List the CRC evaluation criteria that must be considered in addition to the change request form guidelines.

Review Quiz

1. What organization holds all property rights, title, and interest in CDT?
   a. Centers for Medicare and Medicaid Services (CMS)
   b. American Dental Association (ADA)
   c. America's Health Insurance Plans
   d. Blue Cross/Blue Shield Association

2. Which of following information is included in the Code?
   a. Dental claim form instructions
   b. Coding-related questions and answers
   c. Tooth numbering systems
   d. All of the above

3. Which of the following CDT service categories include professional visits?
   a. Diagnostic D0100–D0999
   b. Preventive D1000–D1999
   c. Adjunctive General Services D9000–D9999
   d. Miscellaneous Services D9910–D9999

4. True or False. Unspecified codes are not available in the Code manual.

5. Which of the following is considered an optional component?
   a. Dental procedure code
   b. Nomenclature
   c. Descriptor
   d. None of the above

6. Who is responsible for maintaining the Code?
   a. Centers for Medicare and Medicaid Services (CMS)
   b. Code Revision Committee (CRC)
   c. Blue Cross Blue Shield Association
   d. None of the above

7. Which of the following is a required component that provides a written definition of a dental procedure code?
   a. Terminology
   b. Descriptor
   c. Nomenclature
   d. Subcategory

8. True or False. A bullet symbol identifies a new procedure code in the current version of the Code.

9. Revisions to the Code are published and effective:
   a. Annually
   b. Biannually
   c. Quarterly
   d. All of the above

10. True or False. Dentists may only complete the code change request forms.

Part II

Other Vocabulary, Terminology, and Classification Systems

Chapter 7

Systematized Nomenclature of Medicine Clinical Terms (SNOMED CT®)

Margaret M. Foley, PhD, RHIA, CCS

Learning Objectives

- To trace the evolution of the Systematized Nomenclature of Medicine Clinical Terms (SNOMED CT)

- To discuss the content coverage of various versions of SNOMED

- To explain the purpose of SNOMED CT

- To describe the content and organizational structure of SNOMED CT

- To define the process for ongoing maintenance and continuing evolution of SNOMED CT

Key Terms

Attributes
Clinical Terms Version 3 (CTV3)
College of American Pathologists (CAP)
Computer-based Patient Record Institute (CPRI)
Concept
Concept orientation
Concept permanence
Controlled medical terminology
Description
Etiology axis
Fully specified name
Granularity
International Classification of Diseases-Oncology (ICD-O)
International Health Terminology Standards Development Organisation (IHTSDO)
IS-A relationships
Logical Observation Identifiers, Names, and Codes (LOINC)
Mapping
Morphology axis
Multiaxial
Nomenclature
Post-coordination
Pre-coordination
Preferred term
Read Codes
Reference terminology
Relationship
Root concept
Semantic
SNOMED
SNOMED CT
Subsets
Terminology
URU principle
Vocabulary

Introduction

The Systematized Nomenclature of Medicine (SNOMED) is a controlled medical terminology with comprehensive coverage of diseases, clinical findings, etiologies, and procedures and outcomes used by physicians, dentists, nurses, allied health professionals, veterinarians, and others. The **International Health Terminology Standards Development Organisation** (IHTSDO) defines **SNOMED** as a "comprehensive clinical **terminology** that provides clinical content and expressivity for clinical reporting which is comprised of concepts, terms, and relationships with the objective of precisely representing clinical information across the scope of health care" (IHTSDO 2008a). As of April 2007, the responsibility for the ownership, maintenance, and distribution of **SNOMED** CT was transferred from the College of American Pathologists to IHTSDO, a nonprofit organization based in Denmark.

SNOMED is designed to capture clinical information for use in an electronic health record (EHR) system (Kudla and Rallins 1998). A project of the National Library of Medicine (NLM), the Unified Medical Language System (UMLS) is the source for the United States license for SNOMED CT. It is available at no charge through the NLM.

This chapter traces the evolution of the various versions of SNOMED. It focuses particularly on the purpose, content, and organizational structure of SNOMED CT, the most recent version, first released in 2002. The process for maintaining SNOMED CT is also discussed.

The Evolution of SNOMED

The **College of American Pathologists** (CAP) published the first edition of **SNOMED** in 1974. SNOMED is based on the Systematized Nomenclature of Pathology (SNOP). CAP published SNOP in 1965 to organize information from surgical pathology reports. Because SNOP was widely used and accepted in the medical community, it was expanded as a **nomenclature** for other specialties.

Numerous versions of SNOMED have been published since 1974. (See table 7.1 on page 108.) The January 2009 release of SNOMED CT includes more than 310,000 active **concepts**, more than 794,000 active English-language **descriptions**, and more than 947,000 **relationships**. Used in countries throughout the world, SNOMED CT is the most comprehensive controlled terminology developed in the world to date.

SNOP

SNOP was built on the premise that a detailed and specific nomenclature is essential to accurately reflect the complexity and diversity of information found in a pathology report (Kudla and Rallins 1998). There was never any requirement to use SNOP, but it was widely adopted by pathologists because of its usefulness in organizing pathology records. Pathology reports are typically free-text descriptions of the gross and microscopic findings in a tissue sample. SNOP gave pathologists the ability to codify pathology findings as accurately and in as much detail as desired without being limited to a predetermined classification.

SNOP was one of the first systems to code diseases on a **multiaxial** basis. The principle is that a disease may be defined by the following characteristics (called axes):

- *Topography:* The part of the body affected by disease

- *Morphology:* A structural change in tissue

- *Etiology:* The cause of the disease or injury

- *Function:* Physiological or chemical disorders and alterations resulting from a disease or injury

SNOP is an alphanumeric coding scheme where the first letter of the code represents the primary characteristic, or the axis, of the element coded.
Example:

Orchitis due to mumps:

T-7800	Testis-NOS
M-4800	Inflammation NOS
E-3250	Mumps virus
F-0414	Mumps

Table 7.1.   Summary of the evolution of SNOMED

Year	Name of Version	Description	Content
1965	SNOP	The Systematized Nomenclature of Pathology is an alphanumeric coding scheme; the first letter of the code represents the axis of the element coded. It was used by pathologists to help them code and organize their reports.	Limited to pathology terms, four axes
1974	SNOMED	First called the Systematized Nomenclature of Human and Veterinary Medicine, SNOMED followed the SNOP coding scheme but coded all diagnoses/procedures.	Clinical terms from all specialties, six axes
1979	SNOMED II	Occupations were added as a seventh axis to aid in epidemiological studies examining the effects of occupation and environment on health.	44,587 records classified in six axes, available in a two-volume set with an alphabetic index
1993	SNOMED Version 3.0, or SNOMED International	The etiology axis was split into four distinct axes, and a linkage modifier axis was added. From 1993 to 1997, this version was updated annually.	130,580 terms classified in eleven axes
1997	SNOMED International Version 3.4	This version enhanced SNOMED Version 3.0 by including mapping to LOINC codes. In addition, more than 32,000 terms were mapped to ICD-9-CM. It is provided on a CD-ROM for incorporation into any database application.	More than 150,000 terms classified in eleven axes
2000	SNOMED RT	With the addition of relational tables, this version is a concept-based reference terminology that could be implemented in the electronic health record (EHR). Whether diseases are coded as single or multiple concepts, it has the capability through description logic to identify them as the same condition.	More than 121,000 concepts linked to more than 190,000 synonym terms and an excess of 340,000 explicit relationships
2002	SNOMED CT	A concept-based clinical terminology, SNOMED CT represents the merger of SNOMED RT and Clinical Terms Version 3 (Read Codes). This version refines the mapping criteria to ICD-9-CM and expands the coverage of primary care concepts.	First release contained approximately 325,000 concepts linked to more than 800,000 descriptions with more than 950,000 semantic relationships between clinical concepts
2007	SNOMED CT	Ownership, maintenance, and distribution transferred to the International Health Terminology Standards Development Organisation (IHTSDO), a non-for-profit association based in Denmark.	July 2007 release contains more than 310,000 concepts, 790,000 active descriptions, and more than 923,000 defining relationships

SNOMED

In 1974, CAP published the Systematized Nomenclature of Human and Veterinary Medicine, which represented a major expansion of SNOP to incorporate other specialties. In this, the original SNOMED, the four axes in SNOP were expanded to six axes. (See table 7.2.) Initially, the four axes in SNOP combined together were organized into a list of diseases, which resulted in a fifth axis called disease. A sixth axis called procedures also was defined.

This version of SNOMED became available in 1977 in electronic media, rather than print format, for use in newly developed mainframe-based medical information systems. With the growing prevalence of computers in the 1970s, the healthcare industry began to recognize the need for a nomenclature that worked well with computerized applications. SNOMED was developed to respond to this need. SNOMED was specifically designed to store all aspects of healthcare information recorded on a patient. Following is an example of the early SNOMED coding scheme:

Acquired mature cataract with low vision:

T-XX700	Crystalline lens
M-51120	Cataract, mature
E-0024	Acquired
F-X0050	Low vision
D-X080	Disease of lens

As this example illustrates, the multiaxial design makes it difficult and time-consuming for individu-

Table 7.2.   Six axes of the first version of SNOMED

Axis	Title	Description
1	Topography	Anatomy or parts/regions of the body arranged hierarchically; includes all tissues, organs, anatomic sites, and structures
2	Morphology	Structural change/abnormality of the tissue/anatomy
3	Etiology	Causes and causal agents of disease, dysfunctions, and morphological alterations that occur in the human body; includes chemicals and drugs that can either attack or cure the body
4	Function	Normal and abnormal functions, functional states, and physiological units of the body and the major organ systems
5	Disease	An organized list of classes of diseases, complex disease entities, and syndromes
6	Procedures	Actions of the healthcare team to prevent or cure a disease, illness, or injury, including: administrative, diagnostic, therapeutic, and preventative procedures

als to assign codes manually. Even this first version was designed for computer storage and automatic encoding of medical text.

SNOMED Version II

CAP published SNOMED Version II in 1979. It includes approximately 44,000 terms and contains a seventh axis called occupation. This axis consists of a classification of occupations from the World Health Organization (WHO) International Labour Office. It was included in SNOMED to enable studies on the effects of occupation and environment on health.

SNOMED II also expanded the **morphology axis** to incorporate the **International Classification of Diseases—Oncology** (ICD-O). In 1976, WHO began a project to adapt the American Cancer Society's Manual of Tumor Nomenclature and Coding system into an international coding system for oncology, and CAP collaborated on the project. Since 1979, the morphology section of ICD-O and sections 8 and 9 of the SNOMED morphology axis have been identical (Kudla and Rallins 1998).

SNOMED Version 3.0

CAP published SNOMED Version 3.0, also called SNOMED International, in 1993. In this version, the **etiology axis** was split into four distinct axes and a new axis for linking concepts was added. SNOMED Version 3.0 had a total of eleven axes.

The new axes added with this version included the following:

- *Living organisms:* This axis includes all types of living organisms, from viruses to mammals and from fungi to higher-level plants of all phylogenetic groups.

- *Chemicals:* Chemicals include common elements and their isotopes, chemical compounds, industrial chemicals, pesticides, plant and animal products, and toxins that affect the health of both man and animals.

- *Physical agents, forces, and activities:* Agents, activities, or forces that may cause injury. Also included are term codes for prostheses, artificial organs, hospital equipment, and devices.

- *Social context:* Social context refers to social conditions and circumstances that may have a bearing on the patient's health and medical condition, including ethnic and religious heritage, family status, economic condition, and so on.

- *General linkage modifiers:* These are terms that link the detailed elements found in each of the other modules in a meaningful way to accurately reflect the medical events they are intended to represent. Terms that relate to the need to modify or qualify the diagnostic entries found in each of the other modules also are included.

Table 7.3.   Comparison of code axes in SNOMED versions

SNOP	Original SNOMED	SNOMED II	SNOMED 3.0
Topography	Topography	Topography	1. Topography
Morphology	Morphology	Morphology	2. Morphology
Etiology	Etiology	Etiology	Etiology was split into: 3. Living organisms 4. Chemicals 5. Physical agents, forces, and activities 6. Social context
Function	Function	Function	7. Function
	Disease	Disease	8. Disease
	Procedures	Procedures	9. Procedures
		Occupation	10. Occupation
			11. General linkage modifiers

SNOMED Version 3.0 contained 130,580 terms. From 1993 through 1997, it was updated annually.

Table 7.3 presents a comparison of code axes in the different versions of SNOMED.

Check Your Understanding 7.1

Instructions: Complete the following exercises on a separate piece of paper.

1. What characteristics of disease processes does the TMEF axis format of SNOP identify?
   a. Toxicity, morphology, and environmental factors
   b. Topography, morphology, etiology, and function
   c. Topography, morbidity, and environmental factors
   d. Topology, morphology, etiology, and function

2. True or False. Unlike the current version of SNOMED, the earlier versions were designed to be printed in books and trained coders assigned codes manually.

3. Which of the following is *not* an axis of disease in SNOMED Version 3.0?
   a. Living organisms
   b. Function
   c. Etiology
   d. Occupation

4. Which version of SNOMED was the first to contain more than 100,000 terms?
   a. SNOMED II
   b. SNOMED Version 3.0
   c. SNOMED International Version 3.4
   d. SNOMED RT

SNOMED International Versions 3.4 and 3.5

CAP released SNOMED International Version 3.4 in 1997. This version contained more than 150,000 terms and was provided on a CD-ROM in an ASCII tab-delimited format for incorporation into any database application. Version 3.4 enhanced SNOMED Version 3.0 by including **mapping** to **Logical Observation Identifiers, Names, and Codes** (LOINC) codes. (See chapter 10.) In addition, more than 32,000 terms were mapped to ICD-9-CM.

SNOMED further expanded its content coverage in Version 3.5, first released in August 1998. In this version, SNOMED gained more than 6,000 new terms, most of them in the disease axis. With this release, SNOMED contained 156,965 terms.

Despite the breadth of coverage of SNOMED up to this point, it had not been widely adopted in electronic health records (EHRs). The main problem with using SNOMED for coding patient information was that it was *too* expressive. The multi-axial system provides multiple ways to represent a concept, yet there was no formal mechanism to indicate equivalent meaning. For example, acute appendicitis can be coded as a single disease term, as a combination of a modifier (acute) and a disease term (appendicitis), or as a combination of a modifier (acute), a morphology term (inflammation), and a topography term (variform appendix). This freedom of expression is desirable at the point of input, but frustrating for system developers attempting to build a system that can recognize medical concepts.

Even before the release of this version of SNOMED International, CAP had begun work to resolve this limitation. It collaborated with Kaiser Permanente to define relationships within SNOMED so that, whether a disease is coded as single or multiple concepts, the computer system would recognize the various combinations as the same condition.

SNOMED RT

CAP worked with a team of physicians and nurses from Kaiser Permanente to develop the Systematized Nomenclature of Medicine Reference Terminology (SNOMED RT). Together, they created description logic by defining relational tables so that no matter which axes were used to describe a medical concept, the system would recognize equivalent concepts. In May 2000, SNOMED RT was introduced to the medical community.

SNOMED RT was a **reference terminology** that groups medical terms as a set of concepts and relationships. A reference terminology for clinical data is defined as a set of concepts and relationships that provides a common reference point for comparisons and aggregation of data about the entire healthcare process, recorded by multiple different individuals, systems, or institutions (Spackman, Campbell, and Cote 1997).

In SNOMED RT, data are organized on the basis of eight relational tables. These relational tables are:

- Concepts
- Concepts history
- Concepts history refer to
- Descriptions
- Descriptions history
- Descriptions history refer to
- Relationships
- Relationships history

These tables provide the framework for organizing data. The concepts table lists every concept that appeared in earlier versions of SNOMED, beginning with version III. Each concept, or **fully specified name** as listed on the table, is given a concept identifier.

Concepts are further identified by various terms or phrases that define them. More than 121,000 concepts have linkages to more than 190,000 terms with unique computer-readable codes. The combination of a concept and a term is a description. Descriptions are given a description ID. In addition to concepts and terms, more than 340,000 relationships exist between and among the terms. A relationship is a type of connection between two terms.

SNOMED RT had a tremendous amount of content and is concept based. It had the potential to standardize medical terms, enabling accurate communication among diverse systems. In addition, it allowed healthcare personnel and organizations to collect and analyze data more effectively, to compare the quality of the healthcare being administered, to develop effective treatment guidelines, and to conduct outcomes research (Kudla and Blakemore 2001).

Following is an example of SNOMED RT codes with the relationships underlined:

Pneumococcal pneumonia (DE-13510)

    <u>Is an</u> infectious disease (DE-13500)

    <u>Is a</u> bacterial disease (DE-10100)

    <u>Is due to</u> streptococcus pneumoniae
        (L-25116)

    <u>Causes</u> inflammation (M-40000)

    <u>Affects</u> lung (T-28000)

SNOMED CT

First released in 2002, the Systematized Nomenclature of Medicine Clinical Terms (SNOMED CT) is the result of merging SNOMED RT with the National Health Service (NHS) terminology, **Clinical Terms Version 3** (CTV3), formerly known as the **Read Codes.** CTV3 is a crown copyright work of the NHS in the United Kingdom. Introduced in the 1980s, its purpose (similar to that of SNOMED) was to facilitate the exchange, retrieval, and analysis of key data in the medical record.

SNOMED RT included elementary mapping to ICD-9-CM. The merging of SNOMED RT with CTV3 allows for refinement of mapping criteria and guidelines. SNOMED CT incorporates all the content from both SNOMED RT and CTV3 into a data structure that originally had an estimated 370,000 concepts with more than a million **semantic** relationships to add meaning.

With nearly double the content of SNOMED version 3.5, SNOMED CT became the most comprehensive, multilingual clinical terminology tool providing the information framework for clinical decision making for the EHR (Brouch 2003).

Convergent Medical Terminology Project

To ensure comparability of data across all its facilities, Kaiser initiated the Convergent Medical Terminology (CMT) project in the late 1970s. The purpose of the project was to build a comprehensive and functional terminology that could be integrated into its clinical information systems using SNOMED as the base.

SNOMED RT was born out of the combined efforts of CAP and the physicians and nurses from the Kaiser Permanente CMT project. Beginning with the disease/diagnoses and procedures axes, they built explicit hierarchies and defined the essential char-

acteristics of each SNOMED term, thus converting SNOMED International into SNOMED-RT.

Merger between SNOMED and Clinical Terms Version 3

In the 1980s, James Read, a family practice physician in England, developed a coded terminology for the recording and retrieval of primary care patient data in a computer. Like SNOMED, the **Read Codes** were based on a strict coding scheme where each term was carefully assigned an identifier that represented its position in a hierarchy.

Whereas SNOMED, with roots in pathology, grew in popularity in pathology departments across the United States, the Read Codes, with roots in primary care, grew in popularity in ambulatory care clinics across the United Kingdom (Kudla and Blakemore 2001).

In the early 1990s, the British government, through its National Health Service (NHS), obtained the rights to the Read Codes and, in 1992, embarked on a three-year project to expand the work from a primary care focus to a comprehensive terminology representing the entire scope of clinical practice.

Development of Clinical Terms Version 3 was a product of the Clinical Terms project. Under the leadership of the NHS Information Authority, the project involved fifty-five clinical specialty working groups in the United Kingdom, representing more than 2,000 individuals from the Royal Medical Colleges, nursing professionals, and allied health professionals. These working groups proposed terms and developed and reviewed the content of what was to become the core terminology for EHRs throughout Britain.

Check Your Understanding 7.2

Instructions: Complete the following exercises on a separate piece of paper.

1. In SNOMED RT, the concept of axes was replaced by:
   a. Relational tables
   b. Reference terminologies
   c. Equivalent meanings
   d. Mapping

2. The combination of a concept and a term in SNOMED RT is called a:
    a. Relationship
    b. Description
    c. Reference
    d. Standardized medical term

3. Which of the following is *not* a relational table in SNOMED RT?
    a. Concepts
    b. Concepts history
    c. Morphology
    d. Relationships

4. True or False. SNOMED RT was the first version of the SNOMED family to include mappings.

5. What is the difference between SNOMED RT and SNOMED CT?

Developer

In April 1999, NHS and CAP announced a historic collaboration to unite SNOMED and CTV3 and create "a unified international terminology that supports the integrated electronic medical record." Shortly after that announcement, representatives from NHS and CAP began work designing and building SNOMED CT (Kudla and Blakemore 2001). First released in January 2002, SNOMED CT combined the strength of SNOMED RT in the basic sciences, laboratory, and specialty medicine, including pathology, with the richness of the United Kingdom's work in primary care.

SNOMED CT was originally maintained and distributed by CAP, a medical specialty organization of board-certified pathologists that held the copyright to SNOMED. However, as of April 2007, the responsibility for the ownership, maintenance, and distribution of SNOMED CT was transferred to IHTSDO, a nonprofit organization based in Denmark. IHTSDO contracts with SNOMED Terminology Solutions (STS), a division of the College of American Pathologists (CAP) to perform the development and maintenance tasks.

Purpose

The general purpose of SNOMED is to index, store, and retrieve information about a patient in an elec-

tronic health record. SNOMED is not a classification. Classifications, by nature, are designed to classify like things together. In contrast, SNOMED is designed to uniquely identify clinical information consistently and in great detail (**granularity**). With SNOMED, the objective is to fully describe all the clinical circumstances of a healthcare encounter in a machine-readable format (that is, in codes).

With a classification system such as ICD-9-CM, a coding professional assigns a code. This is not done with SNOMED. SNOMED CT codes are embedded in the EHR system and work behind the scenes to code the clinical language used in the health record. For example, the entire hospital stay for the birth of a healthy baby is represented by a couple of ICD-9-CM codes. In contrast, there are SNOMED CT codes for the finite detail of the normal newborn hospital stay. An Apgar score, a small subset of clinical information collected at birth, is not coded at all in ICD-9-CM but would be represented by separate SNOMED CT codes for the cardiac score, respiratory score, muscle tone, reflex, response, and color.

In a study conducted to assess the feasibility of automated coding in SNOMED using natural language processing, an expert trained in controlled medical terminologies and SNOMED coding took approximately sixty hours to manually assign SNOMED RT codes to one discharge summary report. A total of 431 clinical concepts were abstracted from a 589-word discharge summary, and 285 SNOMED RT codes were used to code the one report (Lussier, Shagina, and Friedman 2001). This example illustrates the breadth of content in SNOMED CT and gives a sense of its purpose embedded within an EHR. It is designed to work in the background to explicitly represent all clinically relevant concepts in machine-readable format. (See figure 7.1 on page 114 for an illustration of SNOMED CT working behind the scenes in an EHR.)

The **Computer-based Patient Record Institute** (CPRI) studied the ability of nomenclatures to capture information for computerized patient records. CPRI no longer exists as a separate entity;

Figure 7.1. SNOMED CT working behind the scenes in an EHR

In the following excerpt from an electronic health record (EHR), a few of the applicable SNOMED CT codes are noted in parentheses to illustrate what SNOMED CT is doing behind the scenes. It is automatically identifying standard terms and tagging them for future reference.

This 85-year- (258707000) old (70753007) female (248152002) was admitted via the emergency room (50849002 ED admission) from the nursing home (42665001) with shortness of breath (267036007), confusion (225440008 onset of confusion), and congestion (85804007). There was no history of (14792006) fever (386661006) or cough (49727002) noted. Patient also has a history of (392521001) senile dementia (15662003) and COPD (13645005)...

Prior to admission, the patient was on the following medications:

Prednisone (116602009), Lasix, Haldol (349874003), and Colace. Patient also has been on lorazepam 0.5mg tablet (377147002) 2x a day as needed for anxiety (48694002). Patient is noted to have a vitamin C deficiency (76169001)...

its mission has been assumed by the Healthcare Information and Management Systems Society (HIMSS). During its existence, CPRI determined that SNOMED is the most comprehensive controlled terminology for coding the contents of the patient record and facilitating the development of computerized patient records (Chute, Cohn, et al. 1996; Campbell et al. 1997). The more recent version, SNOMED CT, is even better suited to fulfill this purpose.

To do this, SNOMED CT must not only contain an incredible amount of content, but it also must be organized in such a way that the underlying meanings of concepts and expressions are represented consistently. The fact that SNOMED CT is a controlled terminology is one of the characteristics that makes it more than just a huge list of coded medical terms. A **controlled medical terminology** (CMT) is a coded **vocabulary** of medical concepts and expressions used in healthcare. *Controlled* means that the content of the terminology is managed carefully to ensure that it is structurally sound, biomedically accurate, and consistent with current practice.

Standardized terminology is needed to facilitate the indexing, storage, and retrieval of patient infor-

mation in an EHR. However, in the field of medicine, two physicians may use two different terms for the same medical condition. This makes it difficult to gather and retrieve information. SNOMED creates a standardized terminology.

A controlled terminology is a key to a functional electronic health record. According to Chris Chute of the Mayo Foundation, "The single greatest obstacle to comparable data remains medical terminology. Failure to adopt and embrace a common terminology will doom outcomes research and data-driven clinical guideline development" (Chute 1994). In Chute's opinion, clinical data gathered without a controlled terminology are not comparable and thus rendered meaningless.

There are many ways to say the same thing in the English language. This certainly applies to medicine. Take, for example, the concept of increased body temperature. In SNOMED CT, the following terms are recognized as synonyms of increased body temperature: fever, pyrexia, hypothermia, febrile. The terms *feverish* and *hyperthermic* also are linked to this concept. If patient data were stored in a computer without a controlled terminology, a search for all patients with the condition "increased body temperature" would miss the numerous cases where this condition was recorded as fever, febrile, and so on. A controlled terminology allows individuals to record data in the patient's record using any one of a variety of synonyms but references the data back to a single primary concept. A versatile computer interface would even allow the individual clinician to use a local or personalized word, such as *temp*, by providing an option that allows the clinician to map this local term as a synonym to the concept of increased body temperature in the controlled terminology. The integration of a controlled clinical terminology such as SNOMED CT into electronic health records provides a comprehensive and functional terminology system.

It is expected that numerous systems, working together in concert, would be required to support an efficient and effective clinical information system and to handle the administrative needs of a healthcare organization. Although ideally suited for clinical purposes, SNOMED CT may not be suitable for certain administrative needs. For example, SNOMED CT would be difficult to use as a reimbursement classification system because of its tremendous amount of content. A classification system such as ICD with its ability to aggregate data is more suitable for claims processing. SNOMED CT is designed for use in the underlying clinical information system to identify and tag data at the point of input so that it can be aggregated and used later for various purposes.

The purpose of SNOMED CT is to enable the consistent recording and documentation of clinical concepts, with clear relationships between concepts, in an EHR. SNOMED CT helps ensure comparability of data records by multiple practitioners across diverse platforms and systems using computer programs.

Check Your Understanding 7.3

Instructions: Complete the following exercises on a separate piece of paper.

1. SNOMED CT resulted from the combination of:
   a. SNOMED RT and Clinical Terms Version 3
   b. SNOMED RT and ICD-9-CM
   c. SNOMED RT and LOINC
   d. SNOMED and the Convergent Medical Terminology

2. True or False. Like other classification systems, SNOMED is designed to fully describe all the clinical circumstances of a healthcare encounter in machine-readable format.

3. What is the difference between a classification system and a controlled medical terminology such as SNOMED?

Content

As illustrated earlier in the example of 285 SNOMED codes needed to capture the clinical detail in one discharge summary, SNOMED provides the terminology needed to code essentially the entire patient medical record. It includes a vast array of clinical concepts beyond diagnoses and procedures. A review of the SNOMED CT codes assigned in figure 7.1 shows the concepts that may be coded in this system. SNOMED CT includes terms that cover diseases, findings, procedures, body structures, pharmacy products, and other concepts that encompass all of healthcare.

In addition, the content of SNOMED CT is very detailed. Whereas a classification system such as ICD may group together certain conditions, SNOMED CT uniquely identifies each condition. (See figure 7.2.)

With this level of detail available, it is not surprising that the size of SNOMED CT far surpasses that of any single classification. As previously stated, SNOMED CT contains more than 315,000 concepts and 806,000 English-language descriptions whereas ICD-9-CM contains about 13,000 diagnosis and 3,000 procedure codes, ICD-10-CM contains about 68,000 diagnosis codes, and ICD-10-PCS contains 87,000 procedure codes.

In describing the content of SNOMED CT, IHTS-DO delineates what is considered part of the core content from additional tools that are considered outside the core content. The core content includes the

Figure 7.2.   ICD-9-CM and SNOMED CT code comparison

ICD-9-CM Code and Inclusion Terms	SNOMED CT Codes and Terms
424.90 Endocarditis valve unspecified, unspecified cause	Endocarditis = 56819008 endocarditis (disorder)
Endocarditis (chronic): NOS	Endocarditis (chronic) = 4851007 chronic endocarditis (disorder)
Endocarditis (valvular)	Valvular endocarditis = 89736004 valvular endocarditis (disorder)
Valvulitis (chronic)	Valvulitis (chronic) = 40964007 chronic cardiac valvulitis (disorder)
Valvular: incompetence, insufficiency, regurgitation, stenosis	

Each of the above conditions is a unique concept in SNOMED CT, whereas only one ICD-9-CM code is used for all of them.

technical specification of SNOMED CT and fully integrated multispecialty clinical content. Specifically, it includes the:

- Concepts table
- Descriptions table
- Relationships table
- History table
- Subsets
- Cross mapping
- Technical reference guide

Mapping

As explained earlier, the comprehensive, granular nature of SNOMED CT makes it ideal for data input into an electronic health record. It is capable of capturing the necessary level of clinical detail required for patient care and clinical decision support. However, this granular detail makes it difficult to use for many administrative purposes, such as claims processing. Automated mapping of SNOMED CT to administrative code sets resolves this difficulty. SNOMED CT provides a technical structure that supports rule-based processing. It is designed to support automated cross mapping to other terminologies or coding schemes. Approximately 96,000 concepts (54,244 disorders and 36,616 findings) in SNOMED CT have been mapped to ICD-9-CM.

A cross-map links the content from one classification or terminology scheme to another. Maps allow data collected for one purpose to be used for another purpose. For example, SNOMED CT mapped to ICD-9-CM facilitates the translation of more granular clinical data into less granular classifications that can be used for administrative and statistical purposes. The map provides an approximation of the closest ICD code or codes that best represent the SNOMED CT concept. This simplifies coding and data-entry processes, which is expected to lower costs and minimize errors.

Maps have been created from SNOMED CT to the following systems:

- Clinical Care Classification (nursing diagnoses, intervention and outcomes)
- ICD-9-CM
- ICD-10
- International Classification of Diseases for Oncology (ICD-O-3)
- Logical Observation Identifiers Names and Codes (LOINC)
- North American Nursing Diagnosis Association (NANDA)
- Nursing Interventions Classifications (NIC)
- Nursing Outcomes Classification (NOC)
- Office of Population Censuses and Surveys Classification of Interventions and Procedures (OPCS-4)
- Omaha System
- Perioperative Nursing Data Set (PNDS)

As mentioned above, a reference terminology is a set of concepts and relationships that provides a common reference point for comparisons and aggregation of data about the entire healthcare process, recorded by multiple different individuals, systems, or institutions (Spackman, Campbell, and Cote 1997). Because of its linkages (mappings) with many other classifications and terminologies and its comprehensive content coverage, SNOMED CT is considered to be a reference terminology.

Subset

A subset is a defined grouping of SNOMED CT concepts, descriptions, and/or relationships that share a common characteristic such as language, specialty, user, or context. Examples of **subsets** available in SNOMED CT include an allergen subset, a CAP Cancer checklist subset, and a U.S. drug extension subset which includes medications approved for use in the United States.

In addition, IHTSDO allows for extensions that build on the core content. The intent of extensions is to meet the national, local, or organizational specialized terminology needs in a format that is compatible with the SNOMED CT core. Tables included in the core content are described in further detail in the SNOMED CT structure section of this chapter.

Recognized Redundancy

Redundancy within a terminology is when the same information can be expressed in two different ways. Synonymous terms (for example, heart attack and myocardial infarction) represented with a single concept code is one way in which SNOMED CT handles redundancy. Because SNOMED CT is so large and comprehensive, it is also possible to represent the same clinical issue with two different SNOMED CT concepts. For example, the concept for the disorder 'angina' and the concept for the clinical finding of 'ischemic chest pain' could be considered clinically equivalent depending upon the context.

SNOMED CT also allows for the pre-coordination and post-coordination of terms. **Pre-coordination** is often used to represent a commonly used clinical term as a single concept; whereas, **post-coordination** is when a combination of concept codes are joined to convey clinical meaning. For example 'fracture of tibia' can be expressed as either a pre-coordinated single concept or as a combination of the concept identifiers: bone structure of femur and clinical finding fracture. A combination of pre-coordinated and post-coordinated concepts is often used to facilitate the capture and representation of clinical documentation. Pre-coordinated concepts are useful when representing issues commonly documented. Post-coordinated concepts allow for the detailed capture of less commonly reported clinical issues. It is important for users of SNOMED CT to be aware that there are multiple ways to express clinical ideas within the terminology and to manage the redundancy when developing EHR systems.

Check Your Understanding 7.4

Instructions: Complete the following exercises on a separate piece of paper.

1. True or False. SNOMED CT is capable of expressing all components of the neonatal Apgar score in coded form.

2. In a controlled medical terminology, all content must meet three of the following criteria. Which of the criteria listed below is *not* a requirement of a controlled vocabulary?
    a. It must be structurally sound.
    b. It must be biomedically accurate.
    c. It must be updated on a regular and specified basis.
    d. It must be consistent with current medical practice.

3. Maps have been created between SNOMED CT and which of the other following terminologies?
    a. ICD-9-CM, ICD-10, and ICD-O
    b. LOINC, ICD-9-CM, CPT, and NOC
    c. NANDA, ICD-9-CM, ICD-10, and CPT
    d. ICD-9-CM, ICD-O, ICD-10-PCS, and ICD-10-CM

Structure

SNOMED was developed at a time when computers were beginning to make inroads in healthcare but were not well established. The coding scheme employed defined axes that enabled humans to easily understand and use the code's hierarchical information in simple computer applications. However, as the number of terms grew and computers were able to handle more complex tasks, the limitations of a code to carry meaning and the potential for misinterpretation became more and more evident. NHS eliminated the use of "meaningful" codes when it introduced CTV3. CAP did the same with the introduction of SNOMED RT. In both SNOMED RT and SNOMED CT, codes do not have embedded meaning and digit restrictions. As a result, even when the knowledge about a concept changes, the SNOMED code remains the same.

All terminology or classification systems use some sort of hierarchical structure to organize the coded information. For example, ICD is organized based on body systems. In ICD-10-CM, for example, codes for diseases of the nervous system are classified in the code range G00–G99. In contrast, SNOMED CT is based on concepts. The terms in SNOMED CT are organized based on the underlying medical concepts they represent.

The structure of SNOMED CT is centered on three elements: concepts, descriptions, and relationships.

Concepts

Concepts are the basic units of SNOMED CT and are defined as unique units of knowledge created by a unique combination of characteristics. In essence, a concept is a specific idea or thought. It may have more than one term associated with it, but it cannot have more than one meaning. In SNOMED CT, a unique identifier is assigned to each concept. For example, the word *cast* can have a number of different meanings. Among other things, it can refer to a rigid material molded to the body, a precipitated product from the kidney tubules found in urine, or, in the United States, the name of a proprietary drug product. Each of these concepts represents a unique expression of thought and is assigned its own unique concept code.

It is important to differentiate between the codes and the names. Codes are machine readable; names are human readable. Following is an example of a concept in SNOMED CT:

Example:

>   129742005 (the code)

>   Spiculated lesion (the name)

Concepts are organized into hierarchies. At the top of the hierarchy are very broad concepts and below are "child" concepts, which are more specialized or specific. Above the top-level concepts is a **root concept** or top-level hierarchy. The root concept incorporates the top-level concepts and the concepts beneath them. A root concept is a single special concept that represents the root of the entire content in SNOMED CT. As one goes down each level of the hierarchy, the concepts become increasingly granular and more specific. (See table 7.4.)

Table 7.4.   Hierarchical structure of SNOMED CT concepts

Organization	Example
Root concept (or main hierarchy)	Clinical finding
19 top-level concepts (upper-level concepts)	Disease: Inflammatory disorder
Subhierarchies (may be several)	Arthritis

There are nineteen top levels or main hierarchies in SNOMED CT, each of which is subdivided into smaller hierarchies. Table 7.5 provides a brief description and examples of elements contained in the top-level hierarchies.

Descriptions

Descriptions are the terms or text for the concept, which has a unique, fully specified name, **preferred term**, or the name in common use, and optional synonym(s). SNOMED CT contains more than 806,000 English-language descriptions or synonyms, which provide flexibility in expressing clinical concepts. All are available in U.S. English, UK English, and Spanish. Translations into several other languages are currently taking place.

Example:

Concept fully specified name:

>   Pain in throat (finding)

Associated descriptions:

>   Sore throat

>   Throat pain

>   Pain in pharynx

>   Throat discomfort

>   Pharyngeal pain

>   Throat soreness

Relationships

Hierarchical relationships organize concepts; role or **attribute** relationships link them. Relationships

Table 7.5. SNOMED CT main hierarchies

Hierarchies	Examples
Clinical finding: • Contains the subhierarchies of Finding and Disease • *R* represents the result of a clinical observation, assessment, or judgment • Important for documenting clinical disorders and examination findings	Finding: Swelling of arm Disease: Pneumonia
Procedure: • Concepts that represent the purposeful activities performed in the provision of healthcare	Biopsy of lung Diagnostic endoscopy Fetal manipulation
Observable entity • Concepts represent a question or procedure which can produce an answer or a result	Gender Tumor size Ability to balance
Body structure • Concepts include both normal and abnormal anatomical structures • Abnormal structures are represented in a subhierarchy as morphologic abnormalities	Lingual thyroid (*body structure*) Neoplasm (*morphologic abnormality*)
Organism • Coverage includes animals, fungi, bacteria, and plants • Concepts represent organisms of etiologic significance in human and animal diseases • Necessary for public health reporting and used in evidence-based infectious disease protocols	Hepatitis C virus *Streptococcus pyogenes* *Acer rubrum* (red maple) *Felis silvestris* (cat)
Substance • Covers a wide range of biological and chemical substances • Includes foods, nutrients, allergens, and materials • Used to record the active chemical constituents of all drug products	Dust Estrogen Hemoglobin antibody Methane Codeine phosphate
Physical object • Concepts include natural and man-made objects • Focus on concepts required for medical injuries	Prosthesis Artificial organs Vena cava filter Colostomy bag
Physical force • Includes motion, friction, electricity, sound, radiation, thermal forces, and air pressure • Other categories are directed at categorizing mechanisms of injury	Fire Gravity Pressure change
Events • Concepts represent occurrences that result in injury • Exclude all procedures and interventions	Flash flood Motor vehicle accident
Environments/geographical locations • Includes all types of environments as well as named locations such as countries, states, and regions	Cameroon Islands of North America Burn center Cancer hospital
Record artifact • Includes items created by an individual for the purpose of providing others with information about events or states	Health record Death certificate

(Continued on next page)

Table 7.5.   (Continued)

Hierarchies	Examples
Social context • Contains social conditions and circumstances significant to healthcare • Includes family and economic status, ethnic and religious heritage, and lifestyle and occupations	Economic status (*social concept*) Asian (*ethnic group*) Clerical supervisor (*occupation*) Donor (*person*) Thief (*lifestyle*) Judaism (*religion/philosophy*)
Situation with explicit context • To represent medical information completely, it is sometimes necessary to attach additional information to a given concept. • If this information changes the concept's meaning, it is known as context. • This category contains concepts that carry context embedded within them.	No family history of stroke Nasal discharge present Aspiration pneumonia resulting from a procedure
Staging and scales • Contains concepts naming assessment scales and tumor staging systems	Glasgow coma scale (*assessment scale*) Alcohol use inventory (*assessment scale*) Dukes staging system (*tumor staging*)
Linkage concept • Contains the link assertion and attribute subhierarchies	Has explanation (link assertion) IS_A (attribute) Associated morphology (attribute)
Pharmaceutical/biological product • Contains drug products	Diazepam 5-mg tablet (product)
Qualifier value • Contains concepts used as values for SNOMED CT attributes	Unilateral (qualifier value) Left (qualifier value) Puncture - action (qualifier value)
Special concept • Concepts that have been retired	Inactive concept
Specimen • Concepts that are obtained for examination or analysis	Urine specimen obtained by clean-catch procedure (specimen) Calculus specimen (specimen)

Source:http://www.ihtsdo.org/fileadmin/user_upload/Docs_01/SNOMED_CT_Publications/SNOMED_CT_User_Guide_20080731.pdf.

are the connections between concepts in SNOMED CT. Every SNOMED CT concept has at least one relationship to another concept. These relationships characterize concepts and give them their meaning. **IS-A relationships** link concepts within a hierarchy. Concepts are always related by IS-A relationship to the concept directly above them. Role relationships link concepts in different hierarchies in order to provide a computer-readable definition of a concept.

IS-A relationships and attribute relationships also are known as Supertype–Subtype relationships and Parent–Child relationships. The SNOMED CT hierarchies consist entirely of these IS-A relationships. Some concepts have more than one IS-A relationship. These concepts have parent concepts in more than one hierarchy, but all parents of a concept are only within one of the main hierarchies.

Attribute relationships, also called role relationships, are properties or characteristics of concepts. **Attributes** are used to characterize and define concepts; they connect concepts together and build relationships. Indeed, they are the bridges between the SNOMED CT main hierarchies (for example, Clinical Finding and Procedure) and supporting hierarchies such as organism, substance, and body structure. The main hierarchies are sometimes referred to as domains.

Each attribute can take on values only from a particular value hierarchy. For example, values for the finding site attribute must come from the body structure hierarchy. The set of allowable values are sometimes referred to as the attribute's range.

Example:
Allergic rhinitis due to pollen

IS-A	Allergic rhinitis
Has-finding-site	Nose
Has-Associated-morphology	Inflammation
Has-Causative-agent	Pollen

Summary of the SNOMED CT Structure

The basic structural elements of SNOMED CT are concepts, descriptions, hierarchies, attributes, and relationships. These elements are necessary to precisely represent and provide clinical information across the scope of healthcare. Understanding the principles behind the SNOMED CT structure is critical to understanding the terminology and its design for use in electronic health records (EHRs). The principles behind the SNOMED CT structure are:

- SNOMED is concept based.

- Each concept represents a unit of meaning.

- Each concept has one or more human language terms that can be used to describe the concept.

- Every concept has interrelationships with other concepts that provide logical, computer-readable definitions. These include hierarchical relationships and clinical attributes.

All concepts in SNOMED CT have formal definitions, explicit representations of the concepts' meanings. A concept's definition consists of its relationships to other concepts, both IS-A relationships and attribute relationships.

IS-A relationships and attribute relationships are known as the defining characteristics of SNOMED CT concepts. IS-A relationships are relationships that link concepts within a hierarchy. Every concept (except the root concept) is assigned at least one hierarchical IS-A relationship. In addition, certain concepts also are assigned attributes to explicitly describe the concept's essential characteristics.

Attribute relationships (or role relationships) link concepts in different hierarchies to provide a computer-readable definition of a concept.

Check Your Understanding 7.5

Instructions: Complete the following exercises on a separate piece of paper.

1. The terms in SNOMED CT are organized based on the underlying _____ that they represent.

2. The function of attribute relationships is to:
   a. Link concepts
   b. Organize concepts
   c. Facilitate mapping to other terminologies
   d. All of the above

3. True or False. A root concept is the most granular division of SNOMED CT.

4. Which of the following is not a main hierarchy in SNOMED CT?
   a. Physical object
   b. Organism
   c. History
   d. Body structure

5. What are the three key elements to the structure of SNOMED CT?

Principles and Guidelines

By the late 1990s, the limitations of existing schemes, based on terms organized with hierarchical codes, were well recognized. Several authors in the medical informatics community published papers laying out formal requirements for a new generation of healthcare terminologies designed for use in the EHR. Nearly twenty requirements in total are outlined in two key papers (Cimino 1998; Campbell et al. 1999). SNOMED RT and SNOMED CT were designed to be compliant with the principles laid out in these scientific papers, including principles for content, structure, and terminology management processes.

Two of the key principles are **concept orientation**, which means concepts are based on meanings and not words, and **concept permanence**, which means that the codes that represent the concept are not reused and thus meanings do not change.

As mentioned earlier, every SNOMED CT concept has a unique identifier (code). These SNOMED CT identifiers (SCTIDs) can be from six to eighteen digits long and are computer readable. They are without embedded meaning and without digit restrictions. They are unique codes, globally, that will not change. This means that if a SNOMED code is entered into a patient record, the meaning is future-proofed. If the knowledge about a concept changes, the meaning of the original SNOMED code will not change. Instead, a new code will be created for the changed concept.

SNOMED contains terminology and codes that allow the recording of data at the appropriate clinical level of detail. The user is not forced to record information at a level of detail that is either too general or too specific. As a guideline, it is preferable to record data at a more specific level if to do so is practical and consistent with clinical practice.

According to IHTSDO, SNOMED CT is developed and maintained with the overlying goal of creating and sustaining semantic interoperability of clinical information. Since 1996, SNOMED modelers have assessed whether content is creating and sustaining semantic interoperability by using the acronym for the **URU principle**. URU refers to:

- **U**nderstandable: The concept must be described and defined in such a way that people can use it easily.

- **R**eproducible: After it is described and defined, the concept must be modeled consistently.

- **U**seful: The concept must be of some actual use in healthcare or a health-related domain.

Maintenance Process

The international version of SNOMED CT which contains the English-language (U.S. and UK) editions is released in January and July of each year. The Spanish edition is released in April and Octo-ber of each year. As of April 2007, the responsibility for the ownership, maintenance, and distribution of SNOMED CT was transferred to IHTSDO. IHTSDO contracts with SNOMED Terminology Solutions (STS), a division of the College of American Pathologists (CAP) to perform the development and maintenance tasks.

The SNOMED CT development process incorporates the efforts of a team of terminologists. A documented scientific process is followed that focuses on understandability, reproducibility, and usefulness. Content is defined and reviewed by multiple clinician editors, with additional experts consulted, as necessary, to review the scientific integrity of the content.

The quality control process is continuously supplemented by feedback from users. These individuals bring expertise in national and international standards, medical informatics, software development and implementation, database licensing, biotechnology, clinical and academic medicine, managed care, laboratory medicine, pharmacy, nursing, education, and database services.

IHTSDO Governance and Structure

When the intellectual property rights for SNOMED CT were transferred from CAP to IHTSDO, the goal of international ownership and governance of the terminology was achieved. The General Assembly is the highest authority of the IHTSDO. It is responsible for "ensuring that the purpose, objects and principles of the association are pursued and that the interests of the IHTSDO are safeguarded" (IHTSDO 2008). A nine-member multinational Management Board has overall responsibility for the management and direction of the IHTSDO.

IHTSDO's four standing committees, which advise the Management Board on their respective areas of responsibility, are: the Content Committee, the Research and Innovation Committee, the Quality Assurance Committee, and the Technical Committee. The Content Committee handles issues related to the definition and maintenance of the clinical content and structure of SNOMED CT, with a focus on users and implementation of the terminology. The Quality Assurance Committee is responsible for compliance with external standards as related to the development and quality assurance of SNOMED CT. The Research and Innovation Committee addresses terminology issues that are on a 3–5 year time horizon and is responsible for testing new and unproven ideas in terminology development. The Technical Committee monitors the technical framework and tools needed for the development and maintenance of SNOMED CT.

Working Groups

As part of its commitment to an open terminology development process, IHTSDO provides a collaborative working space and sponsors two types of work groups: special interest groups (SIGs) and project groups (PGs). Open participation on these groups is encouraged. The working groups vary in scope, ranging from providing input about the direction of the terminology to a detailed review of specific nomenclature domains. For example, a domain-specific working group (for example, nursing, pharmacy, anesthesiology, mappings) may focus on information needs for a particular clinical area and provide advice on the scope of coverage, the creation of hierarchies, semantic structure, and scientific accuracy of the content for the purpose specified.

Working groups that are currently planned or active include:

- Special Interest Groups
  - —Anesthesia
  - —Concept Model
  - —Education
  - —International Pathology and Laboratory Medicine
  - —Mapping
  - —Nursing
  - —Pharmacy
  - —Primary Care
  - —Translation

- Project Groups–Anatomy Model
  - —Collaborative Working
  - —Education
  - —Enhanced Release Format Interchange
  - —Event, Condition, and Episode Model
  - —Format and Reference Sets
  - —Machine and Human Readable Concept Model
  - —Mapping SNOMED CT to ICD-10
  - —Mapping Standard Project
  - —Observable and Investigation Model
  - —Organism and Infectious Disease Model
  - —Pharmacy Naming and Editorial Rules
  - —Request Submission
  - —Substance Hierarchy Redesign
  - —Translation Standard Processes

In addition, the users group meets yearly to learn about new applications relating to SNOMED CT and to share ideas and implementation experiences.

Check Your Understanding 7.6

Instructions: Complete the following exercises on a separate piece of paper.

1. True or False. SNOMED CT codes have embedded meaning, but no digit restrictions.

2. SNOMED CT is updated on a regular basis. For the United Kingdom and United States, updates are provided:
   a. Every January
   b. Every June
   c. Every January and July
   d. October 1 of each year

3. True or False. To ensure that SNOMED CT remains useful, development must involve diverse clinical groups as well as medical informatics experts.

4. What are the responsibilities of SNOMED Terminology Solutions?

Summary

SNOMED, which is currently maintained and distributed by the IHTSDO, has evolved through multiple versions since 1974 to the present. It has grown from a multiaxial system of fewer than 40,000 codes to a relational, concept-based system with more than 315,000 active concepts and more than 806,000 English-language descriptions. Today, the foundation of SNOMED CT is concepts. All the terms in SNOMED CT are organized based on the underlying medical concept that they represent. SNOMED CT may include multiple descriptions for each concept, and concepts are organized by defined relationships, including hierarchical relationships and role or attribute relationships.

Although the content has evolved and grown, its purpose has always focused on clinical data retrieval. SNOMED is designed to index, store, and retrieve information about a patient in an electronic health record. SNOMED is not a classification. Classifications, by nature, are designed to classify like things together. In contrast, SNOMED is designed to uniquely identify clinical information consistently and in great detail. With SNOMED, the objective is to fully describe all the clinical circumstances of a healthcare encounter in a machine-readable format. SNOMED CT helps ensure comparability of data records by multiple practitioners across diverse platforms and systems using computer programs. It is the most comprehensive controlled terminology developed in the world to date.

References

Brouch, Kathy. 2004 (January). Speaker: SNOMED promises to change HIM practice (convention wrap-up). *Journal of the American Health Information Management Association* 75(1):66–67.

Brouch, Kathy. 2003 (July/August). AHIMA project offers insights into SNOMED, ICD-9-CM mapping process. *Journal of the American Health Information Management Association* 74(7):52–55.

Brown, Steven H., Brent A. Bauer, et al. 2003. Coverage of oncology drug indications, concepts, and compositional semantics by SNOMED CT. AMIA 2003 Symposium Proceedings, 115–119.

Campbell, J. R., R. Carpenter, et al. 1997. Phase II evaluation of clinical coding schemes: Completeness, taxonomy, mapping, definitions, and clarity. *Journal of American Medical Informatics Association* 4:238–251.

Campbell, K. E., B. Hochhalter, J. Slaughter, and J. Mattison. 1999 (December). Enterprise issues pertaining to implementing controlled terminologies. IMIA WG 6 Conference, Phoenix, AZ.

Chute, C., et al. 1994 (April 26). Multi-institutional test bed for clinical vocabulary. Grant application to U.S. Department of Health and Human Services. Also found in the testimony of Kent A. Spackman, M.D. http://www.ncvhs.hhs.gov/981208tc.htm.

Chute, Christopher G., Simon Cohn, et al. 1996. The content coverage of clinical classifications. *Journal of the American Medical Informatics Association* 3:224–233.

Cimino, J. J. 1996. Review paper: Coding systems in health care. *Methods of Information in Medicine* 35:273–284.

Cimino, J. J. 1998. Desiderata for controlled medical vocabularies in the twenty-first century. *Methods of Information in Medicine* 37(4–5):394–403.

Department of Health and Human Services. 2008. HIPAA Administrative Simplification: Modifications to Medical Data Code Set Standards to Adopt ICD-10CM and ICD-10-PCS. *Federal Register* 73(164):49796–49832.

Dougherty, Michelle. 2003 (November). Standard terminology helps advance EHR. *Journal of the American Health Information Management Association* 74(10):59–60.

Fenton, Susan. 2000 (November). Clinical vocabularies and terminologies: Impact on the future of health information management. *Topics in Health Information Management* 21(2):74–80.

Huffman, Edna. 1990. *Medical Record Management.* Berwyn, IL: Physicians' Record Co.

Imel, Margo. 2002. A closer look: The SNOMED clinical terms to ICD-9-CM mapping. *Journal of the American Health Information Management Association* 73(6):66–69.

International Health Terminology Standards Development Organisation. 2008. http://www.ihtsdo.org/.

International Health Terminology Standards Development Organisation. 2008a. SNOMED CT User Guide—July 2008 International Release. http://www.ihtsdo.org/fileadmin/user_upload/Docs_01/SNOMED_CT_Publications/SNOMED_CT_User_Guide_20080731.pdf.

International Health Terminology Standards Development Organisation. 2008b. *Second 2008 International Release of SNOMED CT Now Available.* http://www.ihtsdo.org/fileadmin/user_upload/Docs_01/News/Second_2008_International_Release_Press_Release.pdf.

International Health Terminology Standards Development Organisation. 2008c. *SNOMED Clinical Terms (SNOMED CT) Core Content: January 2008 International Release.* http://www.ihtsdo.org/snomed-ct/snomed-ct0/different-languages/. http://www.cap.org/apps/docs/snomed/documents/january_2008_release.pdf

International Health Terminology Standards Development Organisation. 2008d. IHTSDO: Different languages. http://www.ihtsdo.org/snomed-ct/snomed-ct0/different-languages/.

International Health Terminology Standards Development Organisation. 2008e. SNOMED CT Technical Reference Guide—

July 2008 International Release. http://www.ihtsdo.org/fileadmin/user_upload/Docs_01/Technical_Docs/SNOMED_CT_Technical_Reference_Guide_20080731.pdf.

International Health Terminology Standards Development Organisation. 2008f. Proposed International Release Schedule for 2008 and 2009. http://www.ihtsdo.org/fileadmin/user_upload/Docs_01/Copenhagen_Apr_2008/Proposed_International-Release-Schedule-for-2008_2009.pdf.

International Health Terminology Standards Development Organisation. 2008g. SNOMED Clinical Terms Editorial Guidelines Version 1.08. http://www.ihtsdo.org/fileadmin/user_upload/Docs_01/Copenhagen_Apr_2008/SNOMED_CT_Style_Guides/IHTSDO_Editorial_Policy-Content_Inclusion_Principles_and_Process-20080501_v1-08.pdf.

Johns, Merida L. 2002. *Health Information Management Technology: An Applied Approach*. Chicago: American Health Information Management Association.

Kudla, Karen M., and Margo Blakemore. 2001. SNOMED takes the next step. *Journal of the American Health Information Management Association* 72(7):62–68.

Kudla, Karen M., and Marjorie Rallins. 1998. SNOMED: A controlled vocabulary for computer-based patient records. *Journal of the American Health Information Management Association* 69(5):40–44.

LaTour, Kathleen and Shirley Eichenwald. 2006. *Health Information Management: Concepts, Principles, and Practice*. Second Edition. Chicago: American Health Information Management Association.

Lussier, Yves, Lyudmila Shagina, and Carol Friedman. 2001. Automating SNOMED coding using medical language understanding: A feasibility study. *Proceedings of the 2001 AMIA Annual Symposium*, Philadelphia.

National Library of Medicine. 2008. SNOMED CT July 31, 2008 release available for download from the UMLSKS. http://www.nlm.nih.gov/research/umls/Snomed/snomed_main.html.

Ryske, Ellen and Margo Imel. 2003. How SNOMED CT will affect health information management. *AHIMA's 2003 National Convention Proceedings*.

Southwick, Karen. 2002 (April). Merging terminologies for a new mother tongue. *CAP Today*. http://www.cap.org/apps/docs/cap_today/feature_stories/snomed_feature.

SNOMED Terminology Solutions. 2007. SNOMED CT Training Class, December 5–6, 2007.

SNOMED Terminology Solutions. 2008. SNOMED CT and Nursing Terminology. http://www.cap.org/apps/docs/snomed/documents/nursing_terminology.pdf.

Spackman, K. A., K. E. Campbell, and R. A. Cote. 1997 (October). SNOMED RT: A reference terminology for healthcare. *Proceedings of the 1997 AMIA Fall Symposium*. Nashville, Tenn. 640–644. http://www.amia.org/pubs/symposia/D004032.PDF.

Vikstrom, A., Y. Skaner, L.E. Strender and G.H. Nilsson. 2007. Mapping the categories of the Swedish primary health care version of ICD-10 to SNOMED CT concepts: Rule development and intercoder reliability in a mapping trial. *BMC Medical Informatics and Decision Making* (7)9.

Wasserman, Henry, and Jerome Wang. 2003. An applied evaluation of SNOMED CT as a clinical vocabulary for the computerized diagnosis and problem list. *AMIA 2003 Symposium Proceedings*. Washington, DC.

Application Exercises

1. Using MEDLINE, find an article that addresses the content coverage of SNOMED CT. After reading the article, write a paragraph or two in response to this question: Is the content of SNOMED CT sufficient to represent all the information in a person's health record?

2. Survey healthcare organizations in your area. Do they have electronic health record systems, or are they in EHR development and implementation? Is SNOMED-CT included in their existing EHR or EHR plans? Why or why not?

3. Download the UMLS Enhanced VA/KP Problem List Subset of SNOMED CT from ftp://ftp1.nci.nih.gov/pub/cacore/EVS/FDA/. Select the Excel formatted option for the FDA_NCIt_Subsets. Identify SNOMED CT concepts which provide a more granular representation of an idea than ICD-9-CM diagnosis codes.

Review Quiz

1. SNOMED was originally developed by what group?
   a. American Medical Association
   b. College of American Pathologists
   c. World Health Organization
   d. American College of Surgeons

2. True or False. SNOMED was specifically designed to capture and organize clinical information for use in the electronic health record environment.

3. True or False. The construction of a single clinical idea through the use of multiple concepts at the time of documentation into an EHR is an example of use of a pre-coordinated concept.

4. In SNOMED Version III, the etiology axis was further divided into what subsections?
   a. Living organisms, chemicals, physical agents, forces and activities, and social context
   b. Bacteria, fungi, viruses, and Rickettsiae
   c. Living organisms, chemicals, physical agents, and history
   d. Bacteria, chemicals, physical agents, and occupational exposures

5. SNOMED International Version 3.4 included mapping to which classification/terminology?
    a. ICD-9-CM
    b. LOINC
    c. CPT
    d. All of the above

6. A _____ for clinical data is defined as a set of concepts and relationships that provides a common reference point for comparison and aggregation of data about the entire healthcare process, recorded by multiple individuals, systems, or institutions.
    a. Clinical classification
    b. Reference terminology
    c. Relational database
    d. Concept history

7. The merger of SNOMED RT and the Read Codes resulted in:
    a. SNOMED International
    b. SNOMED CT
    c. CTV3
    d. None of the above

8. Read Codes were primarily used in what setting?
    a. Pathology departments in the United States
    b. Pathology departments in the United Kingdom
    c. Ambulatory care clinics in the United Kingdom
    d. Ambulatory care clinics in the United States

9. Because of its tremendous amount of content, SNOMED CT is a poor choice for what function?
    a. Reimbursement
    b. Medical research
    c. Application in the EHR environment
    d. Documentation of clinical concepts

10. The URU principle requires that all SNOMED concepts be:
    a. Uniform, reproducible, useful
    b. Understandable, relevant, uniform
    c. Understandable, reproducible, useful
    d. Understandable, reproducible, uniform

11. What are the three key elements of SNOMED CT?
    a. Attributes, concepts, and codes
    b. Codes, concepts, and hierarchies
    c. Concepts, descriptions, and relationships
    d. Descriptions, relationships, and identifiers

12. Which of the following is *not* a part of the core content of SNOMED CT?
    a. Extensions
    b. Relationships table
    c. ICD-9-CM mapping
    d. Concepts table

13. SNOMED CT is composed of ____ main hierarchies.
    a. 15
    b. 27
    c. 18
    d. 100

14. A motor vehicle accident is an example from which SNOMED CT hierarchy?
    a. Physical force
    b. Event
    c. Context-dependent category
    d. Observable entity

15. True or False. Every SNOMED CT concept has at least one relationship to another concept.

16. The highest level of concept in SNOMED CT is the:
    a. Root concept
    b. Upper-level concept
    c. Subhierarchy
    d. Concept

17. Which of the following is *not* an example from the hierarchy "social context"?
    a. Economic status
    b. Gender
    c. Occupation
    d. Ethnic group

18. True or False. The association responsible for the development and maintenance of SNOMED CT is the IHTSDO.

19. At the time this book was published, how many unique concepts were in SNOMED CT?
    a. More than 190,000
    b. Over 315,000
    c. Over 900,000
    d. More than a million

20. Which of the following is the unique text assigned to a concept in SNOMED CT that completely describes that concept?
    a. Standard phrase
    b. Fully specified name
    c. Common description
    d. Unique identifier

Chapter 8

MEDCIN●

Margaret M. Foley, PhD, RHIA, CCS

Learning Objectives

- To review the development and purpose of MEDCIN

- To describe the use of MEDCIN as an interface terminology

- To identify and describe MEDCIN content

Key Terms

Clinical hierarchy
Clinical proposition
Interface terminology
Intelligent prompting®
MEDCIN

Introduction

This chapter discusses **MEDCIN**, a proprietary clinical terminology developed to facilitate clinician documentation within an electronic health record (EHR) system. The content of MEDCIN, its role as an interface terminology, and other features of its application are discussed.

Developer

MEDCIN was developed by Peter S. Goltra to provide a "common base for creating computer programs for acquisition, review, and transmission of medical information independent of language" (Goltra 1997, vii). Refinement of the data model and field-testing occupied most of the period from its inception in 1978 through 1983. It is a proprietary terminology owned by Medicomp Systems, Inc. EHR vendors obtain licenses to use MEDCIN within their software products. As of 2008, MEDCIN is used in 14 electronic health record systems, including the Department of Defense Armed Forces Health Longitudinal Technology Application (AHLTA) system. MEDCIN has been included as a source terminology in the Unified Medical Language System (UMLS) Metathesaurus since November 2008 (UMLS Customer Support 2008).

Purpose

MEDCIN was specifically designed to provide an intelligent clinical database for documentation by the clinician at the time of care. As such, it has been adopted by a number of EHR developers and, as noted above, by the U.S. Department of Defense for use in its electronic health record systems. It was specifically designed for point-of-service documentation. Essentially, MEDCIN is able to produce the health record based on clinician selection of data elements. *Interface terminology* has been defined as "a systemic collection of health-care-related phrases (terms) that supports clinicians' entry of patient-related information into computer programs such as clinical 'note capture' and decision support tools" (Rosenbloom et al. 2006). MEDCIN's focus on facilitating data capture and ease-of-use by clinicians is why MEDCIN is considered to be an interface terminology (Bowman 2005; Fraser 2005).

Content

MEDCIN content is extensive and includes more than 250,000 clinical data elements, including symptoms, history, physical examination, tests, diagnoses, and therapies. In addition, MEDCIN provides a table of more than 600,000 synonyms and other ways of expression. Each data element is translated into a unique three-, four-, or five-digit number. As with many terminologies, the actual code numbers have no inherent meaning (for example, code number does not indicate related body system) except to represent the data element.

Each MEDCIN data element is a **clinical proposition**, which is defined as "a phrase containing a unique intellectual clinical content. For example 'chest pain' is a clinically useful concept. The term 'chest' defines an anatomical location. 'Chest' does not contain any clinical content but it has semantic relationships with other terms referring to the chest. It can thus be a term in an 'atomic' reference terminology but it is not useful in a clinical setting" (Medicomp 2008).

MEDCIN content addresses various aspects of health record documentation: symptoms; history; physical examination; tests; diagnoses, syndromes, and conditions; and therapy and management.

Symptoms

Symptoms included in MEDCIN are grouped into the following categories:

Systemic

Head

Eyes

Otorhinolaryngeal

Neck

Breasts

Cardiovascular

Pulmonary

Gastrointestinal

Genitourinary

Endocrine

Skin

Hematologic

Musculoskeletal

Neurological

Psychiatric

Examples of symptoms represented by MEDCIN data elements include the following:

Bony lump that doesn't go away (musculoskeletal symptoms) 955

Generalized convulsions (neurological symptoms) 660

Nervous or anxious from anticipation of separation (psychological symptoms) 1457

In addition to capturing symptom-specific information, MEDCIN data elements are available to identify the source of the information, for example: the patient (2063), the spouse (2064), a maternal grandmother (2423), another physician (2067), and so forth. Unique codes are also available to identify cases in which "symptoms reported are inconsistent or changeable" (1347) and when a patient is "in too much discomfort to answer questions" (1507) (Goltra 1997, 31).

History

MEDCIN provides the following categories for history findings:

Social

Family

Travel

Environmental exposure

Pregnancy

Medical, surgical

Pediatric

Trauma

Examples of history findings include:

Smoking of cigarettes (social history) 3801

Exposure to fiberglass (environmental exposure history) 3952

Currently taking medication for diabetes (medical and surgical history) 4208

Physical Findings

Physical examination findings can be collected for the following:

Vital signs

General appearance

Head

Eyes

Otorhinolaryngeal

Neck

Lymph nodes

Chest

Breasts

Cardiovascular

Lungs

Abdomen

Rectal

Genitourinary

Skin

Hair

Nails

Musculoskeletal

Neurological

Obstetrical

Developmental milestones

Adolescent sexual maturation

Examples of physical examination findings include:

Respiration rate 6021

Pupil not reactive to light, by direct illumination, unilateral, on the right side 6516

Diminished S1 heart sound 7147

Ulcer on the plantar aspect of the right foot 9774

Developmental assessment, 2–4 week milestones, responds to sound 9873

Tests

The following are the different categories of test that can be represented through MEDCIN data elements:

Hematology

Blood gas analysis

Blood chemistry

Laboratory-based chemistry

Laboratory-based studies

Surgical studies

Imaging

Pathology

Microbiology

Examples of tests represented in MEDCIN include:

Wide slurred QRS on EKG 13371

ACTH level 12715

Allergy sensitivity testing, patch testing, alder tree, induration of ___ mm 81638

Echocardiogram, aortic valve, unicuspid 20140

X-ray findings to the proximal phalanx of the right second toe 83871

Diagnoses, Syndromes, and Conditions

Diagnoses, syndromes, and conditions represent a large portion of the MEDCIN terminology. These data elements represent disorders for many clinical specialties, including:

Ophthalmology

Otorhinolaryngology

Cardiology

Pulmonary medicine

Gastroenterology

Nephrology

Urology

Gynecology

Obstetrics

Pediatrics

Metabolic disorders

Endocrinology

Dermatology

Rheumatology

Orthopedics

Neurology

Psychiatry

Infectious diseases

Hematology

Immunology

Oncology

Environmental disorders

Examples of diagnoses, syndromes and conditions include:

Cardiac neurosis 35996

Chronic interstitial cystitis 34183

Sprain of the lumbosacral ligament 37241

Adenocarcinoma of the tail of the pancreas 35497

Accident involving a motor vehicle, collision with another motor vehicle on the road 35034

Therapy and Management

The therapy and management section of the MED-CIN system includes the following categories:

Evaluation and management

Office services

Medications, vaccines

Anesthesia

Office and laboratory procedures

Surgery

Transfusions, transplantation

Radiation

Disposition of patient

Medical supplies and equipment

Examples of therapy and management data elements include:

Simple repair of supratentorial AV malformation 45112

Incision and drainage of finger abscess 70046

Renal artery atherectomy, with radiological supervision and interpretation 49893

Mechanical vitrectomy by pars plana approach 49339

Anesthesia for procedures of veins, lower leg, ankle and foot 43180

Acetaminophen + Diphenhydramine 48618

MEDCIN also allows for the entry of free text if no code number exists for the clinical entity being described. Clinical maps have been developed by Medicomp which link MEDCIN content as the source terminology to: ICD-9-CM, CPT-4, LOINC, RxNorm, and SNOMED-CT (Medicomp 2008).

Check Your Understanding 8.1

1. True or False. MEDCIN is a proprietary terminology owned and maintained by the American Medical Association.

2. MEDCIN was developed specifically to accomplish which of the following goals?
    a. To provide a common base for creating computer programs for the review of medical information
    b. To make possible point-of-service clinical charting
    c. To simplify the transmission of medical information among providers
    d. All of the above

3. Which of the following are not included in the therapy and management section of MEDCIN?
    a. Medications
    b. Diagnostic tests
    c. Surgery
    d. Medical supplies and equipment

Features of the Terminology

Since its inception, a major focus of MEDCIN development has been relevance to the clinician. Features of MEDCIN directed at this aim include: identification of medical relationships and clinical hierarchies, clinically precise phrasing, clinical alerts, **intelligent prompting**, automated narrative note generation, and computer-assisted coding. To facilitate these functionalities, each MEDCIN term has an associated property record containing items such as relevant value ranges, units for test results, laterality flags, control for narrative presentation, and cross-references to external code sets.

Medical Relationships and Clinical Hierarchies

MEDCIN's presentation engine identifies medical relationships through multiple hierarchies for each MEDCIN term. MEDCIN includes millions of these medical relationships. For example, chest pain is related to fever in the diagnosis of bacterial pericarditis, but not in the diagnosis of angina. The **clinical hierarchy** leads clinicians to document from less detail to more precision. The clinical hierarchical structure is also designed so that clinical properties associated with less specific concepts also apply to the more specific levels in the hierarchy. Examples of how some musculoskeletal symptoms are arranged in MEDCIN are presented below:

957	joint swelling
958	location
959	hand
1917	fingers
1931	of the right hand
2079	thumb
2194	MCP
2196	IP
2080	index finger
2200	MCP
2198	PIP
2202	DIP
...	
1935	of the fingers of both hands
960	wrist
1940	right
1942	left
1944	bilateral
961	elbow
...	
967	occurring
968	in only one joint
969	in more than one joint
970	suddenly
971	a chronic condition
972	moving from joint to joint
973	localized joint stiffness
974	location

Many clinical hierarchies exist in MEDCIN, defined by the linkage of MEDCIN data elements to diagnoses in the terminology. Because each data element has its own concept hierarchy, concept hierarchies also exist in multiple clinical hierarchies. For example, difficulty breathing and its hierarchy are linked to bilateral ankle swelling and its hierarchy in the diagnostic index of congestive heart failure. This particular multiple hierarchy would not exist for asthma because ankle swelling is not a feature of asthma. These clinical hierarchies group together the data elements likely to appear in a given clinical scenario.

Clinically Precise Phrasing

How words are combined in MEDCIN to create the clinical propositions is also key to how MEDCIN is relevant at the point of care. Consider these two similarly worded MEDCIN data elements:

- Wheezing that is worse during cold weather

- Wheezing that is worse with a cold

Although these two phrases are composed of many of the same words, they have very different clinical implications. The individual words do not contain any clinical content but they do convey clinical meaning when considering their relationships with the other terms in the phrase. At the point of care, differences in the clinical meaning, such as in the two above expressions, are crucial to healthcare providers. The ability of the MEDCIN terminology to recognize these types of medically-related relationships is what distinguishes it from other reference terminologies.

Clinical Alerts

MEDCIN's clinical alerts tables consist of clinical finding that, when present, may constitute a danger to the patient. The alerts function in real time and are scaled from 1 (mild) to 4 (possible death or organ failure). MEDCIN encoded symptoms, history, physical exam, tests, diagnoses, and therapy data are all used in alert evaluation. Drug reference information is also integrated into the clinical alert feature. Users are able to control which levels of alerts are automatically displayed and where within the workflow they appear. The alerts are based upon recommendations for alert capability from the Institute of Medicine. The clinical alerts are published on the National Institutes of Health Web site at http://www.nlm.nih.gov/databases/alerts/clinical_alerts.html.

Intelligent Prompting

Intelligent prompting tables and forms provide a means for displaying only clinically relevant items, thus avoiding the problem of overwhelming a user with too much information. Items displayed vary depending on a patient's age, sex, medical history, and other complaints. This enables relevant items to be documented quickly without having to manually exclude those that are not relevant. For example, a 12-year-old patient with a cough of acute onset will have a different clinical presentation than a 65-year-old patient with a cough and a history of smoking, emphysema, and lung cancer. The search engine presents different data elements appropriate to the particular clinical setting. History, physical, and laboratory data entered are bundled and linked to diagnosis and treatment plans so that the entire encounter is presented to the clinician as a coherent unit.

Examples of clinical relevance are seen in the following types of prompts that occur with the entry of the diagnosis "asthma". There are 279 direct links, each weighted as to sensitivity and specificity as part of the diagnostic matrix included as part of the MEDCIN knowledge base.

- *Symptoms:* Sinus pain, itching of the eyes, nasal discharge, chest tightness, feeling congested in the chest, difficulty breathing, recurrent episodes of difficulty breathing, awakening at night short of breath, cough, coughing up blood, wheezing, wheezing recurring intermittently (plus fifty-four more symptoms not listed here)

- *History:* Prior use of corticosteroids for asthma; previous hospitalization or emergency room visit for a pulmonary problem; protracted upper respiratory infection; exposure to cigarette smoke, dust mites, animal dander, roach antigen; recent contact with pets or other animals; smoking; wood-burning space heater as house heating source; seasonal recurrence of symptoms; history of sinusitis, nasal polyps, allergic rhinitis, urticaria; family history of hay fever, asthma, status asthmaticus, atopic eczematous dermatitis (and twenty-seven other history elements)

- *Physical examination:* Respiratory rate, tachypnea, pulse rate, blood pressure, pulsus paradoxus, intranasal polyp, percussion low diaphragm, percussion hyperresonance, auscultation wheezing, auscultation prolonged expiratory time (plus forty others)

- *Tests:* CBC, WBC, spirometry, pulse oximetry, chest x-ray

- *Therapy:* Environmental control measures, abstinence from smoking, avoidance of exposure to allergens, avoidance of exposure triggers, antihistamines, anti-inflammatory inhaled steroids, anti-inflammatory steroids, antiasthmatics, bronchodilators (plus twenty-eight others)

Automated Narrative Note Generation

Entry of documentation in a MEDCIN-enabled EHR is template driven. Templates are developed for different clinical topics and customize data collection relevant to the topic. Examples of topics for which templates have been developed include: back pain intake, adult upper respiratory infection, and diabetes screening. Users may select from an existing library of templates or develop their own. Output is often expressed as a narrative note. For example, menu driven documentation in the review of systems in which negative worsening vision and negative blurry vision were clicked (selected) can be reported as the following narrative: "Eye symptoms: No worsening vision and no blurred vision" (Medicomp 2008).

Computer-Assisted Coding of Evaluation and Management (E/M) Codes

MEDCIN has a software tool that uses the various MEDCIN data elements collected to automatically generate an E/M code for an encounter (Flanagan and Doyle 2006). The MEDCIN E/M tables have been developed for use with both the 1995 and the 1997 documentation guidelines from the Centers for Medicare and Medicaid Services (CMS). For evaluation of the physical examination performed, the more than 85,000 physical findings in MEDCIN have been individually reviewed with respect to each medical specialty to determine whether they satisfy the requirements for that medical specialty. The more than 43,000 diagnoses in MEDCIN have been reviewed against the risk and complexity guidelines. Risk codes ranging from 1 (mild) to 4 (possible death or organ failure) have been assigned. Complexity codes ranging from 1 (simple, straightforward) to 4 (complex, requiring extensive management) also have been assigned. This information has been conservatively combined with other factors to generate an E/M code that can be overridden by the user. All the information used is displayed for users to review.

Check Your Understanding 8.2

1. True or False. Intelligent prompting ensures that only clinically relevant information will be presented to the clinician for documentation.

2. Which of the following would probably not be presented as a history finding in a patient who presents with abdominal pain?
   a. Prior use of aspirin-containing medications
   b. History of recent foreign travel
   c. Family history of asthma
   d. Recent unusual foods

3. Evaluation and management coding in MEDCIN utilizes what set(s) of guidelines?
   a. AMA's 1995 and 1997 guidelines
   b. AMA's 1997 guidelines
   c. AMA's 1995 guidelines
   d. A proprietary set of guidelines developed by MEDCIN

Strengths and Weaknesses of MEDCIN

Published evaluations of the MEDCIN clinical terminology are limited. An analysis of MEDCIN prepared for the National Committee on Vital and Health Statistics (NCVHS) by a primary care physician who used MEDCIN within an EHR identified both strengths and weaknesses of the system. Strengths of MEDCIN included its usefulness at the point of care, by prompting for the capture of clinically relevant data in a manner that made sense to the physician, and extensive clinical reporting capabilities. Peterson also identified the intervening role of the EHR vendor as a weakness of MEDCIN. For example, the EHR vendor did not always act on MEDCIN updates in a timely manner, and training directly from Medicomp (MEDCIN owner) was difficult for the end-user to obtain. An additional weakness identified was that MEDCIN was slow to update the terminology with new clinical information (Peterson 2003).

A study comparing the ability of MEDCIN and SNOMED CT to represent concepts and interface terms for a general medical examination template found that SNOMED CT significantly outperformed MEDCIN in representing concepts (83% vs. 25% $p < 0.001$). Some of the performance difference was attributed to MEDCIN lacking a mechanism for the post-coordination of clinical terms captured. This study evaluated concept representation only and did not address other aspects of interface terminologies such as usefulness of clinical linkages (Brown et. al. 2007).

Process for Revision and Updates

MEDCIN is updated continually based on the recommendations of a group of consulting editors from Cornell, Harvard, Johns Hopkins, and other major medical centers, with substantial input from user community-based physicians. Updated data files are supplied to licensed users at least twice per year.

Summary

MEDCIN is a proprietary clinical terminology developed by Peter S. Goltra to provide a common base for creating computer programs for the acquisition, review, and transmission of medical information independent of language. This comprehensive terminology is capable of encoding essentially an entire health record, including terms for symptoms, history, physical findings, tests, syndromes and diagnoses, and therapy and management. It is updated continuously and has been adopted as the underlying terminology for several electronic health record systems.

References

Bowman, Sue. 2005. Coordination of SNOMED-CT and ICD-10: Getting the most out of electronic health record systems. *Perspectives in Health Information Management.*

Brown, Steven H., S. Trent Rosenbloom, Brent A. Bauer, Dietlind Wahner-Roedler, David A. Froehling, Kent R. Bailey, Michael J. Lincoln, Diane Montella, Elliot M. Fielstein, and Peter L. Elkin. 2007. American Medical Informatics Association Symposium. Paper read at AMIA 2007 Annual Symposium, November 10–14, 2007, at Chicago.

Flanagan, James R., and Karen Doyle. 2006. Computer-assisted coding: What's here, what's ahead. *Journal of the American Health Information Management Association* 77(7):36–40.

Fraser, Greg. 2005. Problem list coding in e-HIM. *Journal of the American Health Information Management Association* 76(7):68–70.

Goltra, Peter S. 1997. *MEDCIN: A New Nomenclature for Clinical Medicine.* New York City: Springer Verlag.

Medicomp Systems, Inc. 2008. http://www.medicomp.com.

Medicomp Systems. Inc. 2008 April. Medcin Products and Pricing. http://www.medicomp.com.

National Institutes of Health Clinical Alerts and Advisories. http://www.nlm.nih.gov/databases/alerts/clinical_alerts.html.

Peterson, Verlyn M. 2003. Testimony for National Committee on Vital and Health Statistics, Subcommittee on Standards and Security. http://ncvhs.hhs.gov/030521tr.htm#peterson.

Rosenbloom, S. T., R. A. Miller, K. B. Johnson, P. L. Elkin, and S. H. Brown. 2006. Interface terminologies: Facilitating direct entry of clinical data into electronic health record systems. *Journal of the American Medical Informatics Association* 13(3):277–88.

Unified Medical Language System Customer Support. 2008. MEDCIN UMLS e-mail. Philadelphia, September 26, 2008.

Application Exercise

Visit the Medicomp Web site at http://www.medicomp.com/index_html.htm. Select Products and scroll down to the link for the Functional Modules PowerPoint presentation. View the presentation, focusing especially on the slides discussing the encounter documentation for the adult upper respiratory infection (URI) patient. Summarize the methods that MEDCIN uses to indicate clinical relevance, including history and physical examination findings, and diagnosis. Summarize the therapies that may be indicated for this condition on the basis of MEDCIN's knowledge engine.

Review Quiz

1. True or False. MEDCIN has a way of documenting the individual providing the information for the clinical history by assignment of a special source of information code.

2. True or False. MEDCIN is considered to be an interface terminology.

3. Within the MEDCIN alerts system, an alert of 4 defines:
    a. A mild potential side effect
    b. A potential side effect that could cause potential death or organ failure
    c. A potential side effect that occurs only in the elderly population
    d. None of the above

4. True or False. The MEDCIN alerts table is based on clinical findings pairs from a combination of history, physical examination, laboratory findings, medications, and other orders.

5. "A phrase containing a unique intellectual clinical content" is the MEDCIN definition of:
    a. A semantic relationship
    b. A clinical proposition
    c. A data element
    d. An intelligent clinical database

6. True or False. In MEDCIN, the code number used to identify a data element in the terminology provides an indication to the nature and clinical meaning of the data element.

7. Diagnoses, syndromes, and conditions in MEDCIN are categorized by:
    a. Body part
    b. Clinical specialty
    c. A combination of a and b
    d. Strict alphabetical order

Chapter 9

Diagnostic and Statistical Manual
of Mental Disorders (DSM)

Karen Kostick, RHIT, CCS, CCS-P

Learning Objectives

- To discuss the development and purpose of the *Diagnostic and Statistical Manual of Mental Disorders* (DSM)

- To identify the party responsible for developing and updating the DSM

- To describe the different types of information in the DSM

- To recognize the different users of the DSM

Key Terms

American Psychiatric Association (APA)
Descriptive text
Diagnostic and Statistical Manual of Mental Disorders (DSM)
Diagnostic classification
Diagnostic criteria
Global Assessment of Functioning (GAF) Scale
International Classification of Diseases, Ninth Revision, Clinical Modification (ICD-9-CM)
International Classification of Diseases, Tenth Revision (ICD-10)
Multiaxial system

Introduction

The *Diagnostic and Statistical Manual of Mental Disorders* (DSM) is the standard classification of mental disorders used by mental health professionals throughout the United States. DSM is used across all types of healthcare settings and strives to meet the needs of various diverse populations. Moreover, it has been translated into numerous foreign languages. This chapter discusses the developer, history, purpose, principles, and maintenance of the DSM.

Developer

The **American Psychiatric Association** (APA) developed and publishes the *Diagnostic and Statistical Manual of Mental Disorders* (DSM). The APA is a medical specialty society consisting of more than 38,000 member physicians in the United States and abroad. The first edition, DSM-I, was published in 1952. There have been four updates since then, the most recent being DSM-IV-TR, published in 2000. The latest publication is often referred to as the DSM or DSM-IV. The APA owns and holds the copyright to the DSM.

History of the DSM

In 1840, the U.S. census began collecting statistics regarding the mental illness of insanity. Forty years later, the U.S. census expanded its statistical collecting to include mania, melancholia, monomania, paresis, dementia, dipsomania, and epilepsy. By the end of the 1800s, inpatient mental health facilities began developing their own unique **diagnostic classification** system for statistical information.

In 1917, the American Medico-Psychological Association (today named the APA) developed a twenty-two-standard classification list for use by U.S. inpatient facilities. By 1935, the revised APA classification list was incorporated into the second edition of the American Medical Association's Standard Classified Nomenclature of Diseases.

The psychiatric classification system was developed for chronic inpatient conditions and did not meet the needs of all healthcare settings. After World War Two, the U.S. Army began developing a classification system to assist in reporting outpatient diagnoses of its servicemen and veterans. This classification system was later modified by the Veterans Administration (VA).

In 1948, the World Health Organization (WHO) included a mental disorder section in the sixth revision of the *International Classification of Diseases, Injuries, and Causes of Death* (ICD-6). Unfortunately, ICD-6 did not meet all the needs of the psychiatric profession, which led to development of the *Diagnostic and Statistical Manual: Mental Disorders* (DSM-I). Table 9.1 (see page 140) summarizes the DSM history.

Purpose

According to the APA, the purpose of the DSM-IV is "to provide clear descriptions of diagnostic categories in order to enable clinicians and investigators to diagnose, communicate about, study, and treat people with various mental disorders" (APA 2000, xxxvii).

Clinical Users of DSM-IV

The DSM-IV is an authoritative guide used by mental health professionals such as practicing psychiatrists, clinical psychologists, and clinical social workers. The manual provides clinicians with common language and standards to assist with psychiatric diagnoses and appropriate treatment plans.

The DSM manual includes an important statement that cautions:"The specified diagnostic criteria for each mental disorder are offered as guidelines for making diagnoses, because it has been demonstrated that the use of such criteria enhances agreement among clinicians and investigators. The proper use of these criteria requires specialized clinical training that provides both a body of knowledge and clinical skills" (APA 2000, xxxvii).

Table 9.1.   History of the DSM

Version	Year	Description
DSM-I	1952	The APA developed and published the first official DSM edition. A key concept in DSM-I included a psychodynamic theory. The psychiatric classification organized mental disorders around presumed pathogenic processes. DSM-I included a glossary of definitions for the mental categories and was recognized as the first classification system for mental disorders to focus on clinical utility.
DSM-II	1968	During the developmental stage for ICD-8, WHO began to seek and receive recommendations from the psychiatric profession in order to have one classification system used across all nations.
DSM-III	1980	The third edition of the DSM represented a major advance in the diagnosis of mental disorders and significantly facilitated empirical research. A symptomatological approach was incorporated rather than categorizing disorders according to their underlying causes. DSM-III included valuable diagnostic criteria for each mental disorder, a multiaxial system for classification, and neutral descriptions of disorders without regard to etiology. DSM-III was accepted on an international level and provided an important diagnostic tool for mental health professionals. ICD-9 was published in 1975.
DSM-III-R	1987	This edition addressed inconsistencies in the DSM-III.
DSM-IV	1994	This revision process refined previous DSM editions and was the result of a special DSM-IV task force that involved more than 1,000 mental health professionals and various professional organizations. Much of the five-year project involved conducting firm, empirical research of evidence through literature reviews, data analysis, and field trials. Numerous changes were made to the classification, to the diagnostic criteria sets, and to the descriptive text based on the high standards established by the task force. Through a working relationship with WHO, this revision also minimized differences between DSM and ICD-10.
DSM-IV-TR (Text Revision)	2000	The DSM-IV-TR edition focused on the descriptive text. Revisions also were made to some criteria sets to correct errors identified in previous editions. In addition, some diagnostic codes were revised to reflect updates to the ICD-9-CM coding system.
DSM-V		The APA expects to release DSM-V in May 2012.

Legal Users of DSM-IV

DSM-IV can be a valuable diagnostic tool for professionals who conduct forensic evaluations for legal issues, including civil, criminal, and correctional or legislative matters. However, the APA cautions legal decision makers with the following information included in the DSM manual:

> When the DSM-IV categories, criteria, and textual descriptions are employed in making legal judgments, there are significant risks that diagnostic information will be misused or misunderstood. These dangers arise because of an imperfect fit between the questions of ultimate concern to the law and the information contained in a clinical diagnosis. In most situations, the clinical diagnosis of a DSM-IV mental disorder is not sufficient to establish the existence for legal purposes of a "mental disorder," "mental disability," "mental disease," or "mental defect." In determining whether an individual meets a specified legal standard (e.g., for competence,

criminal responsibility, or disability), additional information is usually required beyond that contained in the DSM-IV diagnosis (APA 2000, xxxii–xxxiii).

Information Management Users of DSM-IV

The DSM-IV is a valuable educational tool used in medical schools and as a reference for conducting research such as clinical trials. The **ICD-9-CM** diagnostic codes incorporated into the DSM-IV system are used to report public health statistics and are required under payer policies. Also, the ICD-9-CM coding classification used in the DSM-IV is recognized as an official code set under the Centers for Medicare and Medicaid Services (CMS) Administration Simplification provision of the Health Insurance Portability and Accountability Act (HIPAA) of 1996.

Check Your Understanding 9.1

Instructions: Complete the following exercises on a separate piece of paper.

1. Which of the following organizations is responsible for development of the DSM?
   a. World Health Organization (WHO)
   b. American Psychiatric Association (APA)
   c. Veterans Administration (VA)
   d. American Medico-Psychological Association

2. True or False. The purpose of DSM-IV is to provide clinicians with a tool to diagnose, communicate about, study, and treat patients with mental disorders.

3. How many updates have been made to the DSM since 1952?
   a. Two
   b. Three
   c. Four
   d. Five

4. True or False. Specialized clinical training is not required in order to use the diagnostic criteria in the DSM.

5. The DSM may be used in which of the following areas?
   a. Criminal evaluations
   b. Education
   c. Clinical trials
   d. All of the above

Content

The DSM-IV publication begins with acknowledgments, historical information, and the revision process related to the DSM-IV and DSM-IV-TR. The first chapter, titled "Use of the Manual," provides user instructions on how to apply coding and reporting procedures in the DSM-IV classification. This chapter also provides instructions and introductory information related to the **diagnostic criteria, descriptive text,** and appendixes.

The next chapter lists the DSM-IV-TR classification followed by instructions on how to use the DSM-IV **multiaxial system** for assessment. Most of the content then lies in the chapters containing the diagnostic criteria and descriptive text for each of the listed mental disorders. The manual also includes several appendixes.

Although the DSM-IV classifies mental disorders, no definition sufficiently specifies exact boundaries for the definition of mental disorder. The APA defines a mental disorder as follows:

In DSM-IV, each of the mental disorders is conceptualized as a clinically significant behavioral or psychological syndrome or pattern that occurs in an individual and that is associated with present distress (e.g., a painful symptom) or disability (i.e., impairment in one or more important areas of functioning) or with a significantly increased risk of suffering death, pain, disability, or an important loss of freedom (APA 2000, xxxi).

Diagnostic Classification

The DSM-IV diagnostic classification section includes a listing of all the mental disorders, diagnostic codes, subtypes, specifiers, and notes that are unique to the DSM-IV system. The classification section currently includes ICD-9-CM diagnostic codes. The ICD-9-CM coding classification system represents all diseases; however, the DSM mainly uses the chapter titled "Mental Disorders" and expands on the ICD-9-CM classification system as necessary. Some common general medical conditions and medication-induced disorders that are classified outside the mental disorders chapter of ICD-9-CM have been selected and are included in an appendix to the DSM-IV.

The DSM-IV includes ICD-9-CM diagnostic codes in several places, including:

- In the classification chapter

- As part of the descriptive text section for each mental health disorder

- In the diagnostic criteria for each disorder

- In the appendixes to alphabetical or numerical listings of DSM-IV diagnoses and codes

Multi-axial System

The DSM-IV manual provides a tool for clinicians to evaluate individuals using a five-level, or axes, clinical assessment. The multiaxial assessment was an innovative feature incorporated into the third edition of DSM in 1980. Each axis refers to a different category of information that can be useful in prognosis and treatment planning for an individual being assessed. A multiaxial model is a valuable clinical communication tool in that it evaluates the biological, psychological, and social issues pertaining to an individual. Use of the multiaxial assessment is not required, but it is encouraged because it facilitates a comprehensive and systematic evaluation. The DSM-IV includes examples for clinicians who choose to report diagnoses in a nonaxial format. Table 9.2 summarizes the DSM-IV multiaxial assessment system.

Axis I reports all the various psychiatric disorders or other conditions in the DSM-IV classification except for personality and mental retardation disorders. These disorders are reported separately on axis II to ensure that they will be given consideration and not overlooked if included with axis I conditions.

Current general medical conditions relevant to axis I conditions are reported on axis III. Medical conditions are included on axis III only when a direct physiological relationship exists between the medical condition and the mental disorder. The purpose of axis III is to encourage a thorough evaluation and to enhance communication among healthcare professionals.

Axis IV reports relevant psychosocial and environmental problems that may affect an individual's diagnosis, treatment, or prognosis. When a psychosocial or environmental problem becomes the primary focus of clinical interest, it should be recorded on axis I.

The clinician's judgment of the individual's overall level of functioning is reported on axis V using the **Global Assessment of Functioning (GAF) Scale.** The GAF scale is a 100-point tool rating overall psychological, social, and occupational functioning of individuals. It excludes physical and environmental impairment. The DSM-IV appendix includes additional functional assessment tools that may be useful in some behavioral healthcare settings.

The DSM-IV classification provides a range of possible categories and includes relevant criteria for axes I–IV. The categories are included in figure 9.1.

DSM-IV Diagnostic Criteria and Descriptive Text

The DSM-IV system organizes mental disorders into sixteen major diagnostic classes and one additional section titled Other Conditions That May Be a Focus of Clinical Attention.

The sixteen major diagnostic classes include:

- Disorders Usually First Diagnosed in Infancy, Childhood, or Adolescence
- Delirium, Dementia, and Amnestic and Other Cognitive Disorders
- Mental Disorders due to General Medical Condition
- Substance-Related Disorders
- Schizophrenia and Other Psychotic Disorders
- Mood Disorders
- Anxiety Disorders
- Somatoform Disorders
- Factitious Disorders

Table 9.2.   DSM-IV multiaxial assessment system

DSM-IV Axis	Examples
Axis I: Clinical Disorders and Other Conditions That May Be a Focus of Clinical Attention	Major clinical depression, general anxiety disorder
Axis II: Personality Disorders and Mental Retardation	Antisocial personality disorder, borderline personality disorder
Axis III: General Medical Conditions	Asthma, diabetes
Axis IV: Psychosocial and Environmental Problems	Home, economic, or insurance problems
Axis V: Global Assessment of Functioning (GAF)	Score 41–50—Serious symptoms or serious impairment in one of the following: social, occupational, or school functioning

Source: DSM-IV-TR, page 42. Reprinted courtesy of the American Psychiatric Association.

Figure 9.1. DSM categories

Axis I: Clinical Disorders and Other Conditions That May Be a Focus of Clinical Attention Disorders Usually First Diagnosed in Infancy, Childhood, or Adolescence (excluding Mental Retardation) Delirium, Dementia, and Amnestic and Other Cognitive Disorders Substance-Related Disorders Schizophrenia and Other Psychotic Disorders Mood Disorders Anxiety Disorders Somatoform Disorders Factitious Disorders Dissociative Disorders Sexual and Gender Identity Disorders Eating Disorders Sleep Disorders Impulse-Control Disorders Not Elsewhere Classified Adjustment Disorders Other Conditions That May Be a Focus of Clinical Attention (for example, occupational problem, adult antisocial behavior, noncompliance with treatment) **Axis II: Personality Disorders and Mental Retardation** Paranoid Personality Disorder Schizoid Personality Disorder Schizotypal Personality Disorder Antisocial Personality Disorder Histrionic Personality Disorder Narcissistic Personality Disorder Avoidant Personality Disorder Dependent Personality Disorder Obsessive-Compulsive Personality Disorder Borderline Personality Disorder Personality Disorder Not Otherwise Specified Mental Retardation	**Axis III: General Medical Conditions** Infectious and Parasitic Diseases Neoplasms Endocrine, Nutritional, and Metabolic Diseases and Immunity Disorders Diseases of the Blood and Blood-Forming Organs Diseases of the Nervous System and Sense Organs Diseases of the Circulatory System Diseases of the Respiratory System Diseases of the Digestive System Diseases of the Genitourinary System Complications of Pregnancy, Childbirth, and the Puerperium Diseases of the Skin and Subcutaneous Tissue Diseases of the Musculoskeletal System and Connective Tissue Congenital Anomalies Certain Conditions Originating in the Perinatal Period Symptoms, Signs, and Ill-Defined Conditions Injury and Poisoning **Axis IV: Psychosocial and Environmental Problems** Problems with primary support group Problems related to the social environment Educational problems Occupational problems Housing problems Economic problems Problems with access to healthcare services Problems related to interaction with the legal system/crime Other psychological and environmental problems **Axis V: Global Assessment of Functioning** Global Assessment of Functioning (GAF) Scale

Source: DSM-IV-TR, pages 370–371. Reprinted courtesy of the American Psychiatric Association.

- Dissociative Disorders

- Sexual and Gender Identity Disorders

- Eating Disorders

- Sleep Disorders

- Impulse-Control Disorders Not Elsewhere Classified

- Adjustment Disorders

- Personality Disorders

Within each of the sixteen major diagnostic classes are listed specified mental disorders. For each mental disorder listed, a set of extensive diagnostic criteria is provided that indicates what symptoms must be present and not present for a patient to meet the qualifications for a particular mental diagnosis. As previously noted, users of the DSM find the diagnostic criteria particularly useful because they provide a summarized description of each disorder. Also, use of the diagnostic criteria has been shown to increase diagnostic reliability.

The DSM-IV descriptive text that accompanies each mental disorder is included under the following headings:

- Diagnostic Features

- Subtypes and/or Specifiers

- Recording Procedures

- Associated Features and Disorders

- Specific Culture, Age, and Gender Features

- Prevalence

- Course

- Familial Pattern

- Differential Diagnosis

The appendixes in DSM-IV include the following:

- Appendix A: Decision Tree for Differential Diagnosis

- Appendix B: Criteria Sets and Axes Provided for Further Study

- Appendix C: Glossary of Technical Terms

- Appendix D: Highlights of Changes in DSM-IV Text Revision

- Appendix E: Alphabetical Listing of DSM-IV-TR Diagnoses and Codes

- Appendix F: Numerical Listing of DSM-IV-TR Diagnoses and Codes

- Appendix G: ICD-9-CM Codes for Selected General Medical Conditions and Medication-Induced Disorders

- Appendix H: DSM-IV Classification (with ICD-10 Codes)

- Appendix I: Outline for Cultural Formulation and Glossary of Culture-Bound Syndromes

- Appendix J: DSM-IV Contributors

- Appendix K: DSM-IV Text Revision Advisors

Check Your Understanding 9.2

Instructions: Complete the following exercises on a separate piece of paper.

1. True or False. For each mental disorder listed, a set of extensive diagnostic criteria is provided that indicates what symptoms must be present and not present for a patient to meet the qualifications for a particular mental diagnosis.

2. The DSM-IV classification section includes which code set?
   a. ICD-9-CM diagnostic codes
   b. ICD-9-CM diagnostic and procedure codes
   c. ICD-10-CM diagnostic codes
   d. ICD-10-CM diagnostic and procedure codes

3. Which of the following axes would a clinician use to report a somatoform disorder?
   a. Axis I
   b. Axis II
   c. Axis III
   d. Axis IV

4. True or False. Specific Culture, Age, and Gender Features are categories included within the DSM-IV descriptive text for each mental disorder.

Principles and Guidelines

Coding and reporting guidelines are found at the front of the manual. Even though ICD-9-CM codes and guidelines for coding and reporting are incorporated into the manual, some of the coding guidelines are specific to the DSM-IV system.

ICD-9-CM Diagnostic Codes

Although each diagnosis listed in the DSM-IV-TR is assigned a valid ICD-9-CM code, some DSM-IV-TR disorders require further specification that cannot be provided within the ICD-9-CM classification system. DSM-IV and ICD-9-CM coding guidelines sometimes differ surrounding the reporting rules in selecting and sequencing primary or first-listed diagnoses and fifth-digit diagnostic code assignments. ICD-9-CM diagnostic code changes that affect the October 2008 DSM-IV-TR codes can be found at http://www.psych.org/MainMenu/Research/DSMIV/DSMIVTR/CodingUpdates/NewCodesforDSMIVTROctober12008.aspx.

Some of the incompatibility between DSM-IV and ICD-9-CM continues to improve as the ICD-9-CM classification system revises indexed terms, adds new disorders to the classification system, includes further specificity to current disorders, and updates clinical terminology used in the DSM-IV classification system. For example, in DSM-IV, code 297.1 is reported for delusional disorder. An ICD-9-CM update revised the index and tabular narrative description for code 297.1. Now delusional disorder in ICD-9-CM is coded according to DSM-IV.

The developers of DSM-IV and ICD-10 worked together, which resulted in ICD-10 chapter 5, Mental and Behavioral Disorders (F01–F99), being compatible with DSM-IV in terms of terminology and structure. Adoption of ICD-10-CM as a HIPAA code set standard will replace outdated terminology in ICD-9-CM with terminology that reflects DSM-IV-compatible terms for mental disorders. If a mental health professional includes a diagnostic term that is not listed in DSM-IV, the most recent ICD-9-CM coding guidelines and latest edition of the classification system should be used to report the diagnostic disorder.

Subtypes, Specifiers, Severity, and Course Specifiers

The DSM-IV-TR subtypes, specifiers, severity, and course specifiers provide additional details to a particular disorder. The additional detailed information is reported either in the assignment of a fourth and fifth digit to the diagnostic codes or by including the narrative description after the name of the disorder. The increased specificity allows the clinician to report the following:

- Unique features of a disorder
- Severity of a disorder
- Status of a disorder

DSM-IV defines subtype as "mutually exclusive and jointly exhaustive phenomenological subgroupings within a diagnosis [that] are indicated by the instruction 'specify type' in the criteria set" (First, Frances, and Pincus 2004, 1). DSM-IV notes that "specifiers are not intended to be mutually or jointly exhaustive and are indicated by the instruction 'specify' or 'specify

if' in the criteria set" (First, Frances, and Pincus 2004, 1). Severity and course specifiers are classified and defined in the manual as mild, moderate, severe, in partial remission, in full remission, and prior history.

Figure 9.2 (see page 146) shows examples taken from the DSM-IV-TR diagnostic category chapters to illustrate how additional specification is reported in the DSM-IV system.

The diagnosis example in the DSM chapter is stated as:

> Major Depressive Disorder, Recurrent, Moderate, With Atypical Features, With Seasonal Pattern, With Full Interepisode Recovery
>
> In the DSM system this diagnosis is coded and reported as:
>
> 296.32, with atypical features, with seasonal pattern, with full interepisode recovery
>
> The code and specifiers are broken down as illustrated below:
>
> 296 = Describes the Major Depressive Disorder
>
> 296.3 = The fourth digit "3" describes the recurrent episode
>
> 296.32 = The fifth digit "2" describes the Moderate severity level
>
> With Atypical Features, With Seasonal Pattern, With Full Interepisode Recovery = Specifiers that are added after the code since they cannot be coded.

Principal and First-Listed Diagnosis

The guidelines contained in DSM note that the principal diagnosis (inpatient setting) or the reason for visit (outpatient setting) is indicated on axis I by listing the diagnosis first. The principal diagnosis or reason for visit is assumed to be axis I unless an axis II diagnosis is followed by "(Principal Diagnosis)" or "(Reason for Visit)." Remaining disorders are listed under the appropriate axes and sequenced according to the amount of clinical attention and treatment given to each disorder.

No Diagnosis

When a diagnosis code is not present for axis I, code V71.09, No Diagnosis or Condition on Axis I, is

Figure 9.2.   Additional specification reporting examples, DSM-IV-TR

Subtype

307.1 Anorexia Nervosa

The following subtypes can be used to specify the presence or absence of regular binge eating or purging during the current episode of anorexia nervosa:

Restricting type: This subtype describes presentation in which weight loss is accomplished primarily through dieting, fasting, or excessive exercise. During the current episode, these individuals have not regularly engaged in binge eating or purging.

Binge-eating/purging type: This subtype is used when the individual has regularly engaged in binge eating or purging (or both) during the current episode. Most individuals with anorexia nervosa who binge eat also purge through self-induced vomiting or the misuse of laxatives, diuretics, or enemas. Some individuals included in this subtype do not binge eat but do regularly purge after the consumption of small amounts of food. It appears that most individuals of the binge-eating/purging type engage in these behaviors at least weekly, but sufficient information is not available to justify the specification of a minimum frequency.

> Subtype Example
> Diagnosis: Anorexia Nervosa, restricting type
> Coded and reported as: 307.1, restricting type

Source: DSM-IV-TR, page 585. Reprinted courtesy of the American Psychiatric Association.

Specifier

300.3 Obsessive-Compulsive Disorder

Specify if:

With poor insight: This specifier can be applied when, for most of the time during the current episode, the individual does not recognize that the obsessions or compulsions are excessive or unreasonable.

> Specifier Example
> Diagnosis: Obsessive Compulsive Disorder
> Coded and reported as: 300.3, with poor insight

Source: DSM-IV-TR, page 458. Reprinted courtesy of the American Psychiatric Association.

Severity

Degrees of Severity of Mental Retardation

Four degrees of severity can be specified, reflecting the level of intellectual impairment: mild, moderate, severe, and profound.

317	Mild Mental Retardation:	IQ level 50–55 to approximately 70
318.0	Moderate Retardation:	IQ level 35–40 to 50–55
318.1	Severe Mental Retardation	IQ level 20–25 to 35–40
318.2	Profound Mental Retardation	IQ level below 20 or 25

> Severity Example
> Diagnosis: Mental Retardation, Moderate
> Coded and reported as: 318.0

Source: DSM-IV-TR, page 42. Reprinted courtesy of the American Psychiatric Association.

(Continued on next page)

Figure 9.2.   (Continued)

Subtype, Severity and Specifier Example

Recording Procedures

The diagnostic codes for major depressive disorder are selected as follows:
1. The first three digits are 296.
2. The fourth digit is either 2 (if there is only a single major depressive episode) or 3 (if there are recurrent major depressive episodes).
3. If the full criteria are currently met for a major depressive episode, the fifth digit indicates the current severity as follows: 1 for mild severity, 2 for moderate severity, 3 for severe without psychotic features, 4 for severe with psychotic features. If the full criteria are not currently met for a major depressive episode, the fifth digit indicates the current clinical status of the major depressive disorder as follows: 5 for partial remission, 6 for full remission. If the severity of the current episode or the current remission status of the disorder is unspecified, the fifth digit is 0. Other specifiers for major depressive disorder cannot be coded.

In recording the name of a diagnosis, terms should be listed in the following order: Major Depressive Disorder, specifiers coded in the fourth digit (for example, Recurrent), specifiers coded in the fifth digit (for example, Mild, Severe with Psychotic Features, In Partial Remission), as many specifiers (without codes) as apply to the current or most recent episode (for example, With Melancholic Features, With Postpartum Onset), and as many specifiers (without codes) as apply to the course of the episodes (for example, With Full Interepisode Recovery).

For example, 296.32, Major Depressive Disorder, Recurrent, Moderate, with Atypical Features, with Seasonal Pattern, with Full Interepisode Recovery.

Source: DSM-IV-TR, pages 370–371. Reprinted courtesy of the American Psychiatric Association.

---

indicated. Code V71.09, No Diagnosis on Axis II, also is indicated when there is no axis II diagnosis.

Not Otherwise Specified Diagnosis

The designated not otherwise specified (NOS) code is used in clinical scenarios where relevant clinical information is unavailable to assess a disorder, the disorder is unable to meet specific diagnostic criteria, the patient's disorder is not classified in the DSM system, or the disorder etiology is uncertain.

Example:

300.9 Unspecified Mental Disorder (nonpsychotic)

312.89 Conduct Disorder, Unspecified Onset

294.8 Dementia NOS

298.9 Psychotic Disorder, Not Otherwise Specified

Uncertain Diagnosis

When a situation arises where clinical information is inadequate and a physician is unable to determine a disorder, code 799.9, Diagnosis or Condition Deferred, is reported on axis I or axis II.

Recurrence and Provisional Diagnosis

The manual provides guidelines for clinicians to use when symptoms indicate that a patient's original disorder has recurred, but the symptoms do not yet meet the full criteria set. The term *provisional* is listed after the diagnosis when a clinician does not have enough information available to diagnose a disorder but feels strongly that all the diagnostic criteria will eventually be met.

Process for Revision and Updates

The DSM provides current clinical knowledge with respect to psychiatric diagnoses; therefore, the manual is revised to meet the needs of the mental health profession. The manual also is updated based on the availability of other diagnostic classification systems. Previous DSM revisions have taken place following revisions to the ICD-9-CM publication based on WHO's *Ninth Revision, International Classification of Diseases* (ICD-9).

The APA Division of Research manages the DSM revision process, and the DSM-IV published in 1994 is the last major revision. As noted at the beginning of the chapter, this revision refined previous DSM editions and was the result of a special DSM-IV Task Force that involved more than a thousand mental health professionals and various professional organizations. Much of the five-year project involved conducting empirical research through literature reviews, data analysis, and field trials. Numerous changes were made to the classification, to the diagnostic criteria sets, and to the descriptive text, based on empirical evidence and the high standards established by the task force. A minor text revision of the DSM-IV, called DSM-IV-TR, was published in 2000.

The APA periodically reprints DSM-IV-TR, and at the time of each printing, the ICD-9-CM diagnostic codes are updated to reflect the annual updates. If users of the DSM-IV-TR have a clinical or other related content request, the APA Division of Research requests that they submit a written notice of the request and the page number in DSM-IV-TR. DSM users can forward their online comments at http://www.psych.org/MainMenu/Research/DSMIV/DSMV/MakeaSuggestion.aspx.

DSM-V

The future manual, DSM-V, is expected to be released in May 2012. More information on activities related to the next DSM revision is available on the APA Web site at http://www.psych.org/dsmv.asp.

Check Your Understanding 9.3

Instructions: Complete the following exercises on a separate piece of paper.

1. True or False. The principal diagnosis or reason for visit is assumed to be axis I unless an axis II diagnosis is followed by "(Principal Diagnosis)" or "(Reason for Visit)."

2. True or False. The ICD-10 diagnostic classification system is not compatible with the DSM-IV in terms of terminology and structure.

3. Which of the following is updated when DSM-IV-TR is periodically reprinted?
   a. Diagnostic ICD-9-CM codes
   b. Diagnostic criteria
   c. Descriptive text
   d. All of the above

4. True or False. Subtypes and specifiers are used in both the DSM-IV system and the ICD-9-CM coding classification system.

5. True or False. Specifiers classify distinct phenomenological subgroupings within a diagnosis.

6. What type of code is reported when the patient's disorder is not classified in the DSM system?
   a. Code V71.09, No Diagnosis or Condition
   b. Code 799.9, Diagnosis or Condition Deferred
   c. The designated not otherwise specified (NOS) code
   d. None of the above

Summary

The history of psychiatric classification systems in the United States can be traced back to the mid-1800s. Today, DSM-IV, published by the American Psychiatric Association, is the U.S. official psychiatric classification system across all behavioral health settings. Mental health professionals rely on DSM-IV diagnostic criteria to assist with defining mental disorders and also to diagnose mental disorders. DSM-IV is unique in that no other healthcare profession has developed such a concise classification of specific disorders with extensive diagnostic criteria sets based on empirical facts. Moreover, DSM-IV is used for clinical education, research, public health statistics, and reimbursement purposes.

References

Albaum-Feinstein, Andrea. 1999. *DSM-IV Crosswalk: Guidelines for Coding Mental Health Information*. Chicago: American Health Information Management Association.

American Psychiatric Association. 2008. http://www.psych.org/.

American Psychiatric Association. 2000. *Diagnostic and Statistical Manual of Mental Disorders, Fourth Edition, Text Revision, DSM-IV-TR*. Washington, D.C.: American Psychiatric Association.

First, Michael B., Allen Frances, and Harold Alan Pincus. 2004. *DSM-IV-TR Guidebook*. Washington, D.C.: American Psychiatric Association.

Application Exercise

The Surgeon General of the U.S. Public Health Service has focused the nation's attention on important public health issues. The reports from this office have heightened America's awareness of significant public health issues and have generated public health initiatives.The first Surgeon General's Report on Mental Health emphasizes that mental illness is a serious public health problem that must be addressed by the nation.

Using the Internet, visit the report *Mental Health: A Report of the Surgeon General* at http://www.surgeongeneral. gov/library/mentalhealth/home.html. Review the entire report, concentrating on the foreword and preface and chapters 1 through 5, and then answer the following questions:

1. Explain the importance of treating and preventing mental disorders and of promoting mental health in the nation.

2. Why is the diagnosis of mental disorders believed to be more difficult than the diagnosis of somatic, or general medical, disorders?

3. In what way is DSM-IV a unique approach for reaching a diagnosis by a professional field?

4. Give examples of where the DSM-IV diagnostic categories are referenced in the surgeon general's report.

5. The *Report of the Surgeon General on Mental Health* is a collaboration between which two federal agencies?

Review Quiz

1. True or False. DSM-IV-TR is the latest edition of the manual.

2. Which of the following DSM editions first incorporated valuable diagnostic criteria, a multi-axial system for classification, and descriptive text for each disorder?
   a. DSM-I
   b. DSM-II
   c. DSM-III
   d. DSM-IV

3. DSM-IV mental disorders are grouped into how many major diagnostic classes?
   a. 14
   b. 15
   c. 16
   d. 17

4. True or False. The ICD-9-CM diagnostic codes incorporated into DSM-IV are not recognized as an official code set under the Administration Simplification provision of the Health Insurance Portability and Accountability Act (HIPAA).

5. True or False. ICD-9-CM Codes for Selected General Medical Conditions and Medication-Induced Disorders are found in one of the DSM-IV appendices.

6. The clinician's judgment of an individual's overall level of functioning is reported on:
   a. Axis II
   b. Axis III
   c. Axis IV
   d. Axis V

7. True or False. Clinicians are required to use the multiaxial assessment because it facilitates a comprehensive and systematic evaluation.

8. The DSM-IV benefits which type of professional?
   a. Practicing psychiatrists
   b. Clinical psychologists
   c. Clinical social workers
   d. All of the above

9. True or False. Medical conditions are only included on axis III when there is a direct physiological relationship between the medical condition and the axis I mental disorder.

10. Which of the following organizations is responsible for updating the current DSM?
    a. World Health Organization
    b. American Psychiatric Association
    c. Centers for Medicare and Medicaid Services
    d. None of the above

Chapter 10

Logical Observation Identifiers, Names, and Codes (LOINC®)

Daniel Vreeman, PT, DPT, MSc

Learning Objectives

- To explain the purpose and function of the LOINC codes

- To describe the approach to developing LOINC

- To define LOINC's relationship to other terminologies and code sets

- To describe who has adopted LOINC

Key Terms

Health Level Seven (HL7)

Logical Observation Identifiers, Names, and Codes (LOINC)

LOINC Committee

Regenstrief Institute, Inc.

Regenstrief LOINC Mapping Assistant (RELMA)

Semantic data model

Introduction

A comprehensive electronic health record (EHR) system must coalesce data from many producing sources in order to provide clinicians with complete information. Both within and among institutions, the disparate source systems often store data with local, idiosyncratic terms and codes to identify clinical observations and measurements. In order to fully understand and process the incoming data, receiving systems are thus forced to either adopt the producers' codes or map their terms to them. As the number of interacting systems increases, this effort becomes increasingly burdensome and raises the barrier to interoperability.

The **Logical Observation Identifiers, Names, and Codes** (LOINC) standard provides a set of universal identifiers for laboratory and clinical observations that can serve as the lingua franca for information exchange between electronic systems. LOINC is an openly developed standard used worldwide to facilitate the exchange and aggregation of clinical results for care delivery, management, public health, and research purposes.

History

LOINC is a terminology standard developed at the **Regenstrief Institute, Inc.,** an internationally-respected, nonprofit, medical research organization associated with Indiana University. Regenstrief Institute initiated the development of LOINC in 1994 by organizing the **LOINC Committee,** a voluntary group of interested experts. In response to the demand for moving electronic clinical data from laboratories and other producers to hospitals, physician offices, payers, and health departments, the LOINC Committee developed a system of universal identifiers for observations inside the messages of healthcare data exchange standards.

LOINC provides identifiers and names for observations, not values. If you think of an observation as a "question" and the observation value as the "an-swer," the LOINC codes are for questions. In many cases, the answer would be a numeric quantity. For example, think of the question "what is my patient's serum potassium level?" LOINC provides a code (2823-3) and formal name (Potassium:SCnc:Pt:Ser/Plas:Qn) for that measurement, and the value would be reported as a numeric quantity, like 3.4 mmol/L. For other kinds of observations, the answers to the question could be coded entities. In general, LOINC does not provide codes for the answers, but they could be drawn from other terminology standards, such as ICD-9-CM or SNOMED CT. If the observation is "which organisms were identified in this patient's blood culture?", possible answers might include *Bacillus anthracis* or *Escherichia coli.* So, LOINC would provide a code (600-7) and formal name (Bacteria identified:Prid:Pt:Bld:Nom:Culture) for the culture observation, and a terminology like SNOMED CT could be used to code the answers, 21927003 and 112283007, respectively.

There are several reasons why the LOINC Committee focused on the standardization of observation identifiers (Huff et al. 1998). By 1994, many electronic systems were beginning to send clinical information as discrete results using messaging standards such as **Health Level Seven** (HL7) or ASTM 1238. Inside these messages, laboratories and clinical systems used local, idiosyncratic names and codes to report procedure results. Installing a new system or connecting to a new interface meant investing large resources in mapping the codes between the sending and all receiving systems. Having a universal standard would mean each system in an exchange would only have to map their local terms to the standard once. Existing terminologies were not granular enough, focused on coding for billing rather than clinical results delivery, or did not fit with the messaging models being used. Because such a standard did not exist and would be immediately useful, the LOINC Committee focused on creating a terminology that would have the appropriate level of granularity for defining the names of observations used in laboratory and clinical information systems.

Developer

Regenstrief Institute, Inc. is the overall steward and developer of the LOINC system. Regenstrief Institute research scientists form a highly respected group of health services researchers linked to one of the largest and most comprehensive medical informatics laboratories in the world.

Over the past three decades, Regenstrief's informaticians have been developing the Regenstrief Medical Record System (RMRS), one of the oldest, largest, and most advanced electronic medical record systems. Regenstrief's informaticians have not only designed and implemented the RMRS, but they have published more controlled trials evaluating the impact of health information technology on quality, efficiency, and costs of care than any other research center in the United States (Chaudhry et al. 2006). Building on the successes of the RMRS, Regenstrief's informaticians developed the Indiana Network for Patient Care (INPC), one of the nation's most successful regional health information exchanges. The INPC links clinical data from nearly all of the major health systems in central Indiana into an aggregated virtual patient record.

Throughout its history, Regenstrief's informaticians have been leaders and active participants in developing informatics standards. Regenstrief investigators organized the first medical informatics effort in 1984, wrote the ASTM and HL7 chapters for orders and observation reporting, and were the lead authors of the unified (USAMP) data HL7 data model, the HL7 version 3 data types, and the proposed HIPAA claims attachments documents. In addition, they have developed the Unified Code for Units of Measure, a standard for representing units of measure that facilitates their unambiguous representation in electronic communications.

Led by Clem McDonald, MD, Regenstrief's informaticians initiated the LOINC effort. As the overall steward for LOINC, Regenstrief maintains the LOINC database and supporting documentation, processes submissions and edits to the content, develops and curates accessory content (descriptions, hierarchies, other attributes, and so forth), develops the **Regenstrief LOINC Mapping Assistant (RELMA)** mapping program, and coordinates LOINC releases. In addition, Regenstrief continues to cultivate the LOINC community worldwide and develop the LOINC Web site at http://loinc.org, which serves as the central resource for promoting, distributing, and teaching LOINC.

LOINC Committee

The LOINC Committee, a voluntary group of interested experts, serves a number of key roles in LOINC development. As a group, the Committee defines the overall naming conventions and policies for the development process. The Committee helps set priorities for new content development. Individual members may also take the lead on the development of naming rules and LOINC names for new subject matter and serve as content experts to answer questions that come up with new submissions.

The LOINC Committee has two primary divisions: the Laboratory LOINC Committee, which deals with observations made on specimens, and the Clinical LOINC Committee, which deals with observations made on patients. A third area of development focuses on proposals for the Health Insurance Portability and Accountability Act (HIPAA) attachments. The HIPAA attachments content is created by the HL7 Attachments Special Interest Group, but Regenstrief provides technical advice and constructs new LOINC codes as required.

Approach to Development

Regenstrief Institute and the LOINC Committee have intentionally shaped LOINC development to be empirical, nimble, and open (Huff et al 1998). Since its inception, new content in LOINC has been added by examining the existing system master files and hundreds of millions of live clinical messages, and in response to requirements of adopters around the world. Because of this

Figure 10.1.   Number of LOINC codes per release

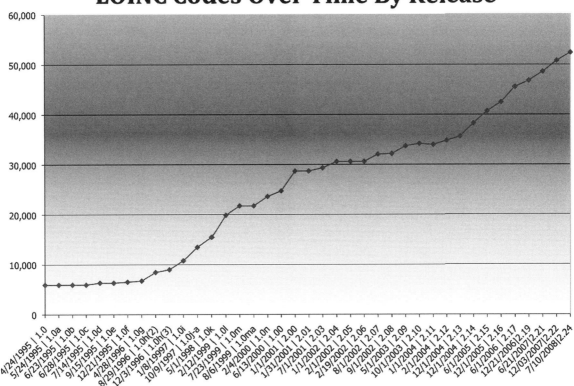

approach, the concepts in LOINC were not created de novo. Rather, they first existed as local terms in a live clinical system, or in the case of the HIPAA attachments and some clinical content, as concepts in published official documents. The LOINC Committee was deliberately organized outside of existing standards development groups to ensure LOINC could always be freely distributed and to avoid the formal balloting procedures typically limiting revisions to two to five years. LOINC needed to be able to respond more quickly to the rapidly evolving growth in the field and among adopters. The LOINC effort has always welcomed suggestions for additions or revisions to the content and has kept its Committee meetings open to the public. Now, after reaching a certain state of maturity, the vast majority of content updates are end-user driven. Focusing development on these principles has helped anchor the vocabulary in immediately relevant domains and contributed to its widespread adoption.

Check Your Understanding 10.1

Instructions: Go to the main LOINC Web site at http://loinc.org, and then answer the following questions on a separate piece of paper.

1.   List three kinds of documentation resources available to learn more about LOINC.

2.   Review the listing of past LOINC Committee meetings. What additional event is often offered with the Laboratory Committee meetings?

Content

In January 2009, Regenstrief Institute released version 2.26 of the LOINC database containing names and codes for 53,344 laboratory and clinical variables. The overall growth of the LOINC database since its first release is shown in figure 10.1.

Laboratory

The laboratory section of LOINC covers the categories of most clinical laboratory testing, including chemistry, urinalysis, hematology, serology, microbiology (including parasitology and virology), toxicology, and molecular genetics. Of the more than 52,000 terms in LOINC version 2.24, nearly 39,000 of them related to laboratory observations. The initial focus of development was on codes for single test observations, not the batteries, panels, or packages that may contain multiple test results. Over time, LOINC has continued to expand coverage for the common and standardized order panels, such as arterial blood gases, hemogram, and differential.

Clinical

The overall domain scope of clinical LOINC is extremely broad. Some of the sections of terms include

- Vital signs

- Hemodynamic measurements

- Fluid intake/output

- Anthropomorphic measures

- Emergency department variables (for example, Data Elements for Emergency Department Systems (DEEDS))

- Respiratory therapy

- Tumor registry

- Patient assessment instruments

- Ophthalmology measurements

- Radiology reports

- EKG

- Cardiac ultrasound

- Obstetrical ultrasound

- Discharge summaries

- History and physical exam findings

- Pathology findings

- Colonoscopy/endoscopy reports

- Clinical documents and sections

Because of its breadth and the early focus on laboratory testing, some observation domains are not yet well represented.

Nursing content is one of the domains with a special focus in Clinical LOINC (Matney 2003). The Clinical LOINC Committee has organized a nursing subcommittee whose mission is to meet the needs for machine-readable clinical, administrative, and regulatory nursing data by providing LOINC codes for observations at key stages of the nursing process, including assessments, goals, and outcomes. In 2002, LOINC received recognition by the American Nurses Association (ANA) Committee for Nursing Practice Information (Thede, 2003). Prior to that time, submission of nursing content for inclusion in LOINC was not well organized, and revisions were slow to progress. Since then, members of the nursing subcommittee have continued collaboration with the ANA and further expansion of the nursing content represented in LOINC.

In addition to nursing, the Clinical LOINC Committee has recently focused special effort into three other domains. First is the definition of terms to represent radiology reports. After a large expansion, two recent evaluations in independent systems (Vreeman and McDonald 2005; Vreeman and McDonald 2006) reported that LOINC provides codes for around 90 percent of diagnostic radiology terms found in hospital radiology systems. In addition, the Committee has been developing and refining a comprehensive framework for representing document and section titles for use in clinical applications and exchange with HL7's Clinical Document Architecture (CDA) standard. Work and analysis in this area has generated several scientific publications (Frazier et al. 2001; Hyun and Bakken 2006; Hyun et al. 2006; Shapiro 2005). Finally, LOINC has developed a formal model for representing standardized patient assessment instruments (for example, surveys and questionnaires) (White and Hauan 2002; Bakken et al. 2003). Recent expansions in this area have led to full representations of patient assessment instruments required by CMS in certain care settings, such as the Minimum Data Set, Outcomes and Assessment Information Set, and the new evolving instrument for post acute care settings, called CARE.

HIPAA Claims Attachments

The HIPAA legislation mandates the adoption of standards for electronically transmitting many healthcare transactions, including claims and claims attachments. A claims attachment is a piece of information the providers attach to a claim to justify it. (The claims attachment standard was given more time to develop than the other nine HIPAA standards.) In September 2005, the U.S. Department of Health and Human Services (HHS) published the Notice of Proposed Rule Making that specifies how the clinical information would be transmitted. The proposal specifies that HL7 messages would be used for the attachment structure, and that LOINC codes would be used to identify the observations requested and returned. For example, a payer who wanted a particular set of results, such as "microbial susceptibility tests," would send a request for LOINC code 18769-0. The care provider's system would respond to that request by sending back the test results in its system, identified by LOINC codes.

The content of the attachments is developed by the HL7 Attachment Group and is supported by Regenstrief and the LOINC Committee. The set of attachments drafted thus far includes: laboratory reports, nonlaboratory clinical reports, ambulance transport, medications, and rehabilitation. Several other areas are currently under development.

Adoption

LOINC has been adopted in many contexts within the United States and supported by various healthcare systems in international communities, including those in Canada, France, Germany, China, Brazil, New Zealand, and Australia.

United States

LOINC has been widely adopted in both the public and private sector. The Centers for Disease Control and Prevention (CDC) has a number of ongoing initiatives under its Public Health Information Network (PHIN) project implementing the Consolidated Health Informatics initiative (CHI) standards, including using HL7 and LOINC. The "questions" in the Data Elements for Emergency Department Systems (DEEDS) emergency room data collection form have all been translated into LOINC codes. The Council of State and Territorial Epidemiologists (CSTE) and the Association of State and Territorial Public Health Laboratory Directors (ASTPHLD), in cooperation with the CDC, use HL7 and LOINC to send information about communicable diseases from laboratories to public health departments automatically. LOINC codes have been created for variables to transmit tumor registry information through a project with the North American Association of Central Cancer Registries (NAACCR) and CDC. Most of the largest commercial laboratories (such as LabCorp, Quest Diagnostics, Mayo Medical Laboratories) and many of the largest healthcare provider organizations (for example, Partners HealthCare of Boston, Intermountain Health Care, Kaiser Permanente, and Aetna Health Care) have adopted LOINC as one of their standard code systems. Quest Diagnostics and LabCorp alone account for close to 35 percent of the nation's nonhospital testing. The American Clinical Laboratory Association (ACLA) has endorsed LOINC as its chosen standard. In addition, LOINC is also included in the National Library of Medicine (NLM)'s Unified Medical Language System Metathesaurus.

LOINC has been specified as a component of numerous clinical data exchange projects and initiatives. LOINC was included as one of the standards for the National Electronic Disease Surveillance System (NEDSS) initiative developed by the CDC. LOINC has been selected for mutual exchange of laboratory data as part of the Federal Health Information Exchange involving the Department of Veterans Affairs, the Department of Defense, and the Indian Health Service. As previously mentioned, it is the coding standard specified in the HIPAA Claims Attachments proposal. The National Committee for Quality Assurance publishes the Healthcare Effectiveness Data and Information Set, which continues using LOINC codes in their quality standards. The Clinical Data Interchange Standards Consortium continues to recommend LOINC in their laboratory specification for the pharmaceutical industry.

The CHI initiative's endorsement solidified a primary role for LOINC in the Federal Health Information Exchange. CHI is a collaborative effort to adopt health information interoperability standards, particularly health vocabulary and messaging standards, for implementation in U.S. federal government systems across agencies. In successive efforts, CHI named LOINC as the adopted standard for the domains of laboratory result names, laboratory test orders, drug section label headers, and for federally-required patient assessment instruments (questions, answers, and forms) including functioning and disability content. In addition, the CHI recommendation for text-based reports specifies use of the Health Level Seven (HL7) Clinical Document Architecture (CDA), which currently recommends the preferential use of LOINC codes for document titles.

International

The international community has adopted LOINC in many contexts. Canada Health Infoway is a group establishing nationwide nomenclature and messaging standards. They adopted LOINC for communicating laboratory results and are in the process of translating much LOINC content into French. Specific projects within this effort have already begun implementing LOINC, including: the electronic Child Health Network (eCHN) which now includes more than 84 hospitals, 42 community care sites, and 500 physician offices; and the Ontario Laboratories Information System, a jurisdictional electronic exchange of laboratory data. The national standards organization of Germany (the Deutche Institute for Normung) has adopted LOINC as a national standard. They provide regular translations of the LOINC documentation translated into German and host a companion LOINC Web site. The European Confederation of Laboratory Medicine has adopted LOINC as a multilingual test directory for clinical laboratorians worldwide. The Assistance Publique-Paris Hospitals in Paris, France, have adopted LOINC and have contributed submissions for many new terms to the database. The Chinese Ministry of Health continues its support of LOINC, with regularly updated translations of the LOINC documentation into Simplified Chinese. LOINC has also been adopted widely by systems in Australia and New Zealand, a Brazilian laboratory integration project in Sao Paulo, various health information exchange projects within Spain, and by the Mexican Institute of Social Security.

Check Your Understanding 10.2

Instructions: Complete the following exercise on a separate piece of paper.

1. In a 2002 article, Herbst called LOINC a "niche vocabulary." What do you think the author means in relation to other vocabulary or terminology systems used in healthcare applications?

2. The LOINC database contains names and codes for which variables?
    a. Laboratory and Pathology
    b. Laboratory and Clinical
    c. Clinical diseases
    d. Clinical and Pathology

3. In which section of LOINC would you find nursing content?

4. Who named LOINC as a standard for the domains of laboratory result names, laboratory test orders, drug section label headers, and for federally required patient assessment instruments (questions, answers, and forms) including functioning and disability content?

Structure

LOINC Naming Conventions

The LOINC vocabulary was developed with an understanding of the structured medical vocabulary and a **semantic data model** (SDM) (Huff et al. 1998). Each record in the LOINC database has a code and formal name that corresponds to a single kind of observation, measurement, or test result. A LOINC code signifies a concept that applies to all tests with equivalent clinical results.

The formal LOINC name models the semantic structure of aggregate or pre-coordinated expressions using the multiaxial representational approach. The LOINC Users' Guide is the definitive source describing the LOINC naming conventions in detail (McDonald et al. 2008). Here we present a summary.

Each LOINC observation name includes as many as six main parts:

- *Component (analyte):* The substance or entity that is measured, evaluated, or observed. Examples include systolic blood pressure, pain onset, and sodium.

- *Kind of property:* The characteristic or attribute of the component that is measured, evaluated, or observed. Examples include length, volume, time stamp, mass, ratio, number, and temperature.

- *Time aspect:* The interval of time over which the observation or measurement was made. Examples include "point in time" and "over a 24-hour time period."

- *System:* The system (context) or specimen type within which the observation was made. Examples include urine, serum, fetus, patient (person), and family.

- *Type of scale:* The scale of the measure. Examples include quantitative (a true numeric measurement), ordinal (a ranked set of options), nominal (for example, E. coli, Staphy-lococcus aureus), or narrative (for example, dictation results from x-rays).

- *Type of method:* The procedure used to make the measurement or observation. Method is only specified when different methodologies would significantly change the interpretation of the result. Method is the only axis that is optional.

LOINC names are called fully specified because they contain entries for each of these axes. By design, LOINC codes were meant for use in the context of clinical data exchange formats like HL7. The LOINC name is not intended to capture all possible information about the testing procedure or the result—only enough to unambiguously identity it. For that reason, several things are specifically *excluded* from the name: the testing instrument and protocol, testing priority (such as STAT), sample volume, and testing location. All of these other aspects can be communicated in other parts of the HL7 message.

Distinct LOINC codes are created for each specimen for which a test kit has been calibrated. So, if an instrument/kit produced one value for each specimen and the test was recommended for use on two specimens (for example, whole blood and cerebrospinal fluid [CSF]), two LOINC codes are needed, one for whole blood and one for CSF. If two or more results per specimen are reported (for example, a control value or a total and a percentage), two or more LOINC codes are needed per supported specimen. However, LOINC concepts are not unique per test manufacturer.

As noted above, the method axis is optional. The method axis is used only when the method distinction makes an important difference in the clinical interpretation of the result. This primarily matters when the other five name axes do not sufficiently distinguish measurements that have important differences in the reference range, sensitivity, or specificity. Whether or not method is specified in the formal name is guided by pragmatics and follows the conventions seen in typical local test names. For this reason, the method is specified at a relatively high level; detailed information about the testing procedure can be sent in other parts of an observation message.

In addition to constructing a fully specified name, LOINC creates a unique code for each concept. LOINC follows sound terminology development practices. LOINC codes themselves have no embedded meaning; they are sequentially assigned, unique numbers that include a MOD10 check digit as a hyphen-separated suffix. Applications can use the check digit to detect common typographic errors when LOINC codes are entered manually. LOINC codes are never deleted from the database. If a term happens to be an error or duplicate, it is flagged in the database as "deprecated."

Examples of LOINC codes and fully specified names are given for laboratory LOINC codes in table 10.1 (see page 160) and for clinical LOINC codes in table 10.2 (see page 160).

LOINC Distribution

LOINC is distributed and made freely available from the LOINC Web site at http://loinc.org. The main LOINC database is distributed in several file formats. New releases of the standard are published twice yearly (typically in June and December), though occasionally additional interim releases are published in response to emergent needs. With each release, a file identifying the changes between versions is also

Table 10.2.   Example clinical LOINC codes and formal LOINC names

LOINC Code	LOINC name (component:property:timing:specimen:scale)
8480-6	Intravascular systolic:Pres:Pt:Arterial system:Qn
8301-4	Body height:Len:Pt:^Patient:Qn:Estimated
28655-9	Discharge summarization note:Find:Pt:{Setting}:Doc: Attending physician
38214-3	Pain severity:Find:Pt:^Patient:Qn:Reported.visual analog score
24801-3	View Merchants:Find:Pt:Knee:Nar:XR

distributed. In addition to the main LOINC database, Regenstrief develops and distributes a software program called the Regenstrief LOINC Mapping Assistant (RELMA) that provides tools for browsing the database, mapping local terminology to the LOINC terms, and reviewing the HIPAA attachments. RELMA is similarly free for use.

The LOINC database and the RELMA program are copyrighted to protect their integrity, but the license permits all commercial and noncommercial uses in perpetuity, at no cost. The full copyright and terms of use are available at: http://loinc.org/terms-of-use. Having the standard copyrighted protects against multiple variants emerging, which would defeat the purpose of a universal standard. LOINC's unrestrictive terms of use ensure a low barrier to widespread adoption.

Database

The LOINC vocabulary is distributed as a single table available in several file formats. The complete table specifications are provided in the LOINC User's Guide (McDonald et al. 2008). Each record in the LOINC table identifies a unique clinical observation and contains the LOINC code, the formal six-part fully specified name, an informal short name, and many other accessory attributes.

RELMA

In addition to the main LOINC table, Regenstrief Institute develops and freely distributes the RELMA program. RELMA contains tools for both browsing the LOINC database and mapping local observation codes to LOINC. Users can import a set of local

Table 10.1.   Example laboratory LOINC codes and formal LOINC names

LOINC Code	LOINC name (component:property:timing:specimen:scale)
2951-2	Sodium:SCnc:Pt:Ser/Plas:Qn
2955-3	Sodium:SCnc:Pt:Urine:Qn
2956-1	Sodium:SRat:24H:Urine:Qn
2164-2	Creatinine renal clearance:VRat:24H: Urine+Ser/Plas:Qn
1514-9	Glucose^2H post 100 g glucose PO:MCnc:Pt: Ser/Plas:Qn
3665-7	Gentamicin^trough:MCnc:Pt:Ser/Plas:Qn
17863-2	Calcium.ionized:MCnc:Pt:Ser/Plas:Qn
2863-9	Albumin:MCnc:Pt:Synv Fld:Qn:Electrophoresis

Figure 10.2.   Main search screen interface of the Regenstrief LOINC Mapping Assistant (RELMA) program, version 3.24

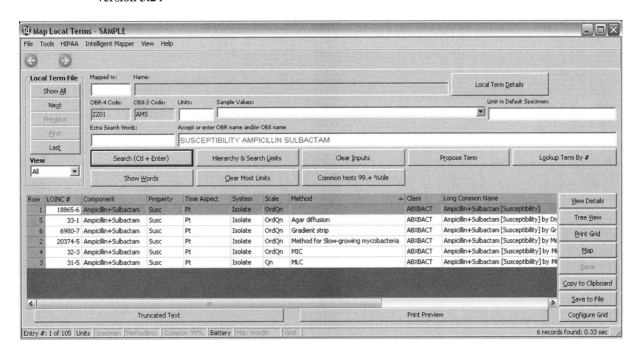

terms for mapping with a text file of their system's master test catalog, or they can use the capabilities within RELMA to generate such a list from a file of HL7 messages. Using real clinical HL7 messages to create the test list has the advantage of being able to include sample values, normal ranges, and other information that is helpful to the mapping process but not always contained in a master test catalog.

The primary interface allows searching and mapping on a term-by-term basis. RELMA contains many features for narrowing searches to find the most appropriate LOINC code, including a set of hierarchies that organize the LOINC concepts. A screenshot of the RELMA search interface is shown in figure 10.2.

In addition to term-by-term searching, RELMA contains an additional program, called Intelligent Mapper, that automatically generates a ranked list of candidate LOINC codes for each local term in a set. Several studies have formally evaluated (Vreeman and McDonald 2005, Vreeman and McDonald 2006) Intelligent Mapper's performance in mapping local radiology terms to LOINC and have demonstrated high accuracy.

As users map their local system terms to LOINC, they will occasionally encounter terms for which no suitable LOINC code exists. RELMA contains a set of tools for proposing additions to the LOINC database. RELMA will create a file of these new term requests that can be sent to Regenstrief for consideration.

Documentation

The LOINC User's Guide is the definitive document about LOINC. It describes the naming conventions and polices in detail. Regenstrief also publishes a User's Manual for RELMA describing its functionality. Along with each LOINC and release, a set of release notes is also published describing the updates and changes since the last version.

All of the LOINC documentation is available on the LOINC Web site. In addition, the Web site contains background information, answers to frequently asked questions, online training materials (in several languages), a bibliography of scientific literature about LOINC, and a community discussion board.

Check Your Understanding 10.3

Instructions: Download the current version of the LOINC user's guide from http://loinc.org and review sections 4.1 and 4.2. Then answer the following questions on a separate piece of paper.

1. Which parts of the formal LOINC name correspond exactly in meaning between laboratory LOINC codes and clinical LOINC codes?

2. What is the advantage of including terms to support atomic result reporting in addition to the pre-coordinated, molecular results?

Community Development

The overall LOINC development effort is largely driven by and for the user community. The vast majority of all new content is created from end-user submissions, and Regenstrief additionally welcomes all public input on existing content within the database. Between 2003 and 2008, requests for new content were contributed by 67 different organizations from 13 countries (Vreeman 2008). A large and continuously growing community of international users generates translations of the LOINC database and documentation into languages other than the source English. Translated terms are distributed with the RELMA program and translated documentation is published on a special section of the LOINC Web site at http://loinc.org/international.

Summary

LOINC is a vocabulary standard developed by the Regenstrief Institute that provides a set of universal identifiers and names for laboratory and other clinical observations. LOINC is an openly developed and freely available standard designed to be used in electronic transactions between independent computer systems. LOINC has been widely adopted, both within the public and private sectors of the United States and internationally. Mapping local observation terms to LOINC provides a bridge across the many islands of health data that currently exist, facilitating the exchange and aggregation of clinical results for care delivery, management, public health, and research purposes.

References

Bakken, S., J.J.Cimino, R. Haskell, R. Kukafka, C. Matsumoto, G.K. Chan, and S.M. Huff. 2000. Evaluation of the clinical LOINC (Logical Observation Identifiers, Names, and Codes) semantic structure as a terminology model for standardized assessment measures. *Journal of the American Medical Informatics Association.* Nov-Dec;7(6):529–538.

Chaudhry, B., J. Wang, S. Wu, M. Maglione, W. Mojica, E. Roth, S.C. Morton, and P.G. Shekelle. 2006. Systematic review: Impact of health information technology on quality, efficiency, and costs of medical care. *Annals of Internal Medicine.* 144(10):742–752.

E-Gov Presidential Initiatives. 2005. http://www.whitehouse.gov/omb/egov/c-3-6-chi.html.

Francis, W.T. Tracy, D. Leavelle, F. Stalling, B. Griffin, P. Maloney, D. Leland, L. Charles, K. Hutchins, and J. Baenziger. 1998. Development of the Logical Observation Identifiers, Names, and Codes (LOINC). *Journal of the Medical Informatics Association,* 73(1):276–292.

Frazier, P., A. Rossi-Mori, R.H. Dolin, L. Alschuler, and S.M. Huff. 2001. The creation of an ontology of clinical document names. *Medinfo,* 10:94–98.

Herbst, M.R. 2002. Another look at LOINC. *Journal of the American Health Information Management Association,* 73(1):56–58.

Huff, S.M., R.A. Rocha, C.J. McDonald, G.J. DeMoor, T. Fiers, W.D. Bidgood, A.W. Forrey, W.G. Francis, W.T. Tracy, D. Leavelle, F. Stalling, B. Griffin, P. Maloney, D. Leland, L. Charles, K. Hutchins, and J. Baenziger.1998. Development of the Logical Observation Identifiers, Names, and Codes (LOINC). *Journal of the Medical Informatics Association,* 73(1):276–292.

Hyun, S. and S. Bakken. 2006. Toward the creation of an ontology for nursing document sections: Mapping Section names to the LOINC semantic model. *AMIA Annual Symposium Proceedings,* 364–368.

Hyun, S., R. Ventura, S.B. Johnson, and S. Bakken. 2006. Is the Health Level 7/LOINC document ontology adequate for representing nursing documents? *Studies in Health Technology and Informatics,* 122:527–531.

Indiana Network for Patient Care (INPC). (http://inpc.org)

Matney, S., S. Bakken, and S.M. Huff. 2003. Representing nursing assessments in clinical information systems using the logical observation identifiers, names, and codes database. *Journal of Biomedical Informatics,* 36 (4-5), 287–293.

Matney, S., J. Ozbolt, and S. Bakken. 2003. Update on Logical Observation Identifiers, Names, and Codes (LOINC). *Online Journal of Nursing Informatics.* http://eaaknowledge.com/ojni/ni/8_1/nurslangup.htm.

McDonald, C., S. Huff, J. Suico, K. Mercer, and D. Vreeman, eds. 2008. Logical Observation Identifiers, Names, and Codes (LOINC) User's Guide. http://loinc.org/downloads.

McDonald, C.J., S.M. Huff, J.G. Suico, G. Hill, D. Leavelle, R. Aller, A. Forrey, K. Mercer, G. DeMoor, J. Hook, W. Williams, J. Case, and P. Maloney. 2003. LOINC, a universal standard for identifying laboratory observations: A 5-year update. *Clinical Chemistry,* 49:624–633.

Shapiro, J.S., S. Bakken, S. Hyun, G.B. Melton, C. Schlegel, and S.B. Johnson. 2005. Document ontology: Supporting narrative documents in electronic health records. *AMIA Annual Symposium Proceedings*, 684–688.

Thede, L.Q. 2003. *Informatics and Nursing: Opportunities and Challenges* (2nd ed.). Philadelphia: Lippincott Williams and Wilkins Publishers.

Vreeman, D.J. and C.J. McDonald. 2005. Automated mapping of local radiology terms to LOINC. *AMIA Annual Symposium Proceedings*, 769–773.

Vreeman, D.J. and C.J. McDonald. 2006 A comparison of Intelligent Mapper and document similarity scores for mapping local radiology terms to LOINC. *AMIA Annual Symposium Proceedings*, 809–813.

Vreeman, D. 2008. Regenstrief Institute internal report.

White, T.M. and M.J. Hauan. 2002. Extending the LOINC conceptual schema to support standardized assessment instruments. *Journal of the American Medical Informatics Association*, Nov-Dec;9(6):586–599.

Application Exercises

1. Go to http://loinc.org/adopters. Explore the listing of organizations that have adopted LOINC. What kinds of institutions are currently using LOINC?

2. Go to http://loinc.org/relma and explore the Web pages concerning this tool designed to work with the LOINC terminology. Then answer the following questions:
   a. What type of computer system is required to use RELMA?
   b. What are its terms of use?

3. Go to http://www.nlm.nih.gov/research/umls/mapping_projects/loinc_to_cpt_map.html. What does this page say about why this mapping project was initiated?

Review Quiz

1. The developer of Logical Observation Identifiers, Names, and Codes (LOINC) system is:
   a. College of American Pathologists
   b. Centers for Medicare and Medicaid Services (CMS)
   c. Regenstrief Institute, Inc.
   d. American Clinical Laboratory Association

2. True or False. LOINC has been named a Consolidated Health Information Informatics Initiative standard for more than one domain.

3. Which of the following is NOT a LOINC axis?
   a. Time aspect
   b. Kind of property
   c. Type of method
   d. Type of test

4. Which LOINC system axis is optional?
   a. Type of method
   b. Kind of property
   c. Component
   d. Type of scale

5. A program for mapping local files to LOINC is:
   a. LOINC database
   b. Regenstrief LOINC Mapping Assistant (RELMA)
   c. HL7
   d. Regenstrief Medical Records System (RMRS)

6. True or False. LOINC provides a standard set of universal names and codes for identifying individual laboratory and clinical results.

7. Which HIPAA standard includes the use of LOINC codes?
   a. Privacy standards
   b. Security standards
   c. Modifications to Electronic Data Transaction Standards and Code Sets
   d. Electronic claim attachment standards

8. The LOINC development process can be characterized as?
   a. Empirical, nimble, proprietary
   b. Empirical, nimble, open
   c. Ontological, nimble, balloted
   d. Ontological, bureaucratic, proprietary

Chapter 11

Drug Terminology Systems

Kathy Giannangelo, MA, RHIA, CCS, CPHIMS, FAHIMA

Learning Objectives

- To describe drug terminologies and drug knowledge bases currently available

- To recognize the developers of drug terminologies and knowledge bases

- To describe the content and organizational structure of RxNorm

- To explain the process for ongoing maintenance and continuing evolution of RxNorm

- To describe the National Drug File Reference Terminology

- To identify the purpose of a drug terminology versus a drug knowledge base

Key Terms

Clinical drug

Concept

Dose form

Drug component

Drug knowledge base (DKB)

e-Prescribing

Formulary

Lexicon

Medical Subjects Headings (MeSH)

National Drug File Reference Terminology (NDF-RT)

Normalized

Physiologic effects

Reference terminology

Routed generic

RxNorm

RxNorm concept unique identifier (RXCUI)

Semantic Branded Drug (SBD)

Semantic normal form (SNF)

SNF clinical formulation (SCD)

SNF drug component (SCDC)

Term type (TTY)

Introduction

Systems to record drug **concepts** and information in a consistent manner are particularly complex. Some of the reasons for this complexity include:

- There are significant maintenance challenges because drugs change frequently, necessitating weekly or monthly updates.

- The systems must address multiple core concepts.

- There are conflicting views on key concepts, appropriate levels of granularity, and where terminology stops and the information model begins.

- It can be difficult to differentiate a drug terminology from a **drug knowledge base.**

This chapter explores and explains some of these complexities. It also introduces the various drug terminologies and drug knowledge bases available at the time of this writing. More detailed information is provided on RxNorm and NDF-RT because RxNorm and a portion of NDF-RT have been recommended as standards for electronic exchange of clinical information throughout the federal government.

Drug Terminologies

According to testimony to the National Committee on Vital and Health Statistics (NCVHS 2003a), the requirements for a drug terminology to be used as a standard in the electronic health record (EHR) are that it must be:

- Maintained by a primary code-assigning authority

- Available for use at little or no cost

- Updated frequently and promptly

- Backwardly compatible with the National Drug Code (NDC) system

- Composed of abstractions at multiple levels of granularity

Drug concepts that must be represented to support common clinical and administrative functions include the following:

- Active ingredients

- **Routed generic**

- **Clinical drug**

- Manufactured drug

- Packaged product

Table 11.1 describes each concept and explains its purpose.

Other concepts addressed by a drug terminology include:

- Therapeutic classification (antihypertensive, beta blocker, ACE inhibitors)

- Form (tablet, liquid, powder)

- Route (inhaled, topical, intravenous, intramuscular)

- Strength (25 mg per 5 ml)

Whether the central, or key, concept of a drug terminology system is based on ingredient or routed

Table 11.1.   Concepts that must be represented to support common clinical and administrative functions

Concept	Description	Purpose
Active ingredients	The chemicals in a drug	Important for allergy checking
Routed generic	Generic name + route of administration	Important for drug-drug-interaction checking
Clinical drug	Routed generic + strength + dosage form	Important for physician order entry
Manufactured drug	Clinical drug + manufacturer + inactive ingredients	Important for medication administration records at the nursing level
Packaged product	Manufactured drug + packaging information	Important for interoperability with pharmacy systems

generic, for example, depends on the purpose of the system. Similarly, different levels of granularity are needed depending on the desired functionality of the particular system.

For instance, testimony at NCVHS indicated that "routed generic" is an appropriate level of abstraction for most decision support functions, but not for order entry. The order-entry function requires more specific and expansive information, including discretely represented trade names, dosage forms, strengths, and so on (2003a).

Additionally, there are differences in inpatient and outpatient medication orders that result in conceptually different database and information needs. For example, a typical inpatient order may be documented as "amoxicillin PO 250 mg, TID." In this order, the physician has not specified strength and form; these details are left up to the pharmacist. However, these details would need to be specified in an outpatient setting, in which case the prescription might read "amoxicillin suspension, 250 mg per 5 ml one teaspoon PO TID."

Further examples of varying levels of granularity are

- Identifying the route as an IV or as a continuous IV infusion

- Identifying the form as a tablet or specifying sustained-release tablet versus enteric-coated tablet

With the many different information needs, it is not surprising that multiple drug terminologies or drug knowledge bases (DKBs) are available. Many are specialized and incompatible. Industry forces moving the EHR forward are demanding a centrally managed and low-cost standard drug terminology for use in the EHR. (See figure 11.1 for uses of a drug terminology.)

As discussed in chapter 7, the Systematized Nomenclature of Medicine (SNOMED) includes a section on pharmaceutical/biological products. This drug section within SNOMED traditionally has existed, for the most part, to support the disease hierarchy

Figure 11.1. Uses of a drug terminology

Drug terminologies are needed for many reasons. For instance, drug terminologies allow:

- Physicians to send prescriptions electronically to pharmacies
- Physicians to use computerized physician order entry systems in the inpatient setting, with communication to the pharmacy and the administering nurse
- Consumers to access personal health records and review or add medications

and to aid in the indexing of certain compounds for basic research. It contains generic ingredient names essentially structured in therapeutic classifications in addition to most of the proprietary names used in the United States, but without product-specific information. In its current form, this section of SNOMED does not meet the needs of a standard drug terminology for an EHR. However, the portion of SNOMED CT for allergy type, allergy severity, and allergy reaction has been named one of the standards used to set requirements for "exchanging" allergy data across the federal health enterprise (CHI 2006).

As discussed in chapter 5, National Drug Codes (NDCs) represent product information, including product name, package size, and manufacturer. However, the information necessary for EHRs, such as all active ingredients, dosage form, strength, and route of administration, is not distributed with NDCs.

NDC codes are useful for electronic exchange of information on the package level. However, if a doctor wants to send a patient's medication list from one hospital to another (noting, for example, that the patient is taking Vioxx 50 mg, PO once daily), a standard drug terminology is needed to make that sort of statement and to transmit it in a manner that can be understood by the receiver.

The move toward adoption and implementation of standard drug terminologies is being partly driven by the interest in medication management and electronic prescribing (**e-prescribing**). CMS, American Health Information Community (AHIC), Healthcare Information Technology Standards Panel (HITSP), and the Certification Commission for Healthcare

Information Technology (CCHIT) have all weighed in on terminology issues related to medication management.

The Standards for e-Prescribing Under Medicare Part D Final Rule, published by CMS, did not name terminology standards even though the pilot test indicated RxNorm had significant potential (DHHS 2008).

In 2007, AHIC created a medication management use case toward their goal of improving medication management to promote patient safety and support relevant aspects of the medication management cycle with better interoperability and efficiency (AHIC 2007). An essential component of this use case was its relation to the federal initiative on e-prescribing. As a follow-up to this work, AHIC has created material to address the identified gaps in the electronic exchange of medication information between electronic health record (EHR), pharmacy, and other related systems as well as e-prescribing and interoperability needs. The plans are for HITSP to utilize the report in their work on standards harmonization.

In addition to the recommendations from AHIC, HITSP also takes into account other work on standards taking place at the federal level. A key factor in the development of HITSP's Medication Management Interoperability Specification (IS), was the e-prescribing federal initiative. The focus of medication management is the information encompassing the acts of prescribing, dispensing, and administering a medication (HITSP 2008). The IS 07 Version 1.1 named several drug terminologies in C32 (HITSP Summary Documents Using HL7 Continuity of Care Document [CCD] Component) and TP43 (HITSP Medication Orders Transaction Package Component). They include the federal drug terminologies defined by HITSP as:

> A set of controlled terminologies and code sets developed and maintained as part of a collaboration between the Food and Drug Administration, National Library of Medicine, Veterans Health Administration, National Cancer Institute and Agency for Healthcare Research and Quality related to medications, including medication proprietary and non-proprietary names, clinical drug code (RxNorm); ingredi-

ent names and Unique Ingredient Identifiers (UNII); routes of administration, dosage forms, and units of presentation from the NCI Thesaurus (NCIt); and certain pharmacological drug classes from the National Drug File Reference Terminology (NDF-RT).

The CCHIT aligned their EHR certification criteria with the AHIC Medication Management use case. A terminology included as a part of the certification road map is RxNorm (CCHIT 2008).

Check Your Understanding 11.1

Instructions: Complete the following exercises on a separate piece of paper.

1. Which of the following concepts is important for nursing medication administration records?
    a. Routed generic
    b. Clinical drug
    c. Manufactured drug
    d. Packaged product

2. True or False. The concept of clinical drug does not include the route of administration.

3. Which of the following concepts includes inactive ingredients?
    a. Routed generic
    b. Clinical drug
    c. Manufactured drug
    d. Packaged product

4. Which of the following is a therapeutic classification of a drug?
    a. Intramuscular
    b. Beta-blocker
    c. Tablet
    d. Inhaled

5. Which of the following concepts is more granular?
    a. Route: IV
        or
        Route: Continuous IV infusion
    b. Form: Tablet
        or
        Form: Enteric-coated tablet

Drug Knowledge Bases

Drug terminologies define a drug but ideally do not include attributes found in a drug knowledge base

(DKB) that enable clinical screening and provide integrated and referential knowledge.

Several years ago, Lau and Lam evaluated existing DKBs and found that they did not meet all the desiderata for a controlled vocabulary. For instance, they were not designed to be concept-based and did not support formal definitions. Also, they were designed to be used in the specific context of pharmacy applications and did not consider other contexts (for instance, a patient-specific context) (Lau and Lam 1999).

Although drug information recorded in a controlled medical terminology supports enterprise-wide and longitudinal EHR applications, DKBs are designed to support specific pharmacy applications. DKBs serve different markets and sets of users. A DKB offers added value through relationships to pricing, indications, adverse effects, drug interactions, allergies, dosing, precautions, and patient education.

Commercial DKBs

First DataBank (a subsidiary of Hearst Corporation), Medi-Span (Wolters-Kluwer Health, Inc.), Micromedex (Thomson Reuters), Multum (Cerner), and Alchemy (Gold Standard) are examples of proprietary, or commercial, products from different pharmaceutical knowledge base providers. All these products support a range of functions and contain terms and/or codes for multiple levels of drug information, including clinical drugs.

These DKBs are available only as part of a larger product and vary considerably in their underlying information models. The systems mentioned above are described in the following subsections.

First DataBank

First DataBank's National Drug Data File Plus (NDDF+) focuses on drug products that have been released in the U.S. market. Everything in NDDF+ is driven by something packaged and identified with an NDC, Universal Product Code, or health-related item code. Attributes are categorized (for example, clinical route, dosage form) and relationships are established.

NDDF+ aggregates the following types of knowledge around a clinical drug concept: indications, drug disease contraindications, side effects, drug–drug and drug–food interactions, and allergy.

NDDF+ is used for a variety of purposes, ranging from profiling patient allergy or patient medications to creating order entries to ambulatory prescribing through order fulfillment, adjudication of claims, and possibly retrospective analysis.

Medi-Span

Medi-Span originated as a monthly drug pricing publication and expanded to include clinical screening data sets and clinical screening application software.

Medi-Span data sets support a wide range of applications, including integrated clinical drug and disease screening, patient profiling, computerized provider order entry to include e-prescribing, billing, claims adjudication, drug dispensing, drug **formulary** creation and maintenance, and retrospective and data warehouse drug analysis.

Micromedex

Micromedex is a wide range of clinical databases, which together comprise a drug information system. The databases include referenced data on dosing, pharmacokinetics, interactions, and clinical applications for investigational and international drugs approved by the Food and Drug Administration (FDA).

Micromedex provides evidence-based clinical information for physicians, pharmacists, and nurses. Some of the Micromedex drug information products are DRUGDEX System for comprehensive drug details; Martindale, an international drug reference; Physicians' Desk Reference (PDR) for information on FDA-approved drugs; and the RED BOOK, which includes drug product, packaging, and pricing.

Multum

Multum's products are based on a lexical foundation that, at the highest view, links packaged drug products, generic formulation concepts, Main Multum Drug Codes (MMDCs), and a generic concept identifier, all grouped into categories. Drug-packaged products coded with NDCs are linked to one MMDC. Each MMDC, in turn, is related to a generic concept identifier for drugs. Concepts are separate from names describing concepts. Thirty-eight thousand drug names at different levels of granularity are included.

Multum has two products that may be used to identify drugs. The Multum **Lexicon** is a minimal data set of seventeen tables. The Vantage Rx Database has 144 tables, including everything in Multum Lexicon plus drug categorization, expanded synonymy, and clinical content.

Alchemy

Alchemy includes a drug database and clinical decision support tools. The database contains drug product and pricing on U.S. approved brand and generic prescription drugs, over-the-counter products, herbals, vitamins and nutritional products, medical devices, and diagnostic kits. Alchemy product data elements are quite extensive. For example, codes (both 10- and 11-digit NDCs), identifiers such as the UPC, inactive and active ingredients, product attributes such as sugar-free, and physical descriptions such as shape, are included (Alchemy 2008).

Some of the uses of the product and pricing files named by Gold Standard for Alchemy are physician order entry, billing, inventory management, and personal health records.

Nonproprietary Drug Terminologies

The pharmaceutical knowledge base providers mentioned above have multiple systems currently in use, and each has taken a slightly different approach to identifying drugs in its unique application. The providers vary in design, naming conventions, and even content coverage based on their perception of market need. For instance, Medi-Span supports the generic product identifier, but the database does not have an enhanced attribute that identifies therapeutic classification. And although First DataBank maintains unique identifiers for all the levels of drug abstrac-

tion, Medi-Span and Multum's generic drug identifiers include the concept of route administration.

To achieve the full potential for EHR applications, a controlled drug terminology is needed that does not duplicate the efforts of knowledge contained in the DKB products. This controlled drug terminology would act as a bridge between commercial DKBs and enterprise-wide systems. For this reason, the federal government undertook two projects to establish and maintain drug terminology standards and code sets. The results of these efforts were Rx-Norm and NDF-RT:

- The National Library of Medicine's **Rx-Norm** is a nonproprietary terminology that represents drugs at the level of granularity needed to support clinical practice.

- The Veterans Administration's **National Drug File Reference Terminology** (NDF-RT) is a nonproprietary drug **reference terminology** that includes drug knowledge and classifies drugs, most notably, by mechanism of action and physiologic effect.

In May 2004, the Departments of Health and Human Services, Defense, and Veterans Affairs announced the adoption of fifteen additional standards agreed to by the Consolidated Health Initiative (CHI) to allow for electronic exchange of clinical information throughout the federal government. A set of federal terminologies related to medications was among the fifteen standards. This set included RxNorm for describing clinical drugs and NDF-RT for specific drug classifications. The portion of NDF-RT that represents the mechanism of action and physiologic effects of drugs was recommended as part of the core set of patient medical record information (PMRI) terminologies because these portions complement, rather than compete with, the capabilities of commercial DKBs developed within the private sector.

The remainder of this chapter focuses on describing RxNorm and NDF-RT in more detail and concludes by describing how drug terminologies and knowledge bases work together in an EHR.

Check Your Understanding 11.2

Instructions: Complete the following exercises on a separate piece of paper.

1. Match each of the following abbreviations with the knowledge base or drug terminology with which it is most associated.

    ___ NDDF+   a. Micromedex
    ___ PDR   b. NDF-RT
    ___ MMDC   c. RxNorm
    ___ NLM   d. First DataBank
    ___ VA   e. Multum

2. Match each of the following descriptions with the knowledge base or drug terminology to which it is most related.

    ___ Useful for drug formulary creation
    ___ Is a wide range of clinical databases
    ___ Products are based on a lexical foundation
    ___ Represents drugs at a granular level to support clinical practice
    ___ Classifies drugs by mechanism of action and physiologic effect
    a. Multum
    b. NDF-RT
    c. RxNorm
    d. Micromedex
    e. Medi-Span

RxNorm

The lack of interoperability among the terminologies used in the proprietary pharmaceutical knowledge bases was the primary motivation for RxNorm's development. For example, a user wishing to use one pharmaceutical knowledge base system for pricing and inventory control and a different system for interaction checking finds it difficult to merge the two systems into a larger environment. This issue was discussed at Health Level 7 (HL7) meetings for several years, with representatives from each of the pharmaceutical knowledge base providers as active participants. It became apparent that interoperability at the clinical drug level might be an achievable goal if a standard clinical drug nomenclature were developed and the terminologies in the various proprietary systems were mapped to it. As a result, the National Library of Medicine (NLM) initiated development of the public domain RxNorm terminology.

The goals of the RxNorm project were to

*   Define a standard for representational form

*   Relate Unified Medical Language System (UMLS) clinical drugs to this standard

*   Facilitate navigation between vocabularies

RxNorm Developer

Development of RxNorm began in late 2001 when the NLM undertook a project to develop a new methodology for identifying clinical drugs in the UMLS. It had long been suspected that there were considerable gaps in the naming of clinical drugs in the UMLS. One of the goals of the RxNorm project was to address these gaps and improve interoperability of existing drug terminologies. Timing was critical as the healthcare industry focused on patient safety related to medications, and there was growing consensus in the HL7 vocabulary technical committee of what a model for clinical drugs should be.

RxNorm Description

RxNorm is a standardized nomenclature for clinical drugs. In RxNorm, a clinical drug is a pharmaceutical product given to, or taken by, a patient, with a therapeutic or diagnostic intent. The RxNorm name of a clinical drug combines its active ingredients, strengths, and form.

RxNorm was developed by creating **semantic normal forms** (SNFs) for clinical drugs, both **drug component** (semantic clinical drug component, or SCDC) and **clinical formulation** (semantic clinical drug, or SCD), found in each of the major sources of names of clinical drugs, including the Veterans Administration's National Drug File (VANDF), Multum, Micromedex, First DataBank, and Medi-Span.

Parsing algorithms were used to create SCDCs or SCDs for about 70 percent of the names in these systems. Where that was not possible (about 30 percent of the names), a UMLS Editor created them (Nelson et al. 2002). The SNFs were edited and then inserted into the Metathesaurus Information Database (MID). As each SNF was inserted, relationships and relationship attributes were added according to predefined definitions. Also, strengths were **normalized** to the smallest number of allowable units. After the data were entered in the MID, duplicates were merged and branded products were linked to generic names. The SNFs, or preferred terms, and the relationships between them together constitute RxNorm.

RxNorm provides standard names for clinical drugs (active ingredient + strength + **dose form**) and for dose forms as administered. It provides links from clinical drugs to their active ingredients, drug components (active ingredient + strength), and some related brand names. To the extent available from the Food and Drug Administration (FDA), NDCs for specific drug products that deliver the clinical drug are stored as attributes of the clinical drug in RxNorm.

In RxNorm, the form is the physical form in which the drug is administered, or is specified to be administered, in a prescription or order. The RxNorm clinical drug name does not refer to the size of the package, the form in which the product was manufactured, or its form when it arrived at the dispensary. The model for RxNorm is based on what a clinician might order and what type of order might be sent to the pharmacy. The dose form is the form in which a drug is administered to a patient, as opposed to the form in which the manufacturer supplied it. It is distinct from the choices the pharmacy might make in fulfilling that order.

RxNorm's standard names for clinical drugs are mapped to the different names of drugs present in many different controlled vocabularies within the UMLS Metathesaurus, including those in commercially available DKBs reviewed earlier in this chapter. This mapping is intended to facilitate interoperability among the computerized systems that record or process data dealing with clinical drugs.

RxNorm Purpose

Because every DKB that is commercially available today follows somewhat different naming conventions, a standardized nomenclature is needed for the smooth exchange of information, not only between organizations, but also within the same organization. For example, a hospital may use one system for ordering and another for inventory management. Still another system might be used to record dose adjustments or to check drug interactions. Several cooperating hospitals might have different systems and find their data incomparable.

A standardized nomenclature that is related to terms from other sources can serve as a means for determining when names from different source vocabularies are synonymous. The goal of RxNorm is to allow various systems using different DKBs to share data efficiently.

RxNorm Content

RxNorm contains the names of prescription and many nonprescription formulations that exist in the United States, including the devices that administer the medications.

It is the intent of RxNorm to cover all prescription medications approved for use in the United States. Prescription medications from other countries may be included as opportunities allow, with a principal consideration being that of an authoritative source of information about these drugs. Over-the-counter (OTC) medications will be added and covered as well when reliable information about them can be found and when they appear to be represented in other UMLS source vocabularies. At the present time, medications, whether prescription or OTC, with more than three active ingredients are not fully represented. In some cases, such as multivitamins, it may not be possible to include all of them within a reasonable time frame.

Radiopharmaceuticals, because of the decay of their strength over time and the requirement that they be ordered and prepared especially for a given time of administration, are listed only as ingredients.

An RxNorm clinical drug name reflects the active ingredients, strength, and dose form comprising that drug. When any of these elements varies, a new RxNorm drug name is created as a separate concept. Thus, an RxNorm name should exist for every strength and dose of every combination of clinically significant active ingredients available in the United States. In addition, each element of the RxNorm clinical drug name is an individual RxNorm term related by formal criteria to the clinical drug name.

As stated earlier, RxNorm is released through the UMLS Metathesaurus. Within the UMLS Metathesaurus, RxNorm terminology contains source vocabularies from the VANDF and from major commercial drug information resources, including First DataBank, Medi-Span, Micromedex, Multum, and Alchemy.

Check Your Understanding 11.3

Instructions: Complete the following exercises on a separate piece of paper.

1. Which of the following is included in the standard name of a clinical drug in RxNorm? (Mark all that apply.)
    a. Active ingredients
    b. Inactive ingredients
    c. Strengths
    d. Form
    e. Route

2. RxNorm was developed by creating semantic normal forms for the clinical drugs found in which of the following systems? (Mark all that apply.)
    a. VANDF
    b. Multum
    c. Micromedex
    d. First DataBank
    e. Medi-Span

3. Which of the following is the preferred term for a clinical drug in RxNorm?
    a. SCD
    b. SCDC
    c. MID
    d. SNF

4. True or False. RxNorm's standard names for clinical drugs are mapped to the various names of drugs present in the UMLS.

5. Which one of the following is *not* included in RxNorm?
    a. Prescription drugs in the United States
    b. Nonprescription drugs in the United States
    c. Prescription medications from other countries
    d. Devices that administer medications

RxNorm Structure

RxNorm follows a standard format in the naming of clinical drugs. Drugs named in disparate ways in various other vocabularies are normalized according to RxNorm's naming conventions.

RxNorm is organized around normalized names for clinical drugs. These names contain information on active ingredients, strengths, and dose forms. (See table 11.2.) The normalized form of the name of a clinical drug may be thought of as being composed of a number of elements, each a concept in its own right. Each element of the normalized form, called the **term type** (TTY), is specifically identified and may include the values listed in table 11.3.

Table 11.2.   Sample of RxNorm dose forms*

Forms	Definitions
Gas for inhalation	A gas that can be breathed into the nose or mouth
Inhalant solution	A finely dispersed liquid medication propelled by gas(es)
Spray	A substance propelled by gas(es)
Nasal spray	A spray intended for use in the nasal cavity
Cream	A homogenous mixture that contains two liquid phases, usually oil in water or water in oil
Nasal cream	A cream intended for use on or in the nasal cavity
Suspension	A nonhomogenous mixture of one or more substances not completely dissolved in a liquid
Injectable suspension	A suspension administered by injection
Capsule	A contained dosage form
Oral capsule	A capsule taken by mouth

* A select few of the dose forms defined in RxNorm are included here to reflect the types of forms that are defined.

Table 11.3.   RxNorm term types

Element	Description	Example
Ingredient (IN)	A compound or moiety that gives the drug its distinctive clinical properties	Fluoxetine
Precise ingredient (PIN)	A specified form of the ingredient that may or may not be clinically active	Fluoxetine hydrochloride
Dose form (DF)	The forms in which drugs may be administered	Oral solution
Semantic clinical drug component (SCDC)	Ingredient plus strength	Fluoxetine 4 mg/ml
Semantic clinical drug form (SCDF)	Ingredient plus dose form	Fluoxetine oral solution
Semantic clinical drug (SCD)	Ingredient plus strength and dose form	Fluoxetine 4 mg/ml oral solution
Brand name (BN)	A proprietary name for a family of products containing a specific active ingredient	Prozac
Semantic branded drug component (SBDC)	Branded ingredient plus strength	Fluoxetine 4 mg/ml (Prozac)
Semantic branded drug form (SBDF)	Branded ingredient plus dose form	Fluoxetine oral solution (Prozac)
Semantic branded drug (SBD)	Ingredient, strength, and dose form plus brand name	Fluoxetine 4 mg/ml oral solution (Prozac)
Synonym (SY)	Synonym of another term type, given for clarity	Prozac 4 mg/ml oral solution

Source: Reprinted courtesy of the National Library of Medicine.

The RxNorm project approached clinical drug representation in a series of steps. The initial effort was to define a semantic normal form (SNF) to represent clinical drugs. SNFs make explicit and/or normalize every active ingredient, strength, unit of measurement, and dosage form for a given clinical drug preparation. Employing both relationships between concepts and attribute-value pairs, the data represent the semantics of a clinical drug concept. SNFs for clinical drugs use standardized (generic) ingredient names, units, and dose forms, in addition to a set of rules for expressing strength in a set of standard units.

Two types of SNFs are created as UMLS concepts for every clinical drug, the **SNF drug component** (SCDC) and the **SNF clinical formulation** (SCD).

The SCDC, consisting of an ingredient and strength:

Form:

> CUI/ShorName/ActiveIngredient/
> PreciseIngredient/Basis/Strength/Units/Notes

Examples:

> C0111111/APAP/Acetaminophen/
> Acetaminophen/B/325/MG/Component
> example#1
> C0123456/Codeine/Codeine Phosphate/
> Codeine/P/30/MG/Component example#2

The SCD, consisting of component(s) (including ingredient and strength) and a dose form:

Form:

> CUI/MetaID/ShortName/Component1/
> Component2/.../OrderableDoseForm/Notes

Example:

> The two SCDCs above can be combined to form the following:

> C0654321/Acetaminophen 325 MG/Codeine
> 30 MG OralCapsule/C0111111/C0123456/
> OralTablet/CF example

RxNorm is organized by **concept.** A concept is a collection of names identical in meaning at this level of abstraction. It serves as a means whereby strings of characters from disparate sources may be taken to name things that are the same. Each concept, or unique meaning, is assigned an RxNorm **concept unique identifier** (RXCUI). An RXCUI always designates the same concept. Drugs whose names map to the same RXCUI are taken to be the same drug or identical as to active ingredients, strengths, and dose forms. Conversely, drugs that differ in any of these particulars are conceptually distinct and will have different RXCUIs. Two drugs, identical in their generic components, may still refer to different concepts when they differ in brand name. (See figure 11.2.)

Within RxNorm, generic and branded normalized forms are related to each other and to the names of their individual components by a well-defined set of named relationships. (See table 11.4.)

In the example in figure 11.2, Acetaminophen 500 MG Oral Tablet is related to Acetaminophen 500 MG Oral Tablet [Tylenol], and both have relationships to Acetaminophen, Acetaminophen 500 MG and Oral Tablet. Also, within the UMLS Metathesaurus, Acetaminophen 500 MG Oral Tablet and Acetaminophen 500 MG Oral Tablet [Tylenol] will each be linked to different names that are used for these entities in other vocabularies.

Relationships between concepts in RxNorm are reciprocal. Each direction of the relationship is represented. A clinical drug consists of components, and the components constitute the clinical drug. (See figure 11.3.)

Figure 11.2. Examples of two distinct concepts

Acetaminophen 500 MG Oral Tablet (for a generic drug name)
Acetaminophen 500 MG Oral Tablet [Tylenol] (for a branded drug name)

Fluoxetine 20 MG Oral Capsule [Prozac]
Fluoxetine 20 MG Oral Capsule [Sarafem]

Table 11.4. RxNorm relationships

Relationship	Definition
constitutes/consists_of	Relationship between an SCD and an SCDC and between an SBD and an SBDC or SCDC
contains/contained_in	Relationship between concepts naming clinical drugs and those naming the devices that dispense them
dose_form_of/has_dose_form	Relationship between a DF and an SCD, SCDF, SBD, or SBDF
form_of/has_form	Relationship between a base ingredient and a precise ingredient
ingredient_of/has_ingredient	Relationship between an IN and an SCDC or SCDF and between a BN and an SBDC, SBD, or SBDF
isa/inverse_isa	Relationship between an SCD and an SCDF and between an SBD and an SBDF
Precise_ingredient_of/has_precise_ingredient	Relationship between an SCDC and a precise ingredient to designate the relationship of the clinical drug to a (usually) nonclinically significant variant of the active ingredient
tradename_of/has_tradename	Relationship between a BN and an IN, between an SBDC and an SCDC, between an SBD and an SCD, or between an SBDF and an SCDF

RxNorm Principles and Guidelines

Specific naming conventions are applied to the term types that are consistent with the definition of each term type. For example, the SCD always contains the active ingredient(s), the strength, and the dose form, in that order. Ingredients named in the SCD, **Semantic Branded Drug** (SBD), and so on are the active ingredients. A distinction is made only for ingredients that have clinical significance. For example, no distinction is made between amoxicillin monosodium salt and amoxicillin potassium salt because the difference is not clinically significant. However, in the case of Penicillin G. Benzathine and Penicillin G. Procaine, the entire compound name is always included as the ingredient.

Figure 11.3. RxNorm concepts and relationships

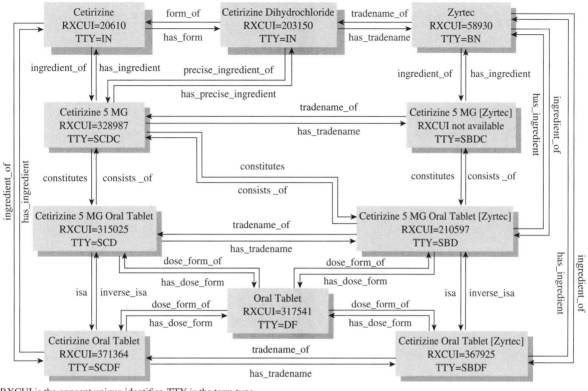

RXCUI is the concept unique identifier. TTY is the term type.
Source: Reprinted courtesy of the National Library of Medicine.

The strengths are based on the active ingredient. In cases where there is more than one active ingredient, a strength will be associated with each ingredient.

Example:

Ascorbic Acid 100 MG/Calcium Carbonate 625 MG/Ferrous Fumarate 122 MG/Folic Acid 1 MG Oral Tablet

In this example, the SCD bears the relationship "consists_of" to each of the several ingredient-strength pairs (essentially SCDCs) separated by slashes.

Only a few units are used in RxNorm in order to standardize the expressions of strength. Where strengths are expressed as ratios, the ratio is given with a denominator value of 1 of the appropriate units. Thus, 100 mg in 5 ml would be expressed as 20 mg/ml. The following units of measurement are used in RxNorm:

MEQ = Milliequivalent

MG = Milligram

ML = Milliliter

MMOL = Millimole

UNT = Unit

% = Used only with gases, otherwise percentages are converted into ratios

The following units appear only in ratios:

ACTUAT = Actuation. Refers to a measured dose per activation of a dispensing devise. For example, in an inhaler, the strength of the clinical drug is given by how much is dispensed with each actuation.

PNU = Protein nitrogen units. Used for allergenic extracts

The following ratios of units have been used in RxNorm:

MEQ/MG

MEQ/ML

MG/ACTUAT

MG/MG

MG/ML

ML/ML

PNU/ML

UNT/MG

UNT/ML

In normalizing terms from other systems to create RxNorm terms, other expressions of units are converted into RxNorm standards. The rules followed are

- Standard conversion factors are used between metric units.

- One liquid ounce is taken to be equivalent to 25 milliliters.

- A grain is 65 milligrams.

When a variable amount of diluent can be used, the minimum amount is used in RxNorm to calculate the concentration that determines the strength. For example, in the case of a drug that can be dissolved in 3 to 5 ml of diluent, RxNorm would use 3 ml. For intravenous solutions, only the initial dilution is used to calculate the strength. For example, a vial containing 50 mg of a drug to be dissolved in 2 ml of water and then added to an IV solution is expressed as having strength of 25 mg/ml.

Strengths are expressed to three significant digits. Thus, nearly equal strengths, which may be expressed differently in different drug vocabularies, are treated as being equivalent. That is, when drug names derived from different source vocabularies would be taken to name the same substance, except for a discrepancy in the strengths, and when the strengths given, upon conversion to common units, are identical to three significant digits, RxNorm treats the names as equivalent and assigns the same RXCUI to each string.

A derivative of RxNorm called RxTerms is available for downloading and testing from the NLM. RxTerms provides drug name information intended for use with e-prescribing and computerized provider order entry (CPOE) applications.

RxNorm Maintenance Process

Drug terminology is constantly changing, with new ingredients, new dosage forms, and new strengths. Additions to the terminology are made as new products are put on the market. The NLM continues to add new clinical drugs and links to additional drug terminologies and to refine the model in response to feedback.

All the RxNorm files are available through the UMLS Knowledge Source Server (UMLSKS). The full set of files will be included in the UMLS Metathesaurus as the primary distribution mechanism. The extraction subsetter of the UMLS, known as MetamorphoSys, can be run to extract an RxNorm subset of the Metathesaurus.

Between releases of the UMLS, RxNorm update files will be made available at the UMLSKS. Updates to RxNorm occurred on a monthly basis until October 2008, when the NLM went to a weekly release. The weekly release is considered to contain new data only and is designed to be used in conjunction with the last full release of RxNorm. A user might choose to obtain the files and add them to the system weekly or monthly. In either case, the files can be viewed as an addition to the existing RxNorm files.

RxNorm Summary

RxNorm is a standard notation for clinical drugs developed by the NLM, the VA, and the FDA, in consultation with the message standards development organization, HL7. It represents drug active ingredients, strength, and dose form and includes various relationships to other drugs, such as equivalencies, trade names, and so on. RxNorm is a nonproprietary terminology that represents drugs at the level of granularity needed to support clinical practice.

Check Your Understanding 11.4

Instructions: Complete the following exercises on a separate piece of paper.

1. Match the following abbreviations with the appropriate description.

   ___ TTY   a. Ingredient plus dose form

   ___ SCD   b. An identifier that is unique for each meaning

   ___ SCDC   c. Ingredient plus strength and dose form

   ___ SCDF   d. Branded ingredient plus dose form

   ___ SBDC   e. Branded ingredient plus strength

   ___ SBDF   f. Element of the normalized form of a clinical drug name

   ___ RXCUI   g. Ingredient plus strength

2. Which of the following statements is true?
   a. In RxNorm, two drugs, identical in their generic components, may still refer to different concepts if they differ in brand name.
   b. More than 100 dose forms are defined in RxNorm.
   c. The SCDC always contains the active ingredient(s), the strength, and the dose form, though not necessarily in that order.
   d. Only dose forms are named in the SCD.

3. Files updating RxNorm are released available _____ through the UMLS.
   a. Weekly
   b. Monthly
   c. Quarterly
   d. Yearly

NDF-RT

The VANDF is a centrally maintained electronic formulary used by every VA medical center nationwide. This national drug file provides standardization of the local drug files in all VA medical facilities. Standardization includes the adoption of new drug no-menclature and drug classification, as well as linking the local drug file entries to data in the national drug files.

For drugs approved by the FDA, the VANDF has provided the VA medical facilities with the ability to access information concerning dosage form, strength and unit, package size and type, manufacturer's trade name, and NDC information. VA facilities have used the VANDF to check drug interactions, manage orders, and send outpatient prescriptions (57 million in 2001) to seven regional automated mail-out pharmacies (Nelson et al. 2002).

The National Drug File–Reference Terminology (NDF-RT) was created from the VANDF to increase functionality, improve quality, and decrease the cost of maintaining the VANDF. Maintenance of the VANDF was largely a manual process, with up to 4,000 NDC-level edits per month. Mapping of drug products in the VANDF to local formularies also was a manual process. To reduce maintenance costs and mapping efforts, the VA decided to create a formal drug reference terminology with imbedded drug knowledge information.

NDF-RT is built on a core of RxNorm. Each NDF-RT entry for a clinical drug or a drug component is linked to its counterpart in RxNorm (although not every drug in RxNorm appears in NDF-RT because not all RxNorm medications are used in the VA health system). RxNorm and NDF-RT were built collaboratively, with NDF-RT adding a more formal representation model and additional types of drug information. NDF-RT augments the RxNorm entries with drug class, mechanism of action, physiologic effect, therapeutic intent, clinical kinetics, and chemical structure.

NDF-RT Content

NDF-RT is the terminology used by FDA and the FedMed collaboration to code these essential pharmacologic properties of medications:

Mechanism of Action

Physiologic Effect

Structural Class

The October 2008 release contains 136,051 concepts.

The NDF-RT contains a novel reference hierarchy to describe the **physiologic effects** (PEs) of drugs. The PE reference hierarchy contains 1,699 concepts arranged in two broad categories: organ-specific and generalized systemic effects. The PE reference hierarchy was originally seeded with candidate concepts extracted from the Chemical Actions subtree of **Medical Subjects Headings** (MeSH), the controlled vocabulary thesaurus of the NLM. These were reviewed, refined, and supplemented by subject matter experts to create the 1,699 concepts currently in the PE reference hierarchy (Rosenbloom et al. 2003).

The concepts in the PE hierarchy are arranged in a tree structure with some concepts residing in multiple branches of the hierarchy. The first level of branching segregates concepts used to describe organ-specific effects from concepts that describe systemic effects. Subsequent branching segregates the individual organs and the organ-specific physiologic processes (such as bronchodilation) from the individual classes of systemic physiologic processes (such as "decreased protein synthesis"). The PE reference hierarchy models intermediary processes that occur as a result of specific molecular interactions leading to intended therapeutic applications (or side effects). Figure 11.4 presents an example of an NDF-RT physiologic effects hierarchy.

Figure 11.4.   NDF-RT physiologic effects hierarchy example

Physiologic effects
    Generalized systemic effects
    Organ-system-specific effects
        Cardiovascular activity alteration
           Cardiac contractility alteration
             Positive inotropy

The concept *positive inotropy* describes a physiologic effect of digoxin. Positive inotropy is a type of cardiac contractility alteration, which is in turn a cardiovascular activity alteration (Rosenbloom 2003).

NDF-RT Maintenance Process

Ongoing development and maintenance of NDF-RT is supported under the VA's Enterprise Reference Terminology project, a major initiative tied to the VA's Health Data Repository and computerized patient record system. The VA plans to maintain NDF-RT so that it remains fully integrated with RxNorm. NDF-RT is disseminated to the public through the UMLS Metathesaurus.

Check Your Understanding 11.5

Instructions: On a separate piece of paper, indicate whether the following statements are true or false.

1. One of the reasons for creating NDF-RT was to control maintenance costs.

2. The VANDF was used to initially populate NDF-RT.

3. NDF-RT was developed by the NLM in consultation with the VA and the FDA.

4. NDF-RT is a drug reference terminology with imbedded drug knowledge.

5. NDF-RT is built on a core of RxNorm.

6. Every drug in RxNorm appears in NDF-RT.

7. All VA drug products are included in NDF-RT.

8. The VA intends to include only drug products from the VA formulary in the NDF-RT.

9. NDF-RT is disseminated to the public through the UMLS Metathesaurus.

Drug Terminology and Drug Knowledge Bases Working Together

RxNorm's standard names for clinical drugs are connected to the varying names of drugs present in many different controlled vocabularies within the UMLS Metathesaurus, including NDF-RT and those in commercially available DKBs. These connections are intended to facilitate interoperability among the

Figure 11.5.   Drug terminologies

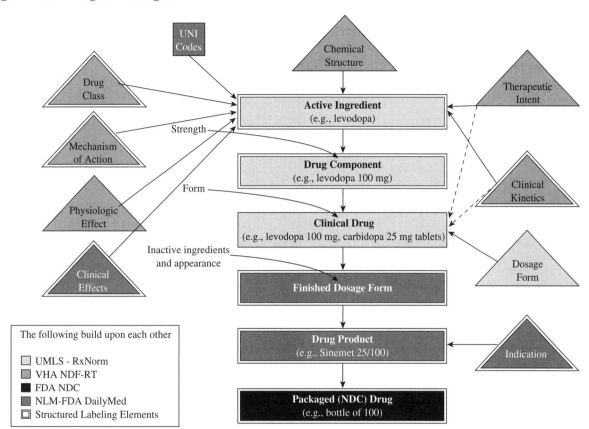

Created by Margaret Amatayakul for NCVHS, 072404

Source: Adapted from U.S. Government Drug Terminology, Randy Levin, MD, Director, Office of Information Management Center for Drug Evaluation and Research, Food and Drug Administration. http://www.ncvhs.gov/040730pl.pdf.

computerized systems that record or process data dealing with clinical drugs.

Figure 11.5 depicts drug information from various sources and illustrates how they build on and interact with each other. Each triangle represents a different level of specificity with respect to information about a particular drug.

Both a controlled terminology of clinical drugs and DKBs are needed to fulfill the myriad clinical and administrative needs related to drug information.

RxNorm is a reference terminology (that is, it has formal definitions, formal relationships, reference taxonomy, and mapping), and does not include drug knowledge. NDF-RT also is a reference terminol-

ogy (it also has formal definitions based on description logic) and includes drug knowledge at the level needed to support pharmacy applications in the VA, primarily disease-based interactions.

Commercial DKBs are not considered reference terminologies (they do not support formal definitions). However, they do include in-depth DKBs based on years of experience and research, including, for example, drug-to-drug interactions with literature references and patient information sheets.

RxNorm serves as a translator for NDF-RT and commercial DKBs, the latter of which are often used in EHR systems as knowledge sources for drug decision support. Each of these systems is useful and may be necessary to achieve fully functional and interoperable EHRs. Because RxNorm and NDF-RT are used more widely and interact with commercial DKBs, the unique functions of each of these systems are expected to become more clearly delineated.

Summary

Drug terminology systems are particularly complex, primarily because they address multiple core concepts and because of the rapid rate of change in drug terms.

Several commercial DKB vendors, such as First DataBank, Medi-Span, Micromedex, and Multum, provide comprehensive drug databases with product-specific information and other encoded knowledge that supports clinical functions pertaining to drug therapy. These drug databases are designed to support specific pharmacy applications but do not necessarily fit the model for a controlled vocabulary.

The National Library of Medicine's RxNorm is a nonproprietary terminology that represents drugs at the level of granularity needed to support clinical practice. RxNorm is mapped to NDF-RT as well as to commercial DKBs, including First DataBank, Medi-Span, Micromedex, and Multum. Thus, RxNorm allows various systems using different DKBs to share data efficiently. It acts as a bridge between DKBs and enterprise-wide systems.

The Veterans Administration's NDF-RT is a reference terminology that includes drug knowledge, particularly disease-based information. NDF-RT was based on the VA's national drug file, an electronic formulary. NDF-RT uses RxNorm as the clinical core but adds a more formal representation model and additional types of drug information. NDF-RT augments the RxNorm entries with drug class, mechanism of action, physiologic effect, therapeutic intent, clinical kinetics, and chemical structure.

Drug terminologies and DKBs each serve a unique purpose. The various commercial DKBs serve different markets and sets of users. To achieve the full potential for EHR applications, multiple systems with unique functions and interoperability are necessary.

References

Alchemy. 2008. Gold Standards. http://www.alchemyrx.com/DrugProduct_PricingFiles.htm.

American Health Information Community. 2008. AHIC Use Cases and Extension/Gaps. http://www.hhs.gov/healthit/usecases/.

American Health Information Community. 2008a. Medication Gaps. http://www.hhs.gov/healthit/usecases/medgaps.html.

Bodenreider, Olivier. 2008. RxNav: Interfaces to drug information sources. Lister Hill National Center for Biomedical Communications, National Library of Medicine. http://mor.nlm.nih.gov/pubs/pres/080801-NLM_BBL.pdf.

Carter, J. S., et al. 2002. Initializing the VA medication reference terminology using UMLS Metathesaurus co-occurrences. In *Proceedings of the 2002 AMIA Annual Symposium*, pp. 116–120. San Antonio, TX: American Medical Informatics Association.

Cimino, James J. 1999. Evaluation of a proposed method for representing drug terminology. In *Proceedings of the 1999 AMIA Annual Symposium*, pp. 47–51. Washington, DC: American Medical Informatics Association.

Certification Commission for Healthcare Information Technology. 2008. Electronic Health Records Criteria. http://www.cchit.org/certify/index.asp.

Consolidated Health Informatics Initiative. 2006. Standards Adoption Recommendation: Allergy. http://www.hhs.gov/healthit/chiinitiative.html.

Department of Health and Human Services. 2008 (April 7). Final Rule on Standards for E-Prescribing Under Medicare Part D and Identification of Backward Compatible Version of Adopted Standard for E-Prescribing and the Medicare Prescription Drug Program. *Federal Register*. http://edocket.access.gpo.gov/2008/pdf/08-1094.pdf.

Healthcare Information Technology Standards Panel. 2008 (August 7). HITSP Medication Management Interoperability Specification. http://www.hitsp.org/ConstructSet_Details.aspx?&PrefixAlpha=1&PrefixNumeric=07.

Kim, Julia M., and Paul Frosdick. 2001. Description of a drug hierarchy in a concept-based reference terminology. In *Proceedings of the 2001 AMIA Annual Symposium*, pp. 314–319.Washington, DC: American Medical Informatics Association.

Lau, L., and S. Lam. 1999. Applying the desiderata for controlled medical vocabularies to drug information databases. In *Proceedings of the 1999 AMIA Annual Symposium,* pp. 97–101. Washington, DC: American Medical Informatics Association.

National Committee on Vital and Health Statistics. 2003a. Meeting minutes of the NCVHS Subcommittee on Standards and Security, August 19-21 and October 30. http://www.ncvhs.hhs.gov/030819mn.htm and http://www.ncvhs.hhs.gov/031030tr.htm, respectively.

National Committee on Vital and Health Statistics. 2003b. Letter to the secretary, recommendations for PMRI terminology standards. http://www.ncvhs.hhs.gov/031105lt3.pdf.

Nelson, Stuart J., et al. 2002. A semantic normal form for clinical drugs in the UMLS: Early experiences with the VANDF. In *Proceedings of the 2002 AMIA Annual Symposium,* pp. 557–561. San Antonio, TX: American Medical Informatics Association.

Rosenbloom, Trent S., et al. 2003. Adequacy of representation of the national drug file reference terminology physiologic effects reference hierarchy for commonly prescribed medications. In *Proceedings of the 2003 AMIA Annual Symposium*, pp. 569–573. Washington, DC: American Medical Informatics Association.

Solomon, W. D., et al. 1999. A reference terminology for drugs. In *Proceedings of the 1999 AMIA Annual Symposium*, pp. 152–156. Washington, DC: American Medical Informatics Association.

Application Exercises

1. Go to http://www.nlm.nih.gov/research/umls/ and find the current size, version, or next release of Rx-Norm.

2. Perform an Internet search for a computerized order entry (CPOE) decision support tool and determine whether a drug terminology or DKB is embedded.

3. Why is a DKB insufficient without a controlled drug terminology?

Review Quiz

1. True or False. Drug terminologies are typically updated twice a year.

2. Which of the following concepts is important for interoperability with pharmacy systems?
   a. Active ingredients
   b. Routed generic
   c. Manufactured drug
   d. Packaged product

3. Which of the following concepts is most important for allergy checking?
   a. Active ingredients
   b. Clinical drug
   c. Routed generic
   d. Manufactured drug

4. True or False. The concept of clinical drug includes the generic name and route of administration.

5. Which of the following is a route of administration of a drug?
   a. Tablet
   b. Liquid
   c. Powder
   d. Inhaled

6. True or False. NDC codes are useful for electronic exchange of information at the package level.

7. Which of the following is a nonproprietary drug reference terminology?
   a. NDF-RT
   b. First DataBank
   c. Medi-Span
   d. Micromedex

8. Which of the following DKBs originated as a monthly drug pricing publication?
   a. First DataBank
   b. Micromedex
   c. Medi-Span
   d. Multum

9. The Consolidated Health Initiative has named a set of drug terminologies among its standards. Which of the following is true in that regard?
   a. NDF-RT was named as a standard for describing clinical drugs.
   b. RxNorm was named as a standard for specific drug classifications.
   c. The portion of NDF-RT that represents a mechanism of action and physiologic effects of drugs was named.
   d. Micromedex was named as a standard for drug reference data.

10. True or False. An NDC is not stored as an attribute of the clinical drug in RxNorm.

11. In RxNorm, the form of a clinical drug is based on which of the following?
    a. The size of the package
    b. How the manufacturer supplied it
    c. What a clinician might order
    d. All of the above

12. Who initiated the development of RxNorm?
    a. HL7
    b. NLM
    c. VA
    d. FDA

13. NDF-RT was created from which of the following?
    a. VANDF
    b. NDC
    c. FDA formulary
    d. RxNorm

14. Reference hierarchies to describe mechanisms of action are included in which system?
    a. RxNorm
    b. NDF-RT
    c. First DataBank
    d. Micromedex

15. Which of the following is a central electronic formulary?
    a. VANDF
    b. NDF-RT
    c. RxNorm
    d. NDC

Chapter 12

Terminologies Used in Nursing Practice

Judith J. Warren, PhD, RN, BC, FAAN, FACMI

Learning Objectives

- To describe the historical evolution of terminology and vocabulary systems associated with the nursing profession

- To recognize the names and purpose of nursing terminologies, including:

    —North American Nursing Diagnosis Association, International (NANDA)

    —Nursing Interventions Classification System (NIC)

    —Nursing Outcomes Classification System (NOC)

    —Clinical Care Classification (CCC)

    —Omaha System

    —International Classification for Nursing Practice (ICNP®)

- To illustrate how selected nursing terminologies compare with other terminologies and vocabularies used in healthcare systems

Key Terms

Comité Européen de Normalisation (CEN), or European Committee for Standardization

Controlled vocabulary

Domain

International Organization for Standardization (ISO)

Likert scale

Nursing informatics

Nursing Information and Data Set Evaluation Center (NIDSEC)

Taxonomy

Introduction

Nurses represent the largest group of organized professionals in many countries, including the United States. Nurse informaticists play a critical role in terminology and classification systems related to nursing care within the healthcare system worldwide. National and international professional associations collaborate on the development of systems created for a variety of nursing purposes.

General medical terminologies fail to represent the broadest clinical concepts needed in nursing care (Shortliffe et al. 2001). The **domain** of **nursing informatics** is gradually merging with other health informatics disciplines to ensure holistic representation of patient information management needs as more electronic data systems are deployed. According to Kathleen A. McCormick, "The open system architecture that the Internet provides is offering additional solutions to the integration of (nursing) vocabularies" (Ball et al. 2000, 110).

This chapter first discusses the history of nursing terminology and vocabulary development and then describes the elements of the key taxonomies currently in use.

History of Nursing-Related Terminology, Vocabulary, and Informatics

Formalized nursing terminology applications began in the late 1970s with the use of computers to support nursing care. One of the first books to describe computers and their relationship to nursing and healthcare was *Using Computers in Nursing*, by Marion Ball and Kathryn Hannah, published in 1984.

In 1991, the American Nurses Association (ANA) formed a committee to review and recognize nursing languages. This work laid the foundation for the growing knowledge of terminology standards for nursing practices. All the terminologies discussed in this chapter have been recognized by the ANA as useful in the support of nursing practice. Work continues to refine nursing terminologies for standards that represent important clinical information generated and/or used by nursing staff for patient care and other administrative functions.

The first terminology systems developed for nursing were called **controlled vocabularies.**

By definition, problems occur in applying a **controlled vocabulary** for too broad a purpose, so the number of nursing terminologies has increased over time. Clearly, there is a need in nursing, as in other areas of healthcare, for a mechanism to resolve problems resulting from the use of diverse terminologies. Thus, work continues to further harmonize nursing terminologies and/or to employ a reference terminology to serve as an interlingua between them (Spackman, Campbell, and Cote 1997).

A number of standards organizations, such as the **Comité Européen de Normalisation,** or **European Committee for Standardization** (CEN), the International Organization for Standardization (ISO), the **International Health Terminology Standards Development Organisation** (IHTSDO), and the U.S. Nursing Terminology Summit, are working collaboratively to achieve greater harmony between nursing terminologies and other vocabularies used in healthcare applications. This work is expected to culminate in greater synchrony as more electronic health record (EHR) systems are used to document and store patient information.

Academic preparation for a career in nursing informatics requires special training in addition to nursing education up to and including master- and doctorate-level degrees with a concentration or specialization in designated domains. Standards for the practice of nursing informatics have been developed for use and a certification examination developed to credential informatics nurses as evidence of competency in this field. Updated in 2008, the *Scope and Standards of Nursing Informatics Practice* is available from the ANA. More information on nursing informatics practice and certification can be found at http://nursingworld.org/books/pdescr .cfm?CNum=3.

Developer, Purpose, Content, Guidelines, and Maintenance for Nursing Terminologies

The developers of nursing terminologies are agencies or professional organizations with an interest in the use of terminology or vocabulary in a specific nursing domain. As each terminology is discussed in subsequent sections of this chapter, the developing body is listed and background information is provided about development and/or maintenance details.

Several of the nursing terminologies discussed in this chapter are listed as source vocabularies in the Unified Medical Language System (UMLS) hosted by the National Library of Medicine (NLM). The most current listing can be found at http://www.nlm.nih.gov/research/umls/sources_by_categories.html.

The ANA, through the Committee for Nursing Practice Information Infrastructure (CNPII), recognizes twelve terminologies to be appropriate for clinical practice. These terminologies are (Warren and Bakken 2002)

- ABC Codes
- Clinical Care Classification (CCC) (formerly Home Health Care Classification [HHCC])
- International Classification for Nursing Practice (ICNP)
- Logical Observation Identifiers, Names, and Codes (LOINC)
- North American Nursing Diagnosis Association, International (NANDA)
- Nursing Interventions Classification (NIC)
- Nursing Management Minimum Data Set (NMMDS)
- Nursing Minimum Data Sets (NMDS)
- Nursing Outcomes Classification (NOC)
- Omaha System
- Perioperative Nursing Dataset
- Systematized Nomenclature of Medicine, Clinical Terminology (SNOMED-CT)

These current terminologies are used in conjunction with the nursing minimum data set and the natural language found in traditional documentation and information management structures. The **Nursing Information and Data Set Evaluation Center** (NIDSEC) requires their use before a vendor's product is recognized as being sensitive to nursing care.

NANDA International

The NANDA classification is a set of nursing diagnoses adopted by the North American Nursing Diagnosis Association, International. This system describes patients' responses to diseases rather than classifying the conditions of diseases and disorders. The NANDA classification is organized around thirteen domains:

- Health promotion
- Nutrition
- Elimination/Exchange
- Activity/Rest
- Perception/Cognition
- Self-perception
- Role relationship
- Sexuality
- Coping/Stress tolerance
- Life principles
- Safety/Protection
- Comfort
- Growth/Development

Within each domain, NANDA lists two or more classes, for example:

Within the Self-perception domain are the following classes: "Self-Concept, Self-Esteem, and Body Image" (NANDA 2007). The diagnoses are classified into the classes. The coding structure is for the nursing diagnoses only, consisting of five digits and carrying no meaning in order to conform with best coding practices.

NANDA International is committed to increasing the visibility of nursing's contribution to patient care by developing, refining, and classifying phenomena of concern to nurses. It is a pioneer in the field of nursing diagnosis classification and standardized language and was the first to be recognized by ANA. This work enables documentation of nursing practice and facilitates aggregation and analysis to build the body of knowledge related to nursing science.

The Vision of NANDA International

For development of the discipline, the NANDA International board believes that

- Nursing diagnosis is seen as an essential component of any professional nursing–client interaction.

- NANDA International is recognized as a major contributor to nursing knowledge development through the identification and use of concepts that are the building blocks of nursing science.

- NANDA International is recognized as the leader in the development and classification of nursing diagnoses (NANDA 2005).

Organization of the NANDA International nursing diagnoses has evolved from an alphabetical listing in the mid-1980s to a conceptual system that guides the classification of nursing diagnoses in a multi-axial **taxonomy.** The NANDA International Taxonomy II is now available in its entirety in the 2007–2008 edition of *NANDA Diagnoses: Definitions and Classification* and is on a two-year update cycle.

The ANA recognizes NANDA as one of the standardized languages of nursing. NANDA also meets the guidelines for information system (IS) vendors in its NIDSEC mentioned earlier. Moreover, NANDA is

- In the NLM's Metathesaurus

- In the Cumulative Index of Nursing and Allied Health Literature (CINAHL)

- One nursing classification system that can be used to meet the Joint Commission standard on uniform data

- Registered in Health Level Seven (HL7)

- Mapped into SNOMED

Several countries outside the United States use NANDA, and it has been translated into a number of languages. NANDA is widely used in major nursing textbooks. It is the foundation of nursing care planning and is most often used in conjunction with NIC and NOC to provide coverage for the nursing care process and plans. More information on NANDA can be found online at http://www.nanda.org.

Check Your Understanding 12.1

Instructions: Complete the following exercises on a separate piece of paper.

1. The first terminology systems developed for nursing were considered
   a. Taxonomies
   b. Controlled vocabularies
   c. Classification systems
   d. Heuristics

2. Formalized terminology in nursing began in which time period?
   a. In the 1990s with the release of the textbook *Using Computers in Nursing*
   b. In the twenty-first century with the routine use of the Internet
   c. In the late 1970s when computers began to be used in some healthcare settings
   d. With implementation of diagnosis-related groups in 1983

Nursing Interventions Classification

The Nursing Interventions Classification (NIC) is a standardized classification of interventions that nurses do on behalf of patients in all care domains.

An intervention is defined as "any treatment, based upon clinical judgment and knowledge, that a nurse performs to enhance patient/client outcomes" (University of Iowa 2009).

NIC has many uses, including those related directly to patient care such as clinical documentation and communication of care across settings, as well as management aspects, including productivity measurement and competency evaluation. Additionally, it has been referenced in textbooks to discuss nursing treatments and utilized by researchers to study the effectiveness of nursing care. NIC also has been implemented in nursing information systems and nursing education programs to structure curricula and to identify competencies of graduating nurses.

NIC is not limited to a specific setting or to only the domain of nursing. This system contains interventions done by other nonphysician providers and thus describes their treatments. The system describes interventions for illness treatment, illness prevention, and health promotion for use with individuals, families, and communities. Included with each intervention is a label name, a definition, a unique number (code), a set of activities to carry out the intervention, and background readings.

The fifth edition of NIC contains 542 interventions organized into thirty classes and seven domains. The domains are

- Physiological: Basic
- Physiological: Complex
- Behavioral
- Safety
- Family
- Health system
- Community

NIC has been on a publication update cycle of approximately every four years since 1992. However, an ongoing process for feedback and review has been established and modifications to existing interventions or proposals for a new intervention are accepted between editions.

The ANA recognizes NIC as one of the standardized languages of nursing. NIC also meets the guidelines for IS vendors in its NIDSEC mentioned earlier. Moreover, NIC is

- In the NLM's Metathesaurus
- In the Cumulative Index of Nursing and Allied Health Literature (CINAHL)
- One nursing classification system that can be used to meet the Joint Commission standard on uniform data
- In Alternative Link's ABC codes used for reimbursement for alternative care providers (see chapter 14 for more information on ABC codes)
- Registered in Health Level Seven (HL7)
- Mapped into SNOMED

Several countries outside the United States have expressed interest in NIC, and it has been translated into a number of languages. For additional information about NIC, go to http://www.nursing.uiowa.edu/excellence/nursing_knowledge/clinical_effectiveness/index.htm.

Nursing Outcomes Classification

The Nursing Outcomes Classification (NOC) is a standardized classification of outcomes developed for use in all settings and with all patient populations. It was developed to evaluate the outcomes of nursing interventions. An outcome is "a measurable individual, family, or community state, behavior, or perception that is measured along a continuum and is responsive to nursing interventions" (University of Iowa 2009).

NOC has many of the same uses as NIC, including clinical documentation, nursing education, and research. Clinical sites are using NOC in their evaluations of nursing practice and educational institutions to structure curricula and teach students clinical evaluation. It is possible to apply NOC across the care continuum to follow patient outcomes over an extended time. However, NOC is not limited to the domain of nursing. Other nonphysician providers may find NOC outcomes valuable in evaluating their interventions.

The third edition of NOC contains 330 outcomes grouped in a coded taxonomy that arranges them within a conceptual framework. The following are included with each outcome:

- A definition

- A list of indicators for evaluating patient status in relation to outcome

- A target outcome rating

- A place to identify the source of data

- A five-point **Likert scale** to measure patient status

- A short list of references used in developing the outcome

Some of the outcomes include an additional measurement scale.

The third edition of NOC describes outcome levels for individuals (311), families (10), and communities (9) grouped into thirty-one classes and seven domains. The domains are

- Functional health

- Physiologic health

- Psychosocial health

- Health knowledge and behavior

- Perceived health

- Family health

- Community health

Included with each outcome is a unique code number that facilitates its use in clinical information systems.

NOC is published every four years. However, regular updates are made for any necessary modifications to existing outcomes or to include new outcomes.

The ANA recognizes NOC as one of the standardized languages of nursing. NOC also meets the guidelines for IS vendors in the ANA's NIDSEC. Additionally, NOC is

- In the NLM's Metathesaurus

- Approved for use by HL7

- Currently being mapped into SNOMED

Several countries outside the United States have expressed interest in NOC, and it has been translated into a number of languages.

NOC's Web address is http://www.nursing.uiowa .edu/excellence/nursing_knowledge/clinical _effectiveness/index.htm

---

Check Your Understanding 12.2

Instructions: Complete the following exercises on a separate piece of paper.

1. Which of the following statements is false?
   a. NOC outcomes are grouped in a coded taxonomy that arranges the outcomes within a conceptual framework.
   b. NIC and NOC are used for the same purpose.
   c. NIC is included in Joint Commission accreditation standards.
   d. NOC is recognized by the ANA as one of the standardized languages of nursing.

2. What is the purpose behind development of the NOC system?
   a. To provide separate reimbursement for nursing care
   b. To create a taxonomy for classifying nursing assessments
   c. To expedite adoption of an EHR specific to nursing care
   d. To evaluate the outcomes of nursing interventions

Clinical Care Classification

Clinical Care Classification (CCC) was previously known as the Home Health Care Classification (HHCC) system. The CCC system consists of two interrelated taxonomies: the CCC of Nursing Diagnoses and Outcomes, and the CCC of Nursing Interventions and Actions. Both taxonomies are classified by care components, or clusters of elements, that represent behavioral, functional, physiological, or psychological care patterns that provide a framework and a unique coding structure for the following purposes (Saba 2005):

- Mapping and linking the two taxonomies to each other and to other health-related classifications

- Assessing, documenting, and classifying patient care in hospitals, home health agencies, ambulatory care clinics, and other healthcare settings

The CCC system came about from the Home Care Project (HCFA No: 17C-98983/3) conducted by Virginia K. Saba and colleagues in 1991 at the Georgetown University School of Nursing. The purpose of the project was to develop a methodology for evaluating and classifying patients to determine what resources are required when providing home health services to the Medicare population.

Current Uses and Status of the CCC System

The two CCC taxonomies are tools that aid documentation of care. This informatics tool serves as a language for nursing and other health services (physical, occupational, and speech therapy; medical social worker; and home health aide) because data capture is enabled at the point of care. Examples of the uses of this system include

- Documentation of integrated care processes

- Classification and tracking of clinical care

- Development of evidence-based practice models

- Analysis of patient profiles and populations

- Prediction of care needs and resources

Use of this system also enables research and education and supports the creation and use of electronic clinical pathways and protocols used in healthcare delivery information systems.

The CCC of Nursing Diagnoses and the CCC of Nursing Interventions were formally "recognized" by the ANA in 1991. The ANA endorsed these terminology tools as nursing taxonomies critical to nursing practice and supported and promoted their use in EHRs. The taxonomies are registered as HL7 languages and integrated into LOINC, SNOMED RT, and NLM's UMLS Metathesaurus. They also are indexed in the CINAHL. In addition, the CCC taxonomies are (Saba 2005)

- The basis for the ICNP developed by the International Council of Nurses (ICN) and are referenced in the Integration of a Reference Terminology Model for Nurses (ISO 18104)

- Approved by the ISO Technical Committee (TC) 215 Working Group 3 Concept Representation

- Approved by home health agencies as Medicare Rules Coverage and Conditions of Participation, and also linked to HCFA Forms 485/486, and the home health prospective payment system (PPS)

- Available in the public domain, even though they are copyrighted (although their use requires written permission)

There is no specific schedule for updates and revisions of the taxonomies. Content will be revised as clinical requirements change in nursing documentation.

For additional information about the CCC system, go to http://www.sabacare.com

Omaha System

The Omaha System was originally developed by the Omaha Visiting Nurses Association (VNA). Practicing clinicians employed by the VNA of Omaha and seven diverse test sites located throughout the United States collected actual patient and family data and submitted them for inclusion in the Omaha System.

Numerous other individuals and groups participated in the research as advisory committee members and consultants. From the beginning of the Omaha System's development, the terms, codes, and definitions were not copyrighted; thus, they are equally accessible to practitioners, administrators, students, faculty, and other potential users.

The Omaha System is a comprehensive practice and documentation tool used by nurses, other healthcare providers, and students from the time of client admission to discharge in the home health setting. The system includes the following components:

- Assessment (Problem Classification Scheme)

- Intervention (Intervention Scheme)

- Outcomes (Problem Rating Scale for Outcomes)

These components provide a structure for documenting client needs and strengths, relating clinician interventions, and measuring client outcomes in a simple, yet comprehensive, manner. When the three components are used together, the Omaha System offers a way to link clinical data to demographic, financial, administrative, and staffing data.

Using the Omaha System is comparable to arranging the diverse pieces of a puzzle into a completed picture. When it is implemented accurately and consistently, the data generated describe client needs, related interventions, and client outcomes, as well as interactions among those data. Automated documentation systems based on the Omaha System provide a powerful information management tool for data collection, aggregation, and analysis (Omaha System 2005).

The Omaha system was one of the first vocabularies recognized by the ANA in 1990. Additionally, it is in the

- NLM's Metathesaurus

- ANSI HISB Inventory of Clinical Information Standards

- Accreditation standards of the Joint Commission

- Community Health Accreditation Program

- SNOMED-CT

The Omaha System is also recognized by HL7.

This system has been used internationally. The pocket guide was translated into Japanese in 1997; other translations are being discussed for the next book. The system's terms, codes, and definitions have been translated into a number of languages.

The terms, codes, and definitions of the Omaha System are not copyrighted. Individuals who use or write about the Omaha System should reference the source. Software based on the Omaha System also must follow copyright laws in order to use the system.

In 2001, a twelve-member Omaha System Advisory Board consisting of representatives from diverse service and educational settings was formed to develop an action plan to review and revise the Omaha System based on comments from survey results of current research and suggestions from users. The goal was to include the revision in the next book about the Omaha System. The most recent edition includes revised terms and definitions, information on how to use the system in diverse settings, and eighteen case studies illustrating terms used in the system (Martin 2004). Currently, there is no scheduled process for updates. See http:// www.omahasystem.org/ for additional information.

Check Your Understanding 12.3

Instructions: Complete the following exercises on a separate piece of paper.

1. The Clinical Care Classification system
   a. Classifies acute care hospital episodes into diagnosis-related groups
   b. Was developed entirely from private funding and is a proprietary system
   c. Is not yet part of the Unified Medical Language System (UMLS)
   d. Resulted from work performed for a home care project initiated by the Centers for Medicare and Medicaid Services (formally the Health Care Financing Administration)

2. A comprehensive practice and documentation tool used by nurses providing home healthcare is called
    a. HHCC (Home Healthcare Classification)
    b. Nursing Intervention for Clinical Care (NICC)
    c. OMAHA System
    d. The last vocabulary system recognized by the ANA

International Classification for Nursing Practice

The **International Classification for Nursing Practice** (ICNP) is a unified nursing language system. It is a compositional terminology for nursing practice that facilitates cross-mapping of local terms and existing terminologies. Cross-mapping allows comparison of nursing data collected using other recognized nursing vocabularies and classification systems. ICNP can be used to represent nursing diagnoses, interventions, and outcomes.

The **International Council of Nurses** (ICN) is a federation of 132 national nurses' associations representing millions of nurses worldwide (http://www.icn.ch). ICN has supported the development of ICNP since 1989 and established the ICNP Programme in 2000. ICNP is copyrighted by ICN. Permission to use, translate, publish, and reproduce the terminology is granted on a case-by-case basis. Some uses require a licensing fee; others are free of charge. The 2005 release of ICNP Version 1.0 was a major change for the terminology. This version was developed using Web ontology language (OWL) in the Protégé software environment to support a unified language and compositional approach. A description logics approach allows for explicit definitions, the possibility of multiple classifications, greater granularity, and sensitivity to variation in language and culture. ICNP Version 1.1, with a new browser and added content, was released in July 2008. ICNP Version 2.0 is scheduled for release in 2009. Table 12.1 lists the release history of ICNP.

ICNP envisions being an integral part of the global information infrastructure informing healthcare practice and policy to improve patient care world-

Table 12.1. ICNP® releases

Title	Date Published/Released
ICNP® Alpha Version	1996
ICNP® Beta Version	1999
ICNP® Beta 2 Version	2001
ICNP® Version 1.0	2005
ICNP® Version 1.1	2008

Source: ICN.

wide. It can serve as a major force to articulate nursing's contribution to health and healthcare globally and promote harmonization with other widely used classifications and the work of standardization groups in health and nursing. (http://www.icn.ch/icnp_ben.htm; accessed 19 November 2008)

ICNP represents nursing concepts used in local, regional, national, and international practice, across specialties, languages, and cultures. Using information about nursing practice, ICNP supports decision making, education, and policy in the areas of patient needs, nursing interventions, health outcomes, and resource utilization. ICNP improves communication in healthcare and encourages nurses to reflect on their own practice and influence improvements in quality of care.

ICNP Version 1.1 is represented in seven axes, all of which describe some aspect of nursing practice. The axes are defined as follows (ICN 2005):

- *Focus:* The area of attention that is relevant to nursing (for example, pain, homelessness, elimination, life expectancy, knowledge)

- *Judgment:* Clinical opinion or determination related to the focus of nursing practice (for example, decreasing level, risk, enhanced, interrupted, abnormal)

- *Means:* A manner or method of accomplishing an intervention (for example, bandage, bladder-training technique, nutritionist service)

- *Action:* An intentional process applied to or performed by a client (for example, educating, changing, administering, monitoring)

- *Time:* The point, period, instance, interval, or duration of an occurrence (for example, admission, childbirth, chronic)

- *Location:* Anatomical and spatial orientation of a diagnosis or intervention (for example, posterior, abdomen, school, community health center)

- *Client:* Subject to which a diagnosis refers and who is the recipient of an intervention (for example, newborn, caregiver, family, community)

Figure 12.1 (see page 196) shows the results of a code search on "intermittent" found in the Time Axis using the ICNP Version 1.1 browser.

Specific guidelines have been recommended in order to create nursing diagnosis, intervention, or outcome statements. According to ICN (2005), when using the 7-Axis Model to compose a diagnosis

- A term from the Focus Axis is required.

- A term from the Judgment Axis is required.

- Additional terms from the Focus, Judgment, and other axes are included, as needed.

Table 12.2 provides an example of a combination of concepts from selected axes for the nursing diagnosis of chronic constipation.

The same guidelines are used to create a nursing outcome.

A different set of guidelines is used when identifying a nursing intervention. The rules for creating a nursing intervention are as follows (ICN 2005):

- A term from the Action Axis is required.

- At least one target term is required. Target terms come from other axes with the exception of the Judgment Axis.

- Additional terms from the Action and other axes are included, as needed.

Table 12.3 provides examples of nursing interventions.

Table 12.2. Nursing diagnosis

Select AXES	Select CONCEPTS
Focus	Constipation
Judgment	Actual
Time	Chronic
Nursing diagnosis: Chronic constipation	

Source: ICN 2005.

To provide nursing professionals with a practical way to use ICNP at the point of care, ICN is collaborating with nurses and specialty organizations to develop ICNP Catalogues or subsets of the terminology. ICNP Catalogues consist of sets of nursing diagnosis, in tervention, and outcome statements for certain specialties or settings, or phenomena that are sensitive to nursing interventions, or health conditions (ICN 2008a). The first catalogue, *Partnering with Individuals and Families to Promote Adherence to Treatment*, was published in 2008 (ICN, 2008b). *Guidelines for ICNP Catalogue Development* were also published in 2008 (ICN 2008a). ICNP Version 1.1 included diagnosis, intervention, and outcome statements with their codes. The repository of these coded, precoordinated statements will continue to grow as more ICNP Catalogues are completed.

Table 12.3. Examples of nursing interventions

SELECT AXES	SELECT CONCEPTS		
Action ⟶	Alleviating	Teaching	Testing
Focus ⟶	Pain	Exercise pattern	Water supply
Client ⟶	Individual	Group	Community
Means ⟶	Cold pack	Instructional materials	Protocol

Interventions:
    Alleviating an individual's pain by applying a cold pack
    Teaching group members about exercise patterns using instructional materials
    Testing the water supply for a community using an established protocol			

Source: ICN 2005.

Figure 12.1.   International Classification for Nursing Practice

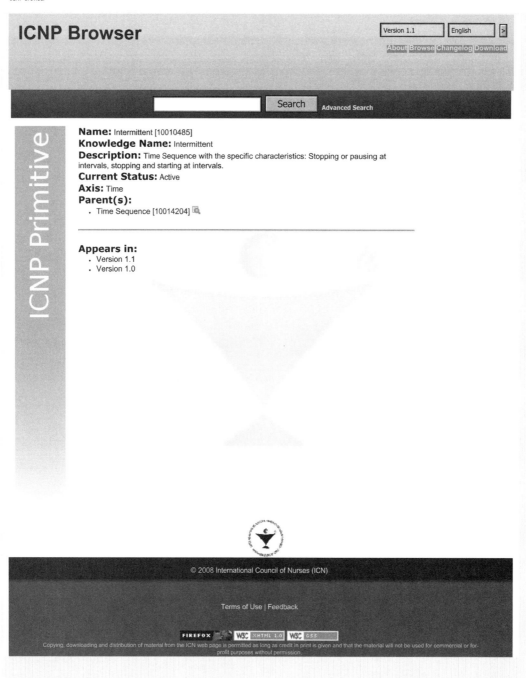

The International Classification for Nursing Practice Programme is responsible for ensuring that ICNP content reflects the domain of nursing. The ICN staff reviews suggestions from nurses worldwide and forwards them to nursing practice expert reviewers and/or technical and informatics experts. These individuals utilize specific criteria to recommend acceptance, rejection, or expanded review of the recommendation to add, modify, or inactivate the concept. The ICN staff uses the recommendations to make a final decision and communicates the results to the person submitting the recommendation.

Recommendations, including new terms and definitions, are accepted through an open process that gives individuals and groups the opportunity to participate in the development of ICNP. There are specific forms on the ICNP Web site for submitting recommendations (ICNF 2008a). The criteria for evaluating each submission are found on the Web site in the forms for reviewers. Figure 12.2 shows the Concept Submission and Review Process.

ICN-Accredited ICNP Research and Development (R&D) Centres support the ongoing development and maintenance of ICNP. The application to be recognized as a Centre can be submitted by nurses in management, education, clinical practice, or research settings. Guidance for application is on the ICNP Web site. The ICNP Consortium is made up of the ICN-accredited R&D Centres. The Consortium meets biennially during the International Council of Nurses Congress (ICNP 2008b).

Check Your Understanding 12.4

Instructions: Complete the following exercises on a separate piece of paper.

1. True or false. The ICN staff is responsible for reviewing the recommendations from the nursing practice expert reviewers.

2. ICNP Version 1.1 was released in what year?
    a. 1996
    b. 2005
    c. 2001
    d. 2008

3. An intentional process applied to or performed by a client is the definition of which axis?
    a. Action
    b. Client
    c. Focus
    d. Judgment

Figure 12.2. ICNP Concept Submission and Review Process Model

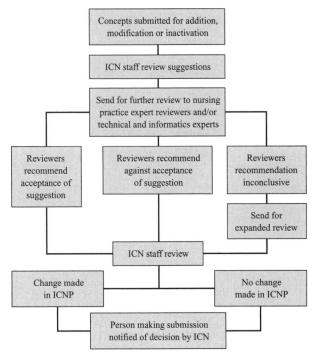

Source: ICN.

Summary

The sets of terms that have been created through professional nursing leadership and specific projects have provided an effective basis for nursing vocabularies in contemporary data systems. More recently, the American Nurses Association has fostered a "recognition" program of classification systems that comprise a Unified Nursing Language System administered through the Committee on Nursing Practice Inforamtion Infrastructure and included in the vendor recognition criteria developed by ANA's NIDSEC. This system evaluates and accredits patient care systems to meet specific requirements. Web sites for this organization include http://www.nursingworld.org/npii and http://www.nursingworld.org/nidsec/. The Web sites provide a listing of the ANA-recognized terminologies that support nursing practice and the recognized patient care products meeting the accreditation standards of this organization.

The nursing profession has been active in the development of standard coding systems to represent clinical concepts needed in nursing care. General terminologies are not adequate for this purpose.

Informatics experts and researchers continue to formulate models of standardized coding and classification systems that integrate nursing vocabulary and terminology with other systems. The systems of the future are expected to include more integrated multidisciplinary concepts of care regarding nursing assessment and care planning.

References

ABC Codes. http://www.alternativelink.com.

American Nurses Association. 2008. *Scope and Standards of Nursing Informatics Practice*. Washington, DC: American Nurses Publishing.

Ball, Marion, et al. 2000. *Nursing Informatics: Where Caring and Technology Meet*, 3rd ed. New York City: Springer-Verlag.

Clinical Care Classification (CCC) (formerly Home Health Care Classification [HHCC]). http://www.sabacare.com.

European Committee for Standardization. 2005. http://www.cenorm.be/cenorm.htm.

Hardiker, Nicholas R., and Anne Casey. 2000. Standards for nursing terminology. *Journal of the American Medical Informatics Association* 7(6):523–28.

International Classification for Nursing Practice (ICNP). http://www.icn.ch.

International Classification for Nursing Practice (ICNP). 2008b. ICN Accredited Centres for ICNP Research & Development. http://icn.ch/icnp_centres.pdf.

International Classification for Nursing Practice (ICNP). 2008a. ICNP Concept Submission and Review Guidelines. http://www.icn.ch/icnp_review.htm.

International Council of Nurses (2005). *International Classification for Nursing Practice—Version 1.0*. Geneva, Switzerland: International Council of Nurses.

International Council of Nurses (2008a). *Guidelines for ICNP Catalogue Development*. Geneva, Switzerland: International Council of Nurses.

International Council of Nurses (2008b). *ICNP Catalogue: Partnering with Individuals and Families to Promote Adherence to Treatment*. Geneva, Switzerland: International Council of Nurses.

International Organization for Standardization. 2005. http://www.iso.org/iso/en/aboutiso/introduction/index.html.

Logical Observation Identifiers, Names, and Codes (LOINC). http://www.loinc.org.

Martin, Karen S. 2004. *The Omaha System: A Key to Practice, Documentation, and Information Management*. St. Louis: Elsevier Saunders.

North American Nursing Diagnosis Association. 2005. http://www.nanda.org.

North American Nursing Diagnosis Association. 2007. *NANDA Diagnoses: Definitions and Classification*. Philadelphia: North American Nursing Diagnosis Association.

Nursing Interventions Classification (NIC). http://www.nursing.uiowa.edu/excellence/nursing_knowledge/clinical_effectiveness/index.htm.

Nursing Management Minimum Data Set (NMMDS). http://www.nursing.umn.edu/ICNP/USANMMDS/home.html.

Nursing Minimum Data Sets (NMDS). http://www.nursing.umn.edu/ICNP/USANMDS/home.html.

Nursing Outcomes Classification (NOC). University of Iowa. http://www.nursing.uiowa.edu/excellence/nursing_knowledge/clinical_effectiveness/index.htm.

Omaha System. 2005. http://www.omahasystem.org/systemo.htm.

Perioperative Nursing Dataset (PNDS). http://www.aorn.org.

Saba, Virginia K. 2005. Clinical care classification system. Sabacare. http://www.sabacare.com.

Shortliffe, Edward, et al. 2001. *Medical Informatics: Computer Applications in Healthcare and Biomedicine*. New York City: Springer-Verlag, 233.

Spackman, K., K. Campbell, and R. Cote. 1997. SNOMED-RT: A reference terminology for healthcare. *Proceedings of the 1997 AMIA Annual Symposium*. Nashville, TN: American Medical Informatics Association.

Systematized Nomenclature of Medicine, Clinical Terminology (SNOMED-CT). http://www.ihtsdo.org.

University of Iowa. 2009. Nursing Interventions Classification (NIC). http://www.nursing.uiowa.edu/centers/cncce/nic/nicoverview.htm.

Warren, J. J. and S. Bakken. (2002). Update on standardized nursing data sets and terminologies. *Journal of the American Health Information Management Association* 73(7), 78–83.

Application Exercise

Go to http://www.minurses.org/prac/SNLOverview.shtml. Review the article, take the post test, and complete the answer sheet.

Review Quiz

1. Each NIC intervention includes all but one of the following:
    a. Five-point Likert scale
    b. Definition
    c. Unique number
    d. Label name

2. Which of the following statements is consistent with the vision of NANDA International?
    a. Intensity of nursing care must be included in the DRG methodology.
    b. Perioperative nursing care is an important area of future research.
    c. Nursing diagnosis is seen as an essential component of any professional nursing–client interaction.
    d. Nursing informatics systems will be subsumed by the acceptance of ICD as a universally recognized reference terminology in the EHR environment.

3. The NIC System includes which of the following?
    a. Interventions for illness prevention
    b. Medication Administration Records (MARs)
    c. Thirty domains with seven classes each
    d. NANDA diagnoses in each NIC

4. The Nursing Information and Data Set Evaluation Center is affiliated with the
    a. American Health Information Management Association (AHIMA)
    b. American Hospital Association (AHA)
    c. American Organization of Nurse Executives (AONE)
    d. American Nurses Association (ANA)

5. Which of the following statements is true about NIC?
    a. Alternative Link has included it in the ABC codes used for reimbursement by alternative care providers.
    b. NIC fails to meet the uniform guidelines for IS vendors required by NIDSEC.
    c. NIC is currently in its twentieth edition because it has been revised annually since 1984.
    d. NIC contains two interrelated taxonomies classified by care components.

6. Which two systems have many of the same uses?
    a. NIC and NOC
    b. NOC and NANDA
    c. NIC and NANDA
    d. NANDA and the Omaha System

7. The NANDA Classification is a
    a. Standardized classification of patient/client outcomes
    b. Set of nursing diagnoses
    c. Standardized classification of interventions
    d. Unified nursing language system into which nursing terminologies can be cross-mapped

8. Which of the following statements is false?
    a. NOC is used to classify outcomes.
    b. NOC is recognized by the ANA as one of the standardized languages of nursing.
    c. NOC may be used in all settings and with all patient populations.
    d. NIC is used for reimbursement of nursing care for Medicare patients.

9. The Clinical Care Classification (CCC) system consists of how many interrelated taxonomies?
    a. Three
    b. Two
    c. Four
    d. Five

10. Which system includes the following components: assessment (Problem Classification Scheme), intervention (Intervention Scheme), and outcomes (Problem Rating Scale for Outcomes)?
    a. NIC
    b. Omaha System
    c. NANDA
    d. NOC

11. A term from the _____ is required to create a nursing diagnosis.
    a. Means Axis
    b. Judgment Axis
    c. Location Axis
    d. Client Axis

12. Which of the following is not one of the seven axes of ICNP?
    a. Focus
    b. Means
    c. Beneficiary
    d. Location

Chapter 13

Derived and Related International Classifications

Ann Zeisset, RHIT, CCS, CCS-P, and
Kathy Giannangelo, MA, RHIA, CCS, CPHIMS, FAHIMA

Learning Objectives

- To identify the World Health Organization family of ICD-derived and -related classifications

- To define the history, use, and purpose of the International Classification of Diseases for Oncology (ICD-O), Third Edition

- To discuss the purpose of a related classification of ICD such as the International Classification of External Causes of Injury (ICECI)

- To identify how classifications such as the International Classification of Primary Care (ICPC) differ from and improve on older systems such as the International Classification of Diseases (ICD)

Key Terms

Derived classification
Differentiation
Histology
International Classification of Diseases for Oncology (ICD-O)
International Classification of External Causes of Injury (ICECI)
International Classification of Primary Care (ICPC)
Morphology
Reasons for encounter (RFE)
Related classification
Rubric
SOAP
Topography
Wonca International Classification Committee (WICC)
World Organization of Family Doctors (Wonca)

Introduction

As discussed in earlier chapters, the World Health Organization (WHO) is a United Nations agency established in 1948 with the objective of working to help people worldwide attain the highest possible level of health. The organization is responsible for the WHO family of international classifications, which includes the International Statistical Classification of Diseases and Related Health Problems (ICD-10). There are several adaptations of the ICD classification system, derived classifications and related classifications.

A **derived classification** is based on a reference classification (ICD, ICF) and may be prepared

- By adopting the reference classification structure and categories, while providing additional detail beyond that provided by the reference classification

- Through rearrangement or aggregation of items from one or more reference classifications (WHO 2008)

A **related classification** partially refers to a reference classification or is associated with the reference classification at specific levels of structure only and describes important aspects of health or the health system not covered by reference or derived classifications (WHO 2008).

This chapter examines the development, purpose, content, structure, principles and guidelines, and process for revision and updates for three adaptations of ICD: the derived classification, the **International Classification of Diseases for Oncology** (ICD-O), and the two related classifications, the **International Classification of External Causes of Injury** (ICECI), and the **International Classification of Primary Care** (ICPC).

Introduction to the International Classification of Diseases for Oncology, Third Edition

ICD-O is a derived classification of ICD, which is used primarily by tumor or cancer registries to code the **topography** (site) and morphology (**histology**) of neoplasms. Over thirty years old, the International Classification of Diseases for Oncology (ICD-O) has undergone several revisions. The current version is the third edition. The topography section of the third edition remains the same as in the second edition, but the morphology section has been revised. This most recent revision primarily involved the addition of new classifications and codes for lymphomas and leukemias.

Developer of ICD-O

WHO published the first edition of ICD-O in 1976. The second edition, a collaboration between WHO and the International Agency for Research on Cancer (IARC), was published in 1990. The second edition was used extensively throughout the world and has been translated into many languages, including Chinese, Czech, French, German, Greek, Italian, Japanese, Portuguese, Russian, Slovak, and Spanish.

Published in 2000, the updated, third edition of ICD-O also was developed by a working party convened by IARC/WHO.

Purpose of ICD-O

The purpose of ICD-O is to provide greater specificity for use by cancer registries and in pathology and other departments specializing in cancer. The topography code describes the site of origin of the neoplasm and uses the same three- and four-character categories as in the neoplasm section of the second chapter of ICD-10. The morphology code describes the characteristics of the tumor itself, including cell type and biologic activity.

Content of ICD-O

ICD-O is based on the structure of ICD-10, but with basic differences. The second chapter of ICD-10, Neoplasms, categorizes the topography and describes the behavior of the neoplasm as follows: malignant, benign, in situ, or uncertain whether malignant or benign. In ICD-10, up to five different categories of codes are needed to describe the

Table 13.1.   ICD-10 Alphabetic Index entries for breast neoplasm

	Malignant, Primary	Malignant, Secondary	In situ	Benign	Uncertain and Unknown
Breast	C50.9	C79.8	D05.9	D24	D48.6

neoplasms of a site. Table 13.1 illustrates how five different codes are used in ICD-10 to describe neoplasm of the breast.

In contrast, ICD-O uses one code for topography, and this code remains the same for all neoplasms of a particular site. The code is based on the malignant neoplasm section of ICD-10. Identification of whether the neoplasm is malignant, benign, in situ, or of uncertain behavior is made by the fifth digit in the morphology code. The other digits of the morphology code describe the type of **morphology** of the neoplasm (for example, adenocarcinoma, carcinoma, squamous cell carcinoma, and so on). Table 13.2 shows how the code stays the same and the morphology code gives the behavior.

Check Your Understanding 13.1

Instructions: Complete the following exercises on a separate piece of paper.

1. What does the topography code in ICD-0 describe?

2. True or False. The morphology code describes the characteristics of the tumor.

3. True or False. ICD-O-2 was used only in the United States.

Table 13.3 shows how the different sections of the second chapter of ICD-10 correspond to the behavior codes in the morphology codes.

Several abbreviations are used throughout the classification, including:

M (morphology)
NOS (not otherwise specified)

Table 13.2.   ICD-O coding of some breast neoplasms

Neoplasm	Code	
Malignant neoplasm of the breast (primary, carcinoma)	C50.9	M-8010/3
In situ neoplasm of breast (carcinoma, intraductal)	C50.9	M-8500/2
Benign neoplasm of breast (adenoma)	C50.9	M-8140/0

Table 13.3.   ICD-O behavior codes and corresponding section of chapter II, ICD-10

Behavior Code	Category	Term
/ 0	D10–D36	Benign neoplasms
/ 1	D37–D48	Neoplasms of uncertain and unknown behavior
/ 2	D00–D09	In situ neoplasms
/ 3	C00-C76, C80–C97	Malignant neoplasms, stated or presumed to be primary
/ 6	C77–C79	Malignant neoplasms, stated or presumed to be secondary

ICD-O (International Classification of Diseases for Oncology)

In ICD-O, NOS appears after topographic and morphologic terms that appear elsewhere in the classification with an additional modifying word or phrase. The NOS is listed first in the Alphabetic Index, followed by the alphabetic listing of modifying words. ICD-O instructs coders to follow a term with NOS when:

-   A topographic or morphologic term is not modified.

-   A topographic or morphologic term has an adjective that does not appear elsewhere.

-   A term is used in a general sense.

Structure and Format of ICD-O

ICD-O consists of the following main sections:

I.   Instructions for Use

II.   Topography: Numerical List

III.   Morphology: Numerical List

IV.   Alphabetic Index

V.   Differences in Morphology Codes between Second and Third Editions

Instructions for Use

The instructions for use section contains an introduction with historical background, differences between ICD-O and ICD-10, the structure and format of ICD-O-3, and coding guidelines for topography and morphology. This section must be read and followed carefully because it contains the guidelines needed to assign codes correctly.

Topography: Numerical List

The topography section is based on the malignant neoplasm chapter in ICD-10. The terms run from C00.0 to C80.9, and a decimal point separates the subdivisions of three-character categories. Figure 13.1 shows the structure of the topography codes.

Figure 13.1.   Structure of topography code

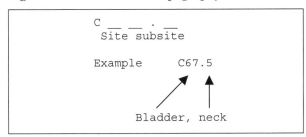

Morphology: Numerical List

Codes in the morphology section have five digits and range from M-8000/0 to M-9989/3. The first four digits of the code give the histology, and the fifth digit, after the slash (/), is the behavior code. The fifth digit indicates whether the tumor is malignant, benign, in situ, or uncertain. Table 13.5 (see page 206) shows an example of the morphology—numerical section.

The behavior refers to the way the tumor acts in the body. A benign tumor can grow in place but does not spread; an in situ behavior indicates the tumor is malignant but still growing in place. Malignant of the primary site indicates the tumor can spread, and metastatic means dissemination from the point of origin and growth at another site. Figure 13.2 (see page 206) illustrates the fifth-digit behavior for morphology codes.

Table 13.4.   Example from the topography—numerical section

	C18	COLON
C18.0		Cecum
C18.1		Appendix
C18.2		Ascending colon
C18.3		Hepatic flexure of colon
C18.4		Transverse colon
C18.5		Splenic flexure of colon
C18.6		Descending colon
C18.7		Sigmoid colon
C18.8		Overlapping lesion of colon
C18.9		Colon, NOS
	C19	RECTOSIGMOID JUNCTION
C19.9		Rectosigmoid junction
	C20	RECTUM
C20.9		Rectum, NOS
	C21	ANUS AND ANAL CANAL
C21.0		Anus, NOS
C21.1		Anal canal
C21.2		Cloacogenic zone
C21.8		Overlapping lesion of rectum, anus, and anal canal

Check Your Understanding 13.2

Instructions: Complete the following exercises on a separate piece of paper.

1. True or False. ICD-O-3 has four main sections.

2. List the type of behavior for the tumors represented by the following codes.
    a. M-8094/3
    b. M-8240/1
    c. M-8010/6
    d. M-8453/2
    e. M-8045/3
    f. M-8371/0

3. What is the topography code in ICD-O-3 for anal canal?

An additional digit is available to identify the histologic grading or **differentiation.** Table 13.6 (see page 206) provides the meanings of this final digit.

The grading codes can be applied to all malignant neoplasms listed in ICD-O when documentation is present that distinguishes the grade or differentiation. For example, to completely code well-differentiated carcinoma, the morphology code would be M-8010/3 1.

Table 13.5.   Example from the morphology—numerical section

880	SOFT TISSUE TUMORS AND SARCOMAS, NOS
8800/3	Soft tissue tumor, benign
8800/9	Sarcoma, NOS
8801/3	Sarcomatosis, NOS
8802/3	Spindle cell sarcoma
8803/3	Giant cell sarcoma
8804/3	Small cell sarcoma
8805/3	Epithelioid sarcoma
8806/3	Undifferentiated sarcoma
8800/3	Desmoplastic small round cell tumor

There is a separate one-digit code for the cell lineage or immunophenotype for lymphoma or leukemias. This is

5   T-cell
6   B-cell
        Pre-B
        B-precursor
7   Null cell
        Non T-non B
8   NK cell
        Natural killer cell
9   Cell type not determined,
        not stated or not applicable

Figure 13.2.   Fifth-digit behavior code for neoplasms

Code	
/0	Benign
/1	Uncertain whether benign or malignant
	Borderline malignancy
	Low malignant potential
	Uncertain malignant potential
/2	Carcinoma in situ
	Intraepithelial
	Noninfiltrating
	Noninvasive
/3	Malignant, primary site
/6	Malignant, metastatic site
	Malignant, secondary site
/9	Malignant, uncertain whether primary or metastatic site

Table 13.6.   Histologic grading or differentiation

Code	Grade	Description
1	I	Well differentiated Differentiated, NOS
2	II	Moderately differentiated Moderately well differentiated Intermediate differentiation
3	III	Poorly differentiated
4	IV	Undifferentiated Anaplastic
9		Grade or differentiation not determined, not stated, or not applicable

Figure 13.3 illustrates the structure of a morphology code.

To completely code with ICD-O, one would use ten characters. The first four indicate the topographic site, the next four give the morphologic type, followed by one digit for behavior and one digit for grade or differentiation. (The M is not calculated in this number). Figure 13.4 provides an example of the structure of a complete code.

Alphabetic Index

The Alphabetic Index is available for use in finding both topography (anatomical sites) and morphology (histologic terms). The terms are interspersed in alphabetical order and are listed under both the noun and the adjective. For example, small cell carcinoma is indexed under Carcinoma, small cell, and under Small cell carcinoma.

By knowing the format of the different codes, it is apparent that the topography codes are identified by the letter *C,* the first character of codes in the

Figure 13.3.   Structure of a morphology code

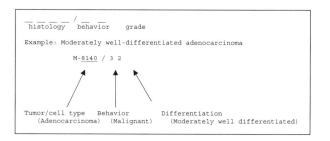

Figure 13.4.   Structure of a complete code

```
Diagnostic term:
Well-differentiated squamous cell carcinoma, lower lobe of the lung

C34.3 M-8070/3 1
```

neoplasms chapter of ICD-10, and the morphology codes begin with the prefix *M-*.

Remember, the first character of ICD-10 codes also may start with the letter *D,* but ICD-O codes are all based on the malignant neoplasm section. The morphology code distinguishes the behavior of the neoplasm in ICD-O.

When topographic (C) and morphologic terms (M) are mixed in the index, they are separated by a space. When three or more terms appear, the term beginning with C or M is in bold type and terms are indented

under it. The NOS term is always listed first under the heading in the index rather than in alphabetical order.

The Alphabetic Index also includes some tumor-like lesions and conditions for which no code is provided; instead, a reference is made to *see SNOMED,* referring the coder to the Systematized Nomenclature of Medicine. The previous versions of ICD-O provided SNOMED codes, but ICD-O-3 omitted them. Figure 13.5 shows the format of the Alphabetic Index of ICD-O.

Differences in Morphology Codes between Second and Third Editions

The section on differences in morphology codes between second and third editions provides the new ICD-O codes, new morphology terms and synonyms, terms that changed morphology codes, terms that changed from tumorlike lesions to neoplasms, terms

Figure 13.5.   Alphabetic Index of ICD-O

	V	
C52.9		Vagina, NOS
C52.9		Vagina, fornix
M-8077 / 2	Vaginal intraepithelial neoplasia, grade III (C52._)	
C52.9		Vaginal vault
C72.5		Vagus nerve
M-8077 / 2	VAIN III (C52._)	
C10.0		Vallecula
C18.0		Valve, ileocecal
C63.1		Vas deferens
	Vascular	
M-8894 / 0	leiomyoma	
M-------	nevus (see SNOMED)	
M-------	spider (see SNOMED)	
C52.9		Vault, vaginal
C49.9		Vein, NOS
C49.5		Vein, iliac
	Vena cava	
C49.4	NOS	
C49.4	abdominal	
C49.4	inferior	
C49.3	superior	
M9122 / 0	Venous hemangioma	
	Ventral surface of tongue	
C02.2	NOS	
C02.2	anterior	
C02.2	anterior 2 / 3	

deleted from ICD-O-3, and terms that changed behavior codes.

Principles and Guidelines for ICD-O

The coding guidelines for topography and morphology available in the ICD-O-3 book. These guidelines consist of Rules A through K. Certain guidelines apply only to topography and some only to morphology, while others apply to both. For example, Rule B. *Prefixes* states: "If a topographic site is modified by a prefix such as peri-, para-, or the like which is not specifically listed in ICD-O, code to the appropriate ill-defined subcategory C76 (ill-defined site), unless the type of tumor indicates origin from a particular tissue (ICD-O-3 2001)."

Another example of a guideline is Rule C. *Tumors involving more than one topographic category or subcategory,* which states: "Use subcategory '.8' when a tumor overlaps the boundaries of two or more categories or subcategories and its point of origin cannot be determined" (ICD-O-3 2001).

After the section listing the guidelines, more detail regarding each rule is provided. The rules are listed again, but with more precise guidelines and examples pertaining to each rule. Rules A through E pertain to topography, and rules F through K deal with morphology.

Process for Revision of and Updates to ICD-O

The third edition of ICD-O was developed by a working party convened by IARC/WHO. A special effort was made in this edition of ICD-O to change as few terms as possible. New terms were added at empty spaces. The topography codes remained the same as in the second edition, but morphology codes were thoroughly reviewed and, where necessary, revised to increase their diagnostic precision and prognostic value. As mentioned earlier, most changes reflected the urgent need to code new diagnoses in leukemia and lymphoma.

Since publication of the hard- and soft-cover version of ICD-O-3 in June 2000, two sets of errata have been created. The first was released May 22, 2001, and the second May 6, 2003. These documents include corrections for a number of errors and discrepancies appearing in the hardcover version.

It is not known at the time of publication if a fourth edition will be developed.

Check Your Understanding 13.3

Instructions: Complete the following exercises on a separate piece of paper.

1. In the code M-8070/3 2, what does the 2 indicate?

2. What immunophenotype code is assigned for leukemia, T-cell?

3. True or False. Only morphology codes are included in the Alphabetic Index.

Introduction to the International Classification of External Causes of Injury

The **International Classification of External Causes of Injury** (ICECI) is a related classification of the WHO Family of International Classifications (WHO-FIC). ICECI has a relationship with ICD-10 chapter XX, External causes of morbidity and mortality. ICECI does not replace the ICD chapter, because it includes external causes and not the injuries. The Centers for Disease Control (CDC) recommends a bridge between the two classifications, not that ICECI replace ICD-10.

Developer of ICECI

The ICECI was developed as a related classification to ICD-10 chapter XX in the WHO-FIC, and the draft creation date was May 1998. The last date change was 2003, with version 1.2 released in 2004. Injury specialists worldwide were coordinated by WHO to assist in the development of ICECI. Some of the countries represented were Australia, United States, Canada, Scandinavia and Western Europe.

Purpose of ICECI

According to WHO, the purpose of ICECI is to "enable classifying external causes of injuries. It is designed to help researchers and prevention practitioners to describe, measure and monitor the occurrence of injuries and to investigate their circumstances of occurrence using an internally agreed classification (WHO 2008)." More detail for injury surveillance and the classification of injury categories was needed than what was available in either ICD-9-CM or ICD-10. The external cause codes from these two systems lack the scope and specificity needed for international comparability, research, and mortality statistics.

Content of ICECI

The content of ICECI is comparable and complementary with ICD-10, because it is based on the existing classification and does not replace the ICD external causes codes. It provides a method to collect more detailed information about a variety of external-cause-related topics. ICECI is arranged in a multiaxial, hierarchical structure and has a modular, "pick and choose" format. This allows various factors to be recorded independently of one another and all or partial use of all modules (ICECI Version 1.2 2004). A traditional index is available and an automated indexing system is in preparation.

ICECI consists of six modules. They are

- Core
- Violence
- Transport
- Place
- Sports
- Occupational

The core module includes seven items:

- Intent
- Mechanism of injury
- Object/substance producing injury
- Place of occurrence
- Activity when injured
- Alcohol use

- Psycho-active drug or substance use

The additional five modules (after the core module) enable the collection of additional information on special topics such as place where the injurious event occurred.

Principles and Guidelines for ICECI

The ICECI must comply with certain underlying principles such as:

- A separate coding axis for each main concept
- Usefulness for injury prevention
- Usability in many types of settings and in many parts of the world
- Comparability with ICD-10
- Compatibility with ICD-10

Process for Revision of and Updates to ICECI

The ICECI updates and revisions occur as experience and assessment result in recommendations for changes, with possible frequency of 1–2 years for minor updates and 5–10 years for major updates (ICECI Version 1.2 2004).

An installation of a Coordination and Maintenance Group was established in 2003. WHO identifies the custodianship and responsibility for maintenance and updating with an international group of experts called the ICECI Coordination and Maintenance Group. Currently three people act as the executive committee of this group (WHO 2008).

Check Your Understanding 13.4

1. True or false. The ICECI provides additional information regarding the occurrence of injury.

2. True or false. ICECI consists of seven modules.

3. Which of the following is part of the core module?
   a. Place of occurrence
   b. Object producing injury
   c. If alcohol was involved
   d. All of the above

Introduction to International Classification of Primary Care

The **International Classification of Primary Care** (ICPC) has been translated into several languages and is used in a number of countries around the world to classify patient data related to general and family practice and primary care. For example, ICPC is required in electronic prescribing systems in the Netherlands (http://www.globalfamilydoctor.com/wicc/icpcstory.html).

In the United States, a variation of ICPC, the Reason for Visit Classification, has been used for twenty years to classify the patient's stated reason for the visit or chief complaint in national ambulatory care surveys (Greenberg and Jones 1997). In addition, a project sponsored by the Agency for Healthcare Research and Quality called the Applied Strategies for Improving Patient Safety is using ICPC as its classification system.

In 2003, WHO recognized the second edition of ICPC as a related classification for the classification of primary care data, and it is considered one of the WHO Family of International Classifications (WHO-FIC). The classification system also has been incorporated into the NLM's Unified Medical Language System (UMLS).

Developer of ICPC

The World Organization of National Colleges, Academics, and Academic Associations of General Practitioners/Family Physicians (Wonca), today known as the **World Organization of Family Doctors** (Wonca), was instrumental in the development of ICPC. Designed by the WONCA Classification Committee (now the **Wonca International Classification Committee** [WICC]), its predecessor, the International Classification of Health Problems in Primary Care (ICHPPC), was first published in 1975, followed by a second edition in 1979 and a third (ICHPPC-2-Defined) in 1983. Although deemed an improvement over the International Classification of Diseases (ICD), this system was still considered inadequate for identifying the patient's reason for encounter and problem list.

Further, the system's insufficiencies were recognized at a WHO conference. The National Center for Health Statistics, the WHO North American Collaborating Center, led an effort to address the identified deficiencies with its development of the Classification of Reasons for Encounter in Primary Care. Under the auspices of WHO, a working party was created, which led to the development of the Reason for Encounter Classification (RFEC). Field trials with members of the WICC were conducted on RFEC, which resulted in the publication of ICPC in 1987. Wonca owns the copyrights to ICPC. Table 13.7 lists the various published versions.

Purpose of ICPC

ICPC enables the labeling of the most prevalent conditions that exist in the community as well as symp-

Table 13.7.   Versions of ICPC

Title	Acronym	Date published/released
International Classification of Primary Care (ICPC)	ICPC-1-v0.0	1987
International Classification of Primary Care (ICPC) Version 2	ICPC-2-v.0.0	1998
International Classification of Primary Care (ICPC) Version 2, Electronic	ICPC-2e-v1.0	2000
International Classification of Primary Care (ICPC) Version 2, Electronic, 2002	ICPC-2e-v2.0	2002
International Classification of Primary Care (ICPC) Version 2, Electronic, 2005, and ICPC Revised Second Edition (ICPC-2-R)	ICPC-2e-v.3.0	2005
International Classification of Primary Care (ICPC) Version 2, Electronic, 2006, and ICPC-2-R including updates	ICPC-2e-v.4.0	2006/currently being tested

toms and complaints. It can classify three important elements of the healthcare encounter: **reasons for encounter** (RFE), diagnosis or problems, and process of care. The RFEs are defined as "the agreed statement of the reason(s) why a patient enters the healthcare system, representing the demand for care by that person" (Wonca 2005).

Reasons why a patient visits a primary care physician might include symptoms or complaints; known diseases; preventive, diagnostic, or administrative services; and specific treatments. Unlike ICD, which identifies the provider's determination, an RFE classification represents the patient's viewpoint for seeing the provider. This is a key element in the healthcare practitioner's decision regarding the patient's diagnosis and its management.

Content of ICPC

The **SOAP** concept was used in the development of ICPC (http://homepages.iol.ie/~bom/ICPC.htm). SOAP is an acronym for a component of the problem-oriented medical record that refers to how each progress note contains documentation relative to subjective observations. ICPC classifies three of the four elements of the problem-oriented medical record SOAP:

S: Subjective observations by the patient of the problem or the reason for encounter

O: Objective observations not classified with ICPC

A: Assessment or diagnosis of the patient's problem

P: Plans or process of care

ICPC consists of a biaxial configuration, chapters, and components. Whereas ICD has different chapter axes, all seventeen ICPC chapters are based on body systems with additional chapters for psychological and social problems. Table 13.8 shows the chapters and their associated alpha characters.

The first character of an ICPC code is the alpha character for the chapter. The next characters in an

ICPC code are two digits, referred to as **rubrics**, and represent the second axis components. Each chapter in ICPC is divided into the following seven components:

- Symptoms and complaints (1–29)
- Diagnostic and preventive procedures (30–49)
- Treatment procedures, medication (50–59)
- Test results (60–61)
- Administrative (62)
- Referral and other reasons for encounter (63–69)
- Diseases (70–99)

For example, D70, a code for gastrointestinal infection, is found in the chapter D(igestive), disease ⟶ component 7: D70.

Table 13.8.   ICPC chapter titles and associated alpha characters

Chapter	Alpha character
General	A
Blood, blood forming organs, lymphatics	B
Digestive	D
Eye	F
Ear	H
Circulatory	K
Musculoskeletal	L
Neurological	N
Psychological	P
Respiratory	R
Skin	S
Metabolic, endocrine, nutrition	T
Urinary	U
Pregnancy, childbearing, family planning	W
Female genital	X
Male genital	Y
Social problems	Z

Principles and Guidelines for ICPC

Some components are uniform throughout all chapters; others are not. The following guidelines for the components are taken from http://www .globalfamilydoctor.com/wicc/icpcstory.html:

- Component 1: Symptoms and complaints: Rubrics in this component describe the problem under management (that is, the problem list) when the condition has not been defined.

- Component 2: Diagnostic screening and prevention: Rubrics in this component are used when there is no underlying pathology for the problem being managed.

- Component 3: Treatment, procedure, and medication: Rubrics in this component should only in rare circumstances be used to identify a problem under management. Instead it is for the naming of processes involved in patient care.

- Component 4: Test results: Rubrics in this component describe problems, which have no pathology.

- Component 5: Administrative: Rubrics in this component also describe problems, which have no pathology.

- Component 7: Diagnoses, diseases: Rubrics in this component are used when a practitioner has enough information to determine a diagnosis. Component 7 has five subgroups: infectious diseases, neoplasms, injuries, congenital anomalies, and other diseases. These subgroups are not numerically uniform across chapters.

- Components 1 and 7 function independently in each of the seventeen chapters. They are used to classify patient RFEs, presenting symptoms, and diagnoses or problems managed.

- Components 2 and 3 are broadly founded on the ICD-9 Procedures in Medicine and the International Classification of Process in Primary Care.

- Components 2 through 6 are common throughout all the chapters, with each rubric equally valid to any body system.

ICPC's structure results in groups of problems being disseminated among chapters rather than found in their own chapters as in ICD. For example, ICD has a separate chapter for injuries. In ICPC, injuries are found in various chapters depending on the body system to which the injury occurred.

Process for Revision of and Updates to ICPC

WICC is responsible for the maintenance of and updates to ICPC. The classification system is currently on an eleven-year full revision cycle, although the maps to other classifications may be revised more often. ICPC-3 work has begun with a target release date of 2011 (WONCANews 2008). Available in both print and electronic forms, a formal license from Wonca is necessary for commercial or national use.

Check Your Understanding 13.5

Instructions: Complete the following exercises on a separate piece of paper.

1. The _____ system led to development of the ICPC.
    a. RFEC
    b. ICHPPC
    c. ICHPPC-2
    d. ICD

2. True or false. The structures of ICPC and ICD are the same.

3. An ICPC code beginning with the letter *L* refers to which body system?
    a. Digestive
    b. Respiratory
    c. Musculoskeletal
    d. Circulatory

4. ICPC-2-v.0.0 was released in what year?
    a. 1996
    b. 1998
    c. 2000
    d. 1987

5. True or false. A full revision to ICPC occurs every eleven years.

Summary

Now in its third edition, the International Classification of Diseases for Oncology (ICD-O) has been used for over thirty years as the standard tool for coding diagnoses of neoplasms in tumor and cancer registries and in pathology laboratories. It is a dual classification with coding systems for both topography and morphology. The topography code describes the site of origin of the neoplasm and uses the same three-character and four-character codes as in the neoplasm chapter of ICD-10. The morphology code describes the characteristics of the tumor itself, including cell type and biologic activity.

ICD-O is under the purview of the heads of the WHO Collaborating Centres for Classification of Disease. The International Association of Cancer Registries (IACR) is an additional resource.

ICD-10 external causes of morbidity and mortality (chapter XX in ICD-10) provides limited detail; therefore a need was identified to provide more information to researchers and prevention practitioners in order to describe, measure, and monitor how and why injuries occur. The International Classification of External Causes of Injury (ICECI) was created to use in surveillance and research regarding the occurrence of injuries internationally.

The International Classification of Primary Care (ICPC) represents a related classification with relatively narrow applications. ICPC is copyrighted by its founding organization and requires a license for use. The Wonca International Classification Committee, developer of ICPC, also maintains and updates this classification.

References

American Burn Association. 2008. International Classification of the External Causes of Injury: ICECI. http://www.ameriburn.org/Research/ICECI_MCTG.pdf.

Centers for Disease Control and Prevention. 2008. International Classification of External Causes of Injuries. http://www.cdc.gov/nchs/ppt/ice/cuernavaca/mulder_netherlands.ppt.

Fritz, A., et al., eds. 2000. *International Classification of Diseases for Oncology,* third edition. Geneva: World Health Organization.

Greenberg, Marjorie S., and Judith M. Jones. 1997. Toward standardization of health information. *Journal of the American Health Information Management Association* 68(2):22–28.

ICECI Coordination and Maintenance Group (2004). International Classification of External Causes of Injuries (ICECI) version 1.2. Consumer Safety Institute, Amsterdam and AIHW National Injury Surveillance Unit, Adelaide. http://www.rivm.nl/who-fic/ICECI/ICECI_1-2_2004July.pdf.

Johns, Merida L., ed. 2007. *Health Information Management Technology.* Chicago: American Health Information Management Association.

LaTour, Kathleen M., and Shirley Eichenwald, eds. 2006. *Health Information Management: Concepts, Principles, and Practice.* Chicago: American Health Information Management Association.

National Center for Health Statistics. 2005. http://www.cdc.gov/nchs/about/otheract/icd9/icfhome.htm.

Norwegian Centre for Informatics in Health and Social Care. 2007. ICPC-2e download. http://www.kith.no/templates/kith_WebPage____1111.aspx.

O'Mahony, Brian. 1997. International classification of primary care (ICPC): Comments and comparisons. Unpublished paper posted on personal Web site at http://homepages.iol.ie/~bom/ICPC.htm.

Wonca International Classification Committee. 2005. http://www.ulb.ac.be/esp/wicc/.

WONCANews. 2008. Wonca. http://www.globalfamilydoctor.com/publications/woncanews/WN%20Aug%2008/index.htm.

World Health Organization. 2000. World Health Organization Meeting of heads of WHO collaborating centres for the classification of diseases. http://www.who.int/classifications/network/en/report2000.pdf.

World Health Organization. 2007. World Health Organization Family of International Classifications: definition, scope and purpose. http://www.who.int/classifications/en/FamilyDocument2007.pdf.

World Health Organization. 2008. http://www.who.int/en.

World Health Organization. 2008a. International Classification of External Causes of Injury (ICECI). http://www.who.int/classifications/icd/adaptations/iceci/en/index.html.

World Organization of Family Doctors. 2005. http://www.globalfamilydoctor.com/wicc/icpcstory.html.

Application Exercises

1. Prepare a short report on who uses ICD-O-3 and how it might provide additional information beyond that obtained in ICD-9-CM.

2. Develop a table or grid that identifies the differences between ICD and ICPC.

Review Quiz

1. Which section remained unchanged in the ICD-O-3 version?

2. In ICD-O-3, how many different categories of codes are used to describe the site?
   a. One
   b. Two
   c. Four
   d. Five

3. True or False. In ICD-10, five different categories of codes are needed to describe all the neoplasms of a site.

4. What is the topography code in ICD-O-3 for descending colon?

5. What does the fifth digit in the morphology code indicate?
   a. Histology
   b. Grading
   c. Behavior
   d. None of the above
   e. All of the above

6. Assign the final two digits for the following statement: Poorly differentiated carcinoma. M-8010/_ _

7. True or false. ICECI is related to chapter XX of ICD-10.

8. Which of the following is not one of the six ICDCI modules?
   a. Violence
   b. Sports
   c. Intent
   d. Occupational

9. The agreed statement of the reason(s) why a patient enters the healthcare system, representing the demand for care by that person, is the definition for which of the following:
   a. Primary diagnosis
   b. Problem list
   c. Process of care
   d. Reasons for encounter

10. ICPC consists of a biaxial configuration, chapters, and _____.
    a. Sections
    b. Components
    c. Subchapters
    d. Titles

11. Which component is addressed by the ICPC-2 code F82, Detached retina?
    a. Component 1
    b. Component 6
    c. Component 7
    d. Component 3

12. Which classification represents the patient's viewpoint for seeing the provider?
    a. RFEC
    b. ICF
    c. ICD
    d. ICHPPC

13. True or False. WICC is responsible for maintenance of and updates to ICPC.

Chapter 14

Other Vocabulary, Terminology, and Classification Systems

Kathy Giannangelo, MA, RHIA, CCS, CPHIMS, FAHIMA
and Ann Zeisset, RHIT, CCS, CCS-P

Learning Objectives

- To discuss the development of some other vocabulary, terminology, and classification systems such as the Universal Medical Device Nomenclature System (UMDNS), the Systematized Nomenclature of Dentistry (SNODENT), ABC codes, and others

- To become familiar with the uses and applications of these systems

- To identify how classifications such as International Classification of Functioning, Disability and Health (ICF) differ from and improve on older systems such as the International Classification of Diseases (ICD)

Key Terms

ABC codes
Complementary and alternative medicine (CAM)
ECRI (formerly the Emergency Care Research Institute)
Generic device group
Global Medical Device Nomenclature (GMDN)
International Classification of Functioning, Disability and Health (ICF)
International Classification of Health Interventions (ICHI)
International Classification of Impairments, Disabilities and Handicaps (ICIDH)
Medical Dictionary for Regulatory Activities (MedDRA)
Morbidity
Mortality
National Center for Health Statistics (NCHS)
Preferred term
Relative value units (RVUs)
Systematized Nomenclature of Dentistry (SNODENT)
Universal Medical Device Nomenclature System (UMDNS)
WHO Family of International Classifications (WHO-FIC)

Introduction

Although some vocabulary, terminology, and classification systems such as ICD (International Classification of Diseases) have been around for a long time, others have emerged only in the past twenty or so years because of changes in the healthcare environment. For example, the government found that Current Procedural Terminology (CPT) did not have the detail needed to identify certain services for such things as supplies. Identifying this gap, the Centers for Medicare and Medicaid Services (CMS) developed a code set called HCPCS Level II to meet the operational needs of the Medicare and Medicaid reimbursement programs. In addition, passage of the Health Insurance Portability and Accountability Act (HIPAA) of 1996 and the identification of standard transaction and code sets has resulted in comments by various organizations noting additional gaps in the current systems. Finally, the movement toward electronic health records (EHRs) also has been an influencing factor in the evolution of, and need for, specific systems.

This chapter examines the following vocabulary, terminology, and classification systems: the **Universal Medical Device Nomenclature System** (UMDNS) and the **Global Medical Device Nomenclature** (GMDN), the **Medical Dictionary for Regulatory Activities** (MedDRA), the **Systematized Nomenclature of Dentistry** (SNODENT)**, ABC Codes**, **International Classification of Functioning, Disability and Health** (ICF), and the **International Classification of Health Interventions** (ICHI).

The latter two, ICF and ICHI, are World Health Organization (WHO) systems. WHO mandates the production of international classifications on health so meaningful and useful frameworks are developed as a common language for use by governments, providers, and consumers. "Internationally endorsed classifications facilitate the storage, retrieval, analysis, and interpretation of data. They also permit the comparison of data within populations over time and between populations at the same point in time

as well as the compilation of nationally consistent data." (WHO 2008h). The purpose of the **WHO Family of International Classifications** (WHO-FIC) is to promote appropriate selection of classifications in the range of settings in the health field across the world. There are three reference classifications approved by WHO-FIC:

- International Classification of Diseases (ICD)
- International Classification of Functioning, Disability, and Health (ICF)
- International Classification of Health Interventions (ICHI)

ICD is discussed in chapters 2 and 13, and ICF and ICHI are included in this chapter.

Introduction to the Universal Medical Device Nomenclature System

The Universal Medical Device Nomenclature System (UMDNS) is a proprietary, standardized, controlled international nomenclature and computer coding system for medical devices and materials, clinical laboratory equipment and in vitro diagnostics, disposables and supplies, selected hospital furniture, casework, and instruments used to test clinical equipment. UMDNS does not provide a classification system for diseases or procedures but, instead, is limited to Universal Medical Device Codes (UMDCs) and UMDNS device terms.

Developer of UMDNS

UMDNS was developed by **ECRI** (formerly the Emergency Care Research Institute), an organization formed in the United States to promote safety, quality, and cost-effectiveness in healthcare to benefit patient care through research, publishing, education, and consultation. The European Union (EU) and a number of other nations have officially adopted it. In addition, the U.S. National Library of Medicine

(NLM) has incorporated UMDNS into its Unified Medical Language System (UMLS).

Purpose of UMDNS

UMDNS was established to classify medical devices for the purposes of indexing, storing, and retrieving device-related information (for example, inventory control and adverse incident tracking). UMDNS terms and the corresponding five-digit codes have been incorporated into publications, databases, medical information systems, hazard alerting systems and other software used by government agencies, healthcare systems, and facilities. Additionally, it is used in ECRI's many databases, which are used to report potential problems with medical devices and other types of items cataloged in UMDNS. The Institute of Medicine's Committee on Data Standards for Patient Safety has recommended UMDNS as one of the core terminologies for the EHR.

Content of UMDNS

UMDNS covers all medical devices, equipment, supplies, disposables, clinical laboratory instrumentation, reagents, test kits, dental instruments and equipment, selected hospital furniture, casework, and instruments used to test medical equipment. Medical devices thus defined include almost any nondrug item used for patient care.

The UMDNS can be obtained from ECRI. The license for its use is free to nonprofit organizations and may be purchased by medical equipment vendors and other for-profit organizations.

UMDNS consists of several thousand five-digit numeric codes and more than 7,500 so-called **preferred terms** (discussed later), as well as thousands of additional entry terms. A complete listing of UMDNS terms and code numbers is available online from http://www.tuvamerica.com/tools/forms/UMDNS.DOC.

Principles and Guidelines for UMDNS

UMDNS classifies medical devices with similar attributes into categories. Each category is identified with a unique five-digit identifier.

ECRI also developed a set of key words that can be used to target the appropriate top-level category. Suppliers assign each of their product lines to a device category. Codes are assigned to product lines only. Individual items cannot be assigned their own UMDNS code. For example, all arthroscopes are assigned code 10-198, regardless of manufacturer, size, and so on.

Devices can be categorized into various subsets on the basis of preferred terms, entry terms, and UMDC codes. A preferred term represents the generic product category, which is a list of preferred concepts (admitted terms) that name the devices in a formal way. The unique five-digit UMDC codes are assigned to the preferred terms. Entry terms are provided as entry points into the UMDNS and also are known as non-preferred terms. Entry terms carry a *see* note directing the user to the appropriate preferred term. Entry terms have no UMDC codes assigned to them.

The following example from the 2008 UMDNS Product Categories Thesaurus illustrates the difference between preferred terms and entry terms:

> Compressed Gas Hoses
> -- *see*
>   Hoses, Compressed Gas
>
> Compresses [10-965]
> -- *Category expanded below*
>
> Compresses, Cold [15-026]
> -- *see also*
>   Bottles, Hot/Cold Water
>   Cold Packs
>   Collars, Ice
>   Ice Bags
>
> Compresses, Gauze [10-966]
> -- *see also*
>   Bandages, Gauze
>   Gauze
>   Sponges, Gauze
>
> Compresses, Moist Heat [10-967]
> -- *see also*
>   Moist Heat Therapy Packs

Compression Clamps
-- *see*
  Clamps

Compression Devices, Radiographic [16-559]

Compression Dressings
-- *see*
  Bandages, Pressure

Compression Stockings
-- *see*
  Stockings, Compression

Compressors [10-971]
-- *Category expanded below*

Compressors, Aspirator
-- *see*
  Aspirators

Compressors, External Cardiac
-- *see*
  Resuscitators, Cardiac

Compressors, External Vascular [17-718]

Compressors, Eye
-- *see*
  Pressure Reducers, Intraocular

As noted, the Thesaurus also includes cross-references in the form of *see* and *see also* notes. As in ICD-9-CM, *see* notes instruct the reader to go elsewhere to find the appropriate code and *see also* notes offer additional instructions that may result in a more precise code assignment.

The nomenclature uses a hierarchy moving from general to more specific terms, with each having a five-digit code. For example, following are codes for angioplasty catheters, hematology analyzers, and drug-dose dispensers.

17-183	Catheters, Vascular, Angioplasty
17-184	Catheters, Vascular, Angioplasty, Balloon
17-185	Catheters, Vascular, Angioplasty, Direct Laser Ablation

17-740	Analyzers, Laboratory, Hematology
17-741	Analyzers, Laboratory, Hematology, Cell Counting, Automated
17-742	Analyzers, Laboratory, Hematology, Cell Counting, Semiautomated

17-752	Unit-Dose Dispensers
17-753	Unit-Dose Dispensers, Pill
17-754	Unit-Dose Dispensers, Pill, Programmable
17-755	Unit-Dose Dispensers, Pill, Manual

More extensive listings can be seen in the entries for beds and forceps.

10-342	Beds
10-345	Beds, Electric, Circular Revolving
10-347	Beds, Electric
10-348	Beds, Electric, Flotation Therapy
10-351	Beds, Electric, Radiography/Fluoroscopy
10-353	Beds, Hydraulic
10-357	Beds, Mechanical
10-360	Beds, Fixed, Orthopedic
10-362	Beds, Fixed, Cradle, Pediatric

11-774	Forceps
11-775	Forceps, Biopsy
11-777	Forceps, Dressing
11-779	Forceps, Laparoscopic
11-780	Forceps, Epilation
11-781	Forceps, Fixation
11-782	Forceps, Gallbladder
11-784	Forceps, Hemostatic
11-785	Forceps, Intestinal
11-787	Forceps, Lung
11-788	Forceps, Obstetric
11-790	Forceps, Specimen
11-791	Forceps, Sponge
11-792	Forceps, Sterilizer Transfer
11-793	Forceps, Stone Manipulation
11-794	Forceps, Suction
11-797	Forceps, Tissue
11-798	Forceps, Utility

Process for Revision of and Updates to UMDNS

ECRI updates UMDNS on a daily basis, but, officially, UMDNS is updated annually. New terms can be added, obsolete terms deleted, and existing terms modified. Anyone can suggest changes to UMDNS. A form for submitting suggestions for additions or changes (in English and Portuguese) can be downloaded from the Internet at http://www.opas.org.br/servico/Arquivos/Sala3920.pdf.

Check Your Understanding 14.1

Instructions: Complete the following exercises on a separate piece of paper.

1. Which of the following concepts is not represented in the UMDNS system?
   a. Medical devices and materials
   b. Surgical procedures
   c. In vitro diagnostics
   d. Hospital furniture

2. True or False. Because of UMDNS's narrow scope, the National Library of Medicine has declined to include it in its Unified Medical Language System.

3. The five-digit UMDC numbers are assigned to _____ terms.
   a. Main
   b. Preferred
   c. Entry
   d. All of the above

4. True or False. Only licensed users of UMDNS can request changes to the nomenclature.

5. Using the information presented in this chapter, assign the appropriate code for radiographic compression devices.
   a. 16-836
   b. 16-559
   c. 18-085
   d. 10-969

Introduction to Global Medical Device Nomenclature

The **Global Medical Device Nomenclature** (GMDN) and UMDNS are very similar in scope; both provide names, definitions, and unique codes for essentially all medical devices and supplies at the **generic device group** level (although device attributes are being considered for GMDN that will significantly increase its level of specificity). Both terminologies are being used internationally, GMDN primarily by regulatory agencies and UMDNS primarily by healthcare institutions.

Developer of GMDN

GMDN was developed by the European Committee for Standardization body (CEN) (also known as the Comité Européen de Normalisation) under a project sponsored by the European Community (EC) and with full participation and parallel acceptance by the International Organization for Standardization (ISO).

GMDN was developed largely through the harmonization of six established medical device terminologies, including a previous version of UMDNS and the terminology used by the Center for Devices and Radiological Health, U.S. Food and Drug Administration (FDA). GMDN is managed and its content maintained by the GMDN Agency, an international maintenance agency, with significant FDA representation.

The six chosen nomenclatures were:

- Classification Names for Medical Devices and in Vitro Diagnostic Products (**CNMD**) was developed by the FDA and is the U.S. official nomenclature.

- European Diagnostic Manufacturers Association in Vitro Diagnostic Product Classification (**EDMA**) is used in Europe.

- International Organization for Standardization (**ISO**) 9999 Technical Aids for Disabled Persons Classification is used internationally.

- Japanese Medical Device Nomenclature (**JF-MDA**) is used in Japan and Southeast Asia.

- Norsk Klassifisering Koding and Nomenklatur (**NKKN**) is a Norwegian Nomenclature used in Norway and parts of Europe.

- Universal Medical Device Nomenclature System (**UMDNS**) was developed by ECRI and is used in the United States, some countries in Europe, and some countries worldwide. As the most complete and widely used terminology, UMDNS was given precedence in the development of GMDN, and whenever a term from the ECRI UMDNS has been used as a term in GMDN, the code number is identical.

Purpose of GMDN

GMDN was developed to allow for the classification of all medical devices put on the market as defined in the three European Directives, which set out safety and performance requirements for medical devices and procedures.

The developers designed the terminology for use by a number of different entities, including:

- Regulatory competent authorities
- Notified bodies and conformity assessment entities
- Accredited test houses
- Manufacturers
- Health authorities
- Purchasing departments in hospitals
- Suppliers/trading/E-commerce
- Clinical engineers/technicians
- Clinical personnel
- Researchers

Content of GMDN

Currently, GMDN is made up of three general levels: device category, generic device group, and device type (GMDN Users Guidance 2008). The first level is divided into twenty categories with sixteen of those active. The device categories are the broadest grouping of devices having common areas of intended use or other common characteristics. The sixteen device categories are as follows:

- 01 Active implantable devices
- 02 Anaesthetic and respiratory devices
- 03 Dental devices
- 04 Electro mechanical medical devices
- 05 Hospital hardware
- 06 In vitro diagnostic devices (IVD)
- 07 Non-active implantable devices
- 08 Ophthalmic and optical devices
- 09 Reusable instruments
- 10 Single use devices
- 11 Assistive products for persons with disability
- 12 Diagnostic and therapeutic radiation devices
- 13 Complementary therapy devices
- 14 Biological-derived devices
- 15 Healthcare facility products and adaptations
- 16 Laboratory equipment

When a new product area needs to be included in this nomenclature, a new category code is allotted and the category developed.

The next hierarchical level of the system is the generic device group, which is the actual nomenclature or naming level by which a product or a group of similar products can be classified using a selected generic descriptor and its unique code. The codes are five digits and do not have any inherent meaning.

While not a part of the nomenclature, the device type is the information (name or designation) provided by the manufacturer that uniquely identifies a specifically produced type of medical device. This unique qualifier is made up of the device's make and model.

Principles and Guidelines for GMDN

GMDN terms are composed of four types associated with the generic device groups (GMDN Users Guidance 2008). These types are:

- The preferred (P) term is used to generically classify a group of medical devices. It is the only one of the four allowed for the purpose of product identification (GMDN Users Guidance 2008).

- The template (T) term is a collective term for grouping similar preferred terms.

- The synonym (S) term is an alternative name to a preferred or template term to which it is linked. Synonym terms do not have definitions.

- The multiple-linked synonym term (MS) is linked to more than one preferred and/or template term.

The preferred term, the template term, the synonym, and the multiple-linked synonym term all occur at the generic device group level.

Another type of term, equivalent (E), is equal in concept to a preferred term, template, synonym, or multiple-linked synonym term. Equivalent terms come from one of the six nomenclatures used to create GMDN and are not active terms.

Preferred Terms

The preferred term is the optimal name selected to represent a generic device group (GMDN User Guidance 2008). The preferred term consists of:

- Term name: The name contains a base concept, the first and principal component of the term, and one or more qualifiers as needed to increase the term's specificity. Qualifiers are separated from base concepts and other qualifiers by commas (for example, Catheter, biliary, manometric—where catheter is the base concept and biliary and manometric are qualifiers).

- An associated definition

- A unique five digit numerical code

- Category or the general medical device family assigned to the term

- Term type identifier such as (P) for preferred term

- Product specifier, a data field, indicating the terms valid for product identification

The base concept can be a single noun (for example, Catheter) or a compound noun (for example, Catheter guide wire).

Template Terms

The template term is a name used to group similar preferred terms and to develop a hierarchy in the nomenclature. A template term is added to the nomenclature when the same base concept occurs in three or more preferred terms. The template term is made up of the common base concept and then the qualifier <specify> separated by a comma. It is possible for a template term to have additional qualifiers between the base concept and the <specify>.

Following are examples of various terms shown in the GMDN User Guidance:

Template

Cardiac catheter, <specify>

Cardiac catheter, balloon <specify>

Preferred

Cardiac catheter, ablative

Cardiac catheter, balloon, intra-aortic

Cardiac catheter, balloon pacing electrode

Cardiac catheter, balloon, pulmonary artery, basic

Synonym

Dinamap for template term sphygmomanometer, electronic, <specify>

Hess-screen for preferred term Campimeter

Process for Revision to and Updates of GMDN

CEN owns the copyright for GMDN but has delegated administration of the terminology to the Maintenance Agency Policy Group (MAPG), an entity of the GMDN Agency. MAPG comprises representation from the FDA as the U.S. regulatory body, the EC, the Japanese Ministry of Health, Labour, and Welfare, as well as up to five nominees approved to represent CEN, five nominees approved to represent ISO interests, and a representative of the Global Harmonization Task Force (GHTF). MAPG updates GMDN at least annually.

Requests for adding a term or modifying an existing one are accepted via a GMDN application found via a link on the GMDN Agency's home page. The GMDN Agency assesses a fee after the submitted material has undergone GMDN review.

Detailed information regarding GMDN is available online at http://www.gmdnagency.com/.

Check Your Understanding 14.2

Instructions: Complete the following exercises on a separate piece of paper.

1. The highest level of classification in GMDN is the:
   a. Category of devices
   b. Generic device group
   c. Preferred term
   d. None of the above

2. True or False. A template term contains a group of similar preferred terms.

3. **Cardiac, catheter,** <specify> is an example of a:
   a. Preferred term
   b. Template term
   c. Synonym term
   d. Equivalent term

4. True or False. Because GMDN is a global nomenclature, it is not covered by copyright laws of any nation.

Introduction to the Medical Dictionary for Regulatory Activities

The Medical Dictionary for Regulatory Activities (MedDRA) is applicable to all phases of drug devel-

opment except animal toxicology and the health effects and malfunctions of devices (MedDRA 2008b).

Developer of MedDRA

MedDRA was developed under the auspices of the **International Conference on Harmonization (ICH) of Technical Requirements for Registration of Pharmaceuticals for Human Use** to complement ICH's ongoing safety, quality, and efficacy harmonization efforts. MedDRA was based on the U.K. Medicines Control Agency's medical terminology and is owned by the International Federation of Pharmaceutical Manufacturers and Associations (MedDRA 2008a). The FDA recommends (though does not require) MedDRA, and the European Union has required MedDRA coding for submissions and safety reporting since January 2003.

Purpose of MedDRA

MedDRA was developed as a tool to be used by pharmaceutical companies in reporting adverse effects and potential adverse effects of medications and other products. It was designed to facilitate medical product regulation and related electronic data interchange.

Content of MedDRA

MedDRA has a hierarchical structure in which lowest-level terms (LLTs) are mapped first to preferred terms (PTs), then to a high-level term (HLT), next to a high-level group term (HLGT), and finally to a system organ class (SOC). This dictionary of terms is currently available in Czech, Dutch, French, German, Japanese, Italian, Portuguese, and Spanish.

Each MedDRA term is assigned an eight-digit code without taxonomic meaning. Initially, codes were assigned alphabetically beginning with 10000001, with new terms assigned sequentially.

MedDRA is a multiple axial system that uses nonindexed codes and includes a five-level hierarchy. In the 11.1 version of MedDRA, the distribution of terms was as follows:

Level	Name	No. of Terms
SOC	System Organ Class	26
HLGT	High-Level Group Term	332
HLT	High-Level Term	1688
PT	Preferred Term	18,209
LLT	Low-Level Term	66,587

Principles and Guidelines for MedDRA

MedDRA terms cover all types of adverse reactions to pharmaceuticals. Embedded within MedDRA are many other coding and reporting systems, including:

- The World Health Organization—Adverse Reaction Terminology (WHO-ART)

- Coding Symbols for a Thesaurus of Adverse Reaction Terms (COSTART)

- International Classification of Diseases, Ninth Revision (ICD-9)

- International Classification of Diseases, Ninth Revision, Clinical Modification (ICD-9-CM)

- Japanese Adverse Reaction Terminology (J-ART)

- Hoechst Adverse Reaction Terminology System (HARTS)

In addition, the *Diagnostic and Statistical Manual of Mental Disorders, Fourth Edition* (DSM-IV) was used as the basis for the psychiatry section. Although MedDRA is used to report adverse effects of drugs, it does not itself contain codes for drugs.

An interesting effect of MedDRA's hierarchical system is that very similar clinical conditions may be indexed and coded quite differently. For example, the terms *hypoglycemia* and *decreased blood sugar* both exist at the PT level but reside in different SOCs. The decreased/increased terms have been placed in the SOC investigations, whereas all the hypo/hyper terms have been placed under their respective body systems. The reason for this is that hyper/hypo terms supposedly represent diagnoses whereas increased/decreased terms represent only laboratory results. For example, "decreased blood sugar" would only be an indication of an occurrence of a decrease in blood sugar, which may not be diagnostic. On the other hand, "hypoglycemia" is considered to mean a decreased blood glucose level indicative of a diagnosis, in this case a decreased blood glucose associated with signs and symptoms such as dizziness. MedDRA authors recognize that the differentiation created between hyper/hypo and increased/decreased is rather fine and is not consistent throughout, even though it is the convention in MedDRA. What is considered diagnostic may depend on the company, clinical trial, or laboratory. This fine distinction in MedDRA could create problems in data retrieval because the same event could be coded differently and thus result in incomplete data retrieval (PSI International 2003).

Rule Out, Possible, Probable Diagnoses

At present, like ICD-9-CM, MedDRA cannot capture concepts such as "suspicion of," "maybe," "possibility of," or "rule out." However, because suspected diagnoses are important data to collect, those reported as "rule out," "possibility of," or "maybe" are to be coded just as if the diagnosis was confirmed, although the coding guidelines may differ depending on the organization's objectives. Guidelines published by ICH include options when sign(s)/symptom(s) and a provisional diagnosis are stated (PSI International 2003).

It is important to stress that no matter how an organization chooses to address a coding issue, the issue needs to be addressed in such a manner to promote uniformity and consistency and thus enable complete data retrieval (PSI International 2003).

Abbreviations Used in MedDRA

As in ICD-9-CM, in MedDRA, NOS stands for "not otherwise specified" and NEC stands for "not elsewhere classified." NOS (for example, in the MedDRA LLT "Pain NOS") indicates that the condition is not included in another LLT (such as "Chest pain" or "Flank pain"). It is often a general term for a condition that has specific instances listed as separate LLTs. The other LLTs may be in multiple SOCs, as the example of different pains indicates.

NEC (for example, in the MedDRA HLGT "Eye disorders NEC") indicates the condition is not classified in any other grouping or within any other SOC under the multi-axial classification schema. Unlike NOS, which is seen exclusively at the LLT level, NEC is usually seen at the HLT or HLGT level to gather preferred terms that are not easily classified under other HLTs or HLGTs.

The HLGT and HLT levels group related terms under them by anatomy, pathology, physiology, etiology, or function. The PT level contains distinct descriptors for medical concepts including symptoms, signs, diseases, diagnoses, therapeutic indication, investigation, surgical or medical procedures, and medical, social, or family characteristics. The LLT level contains synonyms, quasi-synonyms, or lexical variants of the PT to which they are linked. Because LLTs accommodate culturally unique terms, each LLT may not have a translation in all languages. An LLT can be linked to only one PT (MedDRA Introductory Guide 2008).

The term "malignant neoplasm of the upper lobe" can be traced through the five levels of the MedDRA system as follows: At the SOC level, the term may be classified on either the etiological axis, Neoplasms benign, malignant and unspecified, or the anatomical axis, Respiratory, thoracic and mediastinal disorders. Selecting the etiological axis leads to the HLGT, Respiratory and mediastinal neoplasms malignant and unspecified; the HLT, Respiratory tract and pleural neoplasms malignant cell type unspecified NEC; the PT, Lung neoplasm malignant; and, finally, the LLT, Malignant neoplasm of upper lobe. If the anatomical axis is selected, the process begins with the SOC, Respiratory, thoracic and mediastinal disorders; the HLGT, Respiratory tract neoplasms; the HLT, Lower respiratory tract neoplasms; and the PT, Lung neoplasm malignant.

In the latter example, the PT was included under two HLT terms. Although a PT can have more than one associated HLT (HLGT and SOC), there is at most one path down through the hierarchy (SOC-HLGT-HLT-PT) to any PT so that counting errors are avoided when querying on the SOC, HLGT, and HLT levels.

Standardized MedDRA Queries

Standardized MedDRA queries (SMQs) are groupings of terms from one or more MedDRA SOCs that relate to a defined medical condition or an area of interest. They are intended to aid in case identification. SMQs were previously known as special search categories. Because one entity can be coded into different SOCs, SMQs allow for easy retrieval of related conditions for study purposes.

The included terms may relate to signs, symptoms, diagnoses, syndromes, physical findings, laboratory and other physiologic test data, and so on related to the medical condition or area of interest (SMQ Introductory Guide 2008).

LLTs that are not subordinate to an included preferred term are excluded.

With the release of MedDRA Version 11.1, there are 67 SMQs. Those most recently added include the following:

- Breast neoplasms, malignant and unspecified
- Cardiomyopathy
- Demyelination
- Hypertension
- Lens disorders
- Optic nerve disorders
- Ovarian neoplasms, malignant and unspecified
- Prostate neoplasms, malignant and unspecified
- Uterine and fallopian tube neoplasms, malignant and unspecified

The terms defined for acute renal failure, for example, are the following:

Acute renal failure, "narrow" terms

Acute pre-renal failure

Anuria

Azotemia

Continuous haemodiafiltration

Dialysis

Hemodialysis

Neonatal anuria

Nephropathy toxic

Oliguria

Peritoneal dialysis

Renal failure

Renal failure acute

Renal failure neonatal

Renal impairment

Renal impairment neonatal

Acute renal failure, "broad" terms

Albuminuria

Blood creatine abnormal

Blood creatinine increased

Blood urea abnormal

Blood urea increased

Blood urea nitrogen/creatinine ratio increased

Creatinine renal clearance abnormal

Creatinine renal clearance decreased

Edema due to renal disease

Glomerular filtration rate abnormal

Glomerular filtration rate decreased

Hypercreatininaemia

Nephritic syndrome

Nephritis

Nephritis interstitial

Protein urine present

Proteinuria

Renal function test abnormal

Renal transplant

Renal tubular disorder

Renal tubular necrosis

Tubulointerstitial nephritis

Urea renal clearance decreased

Urine output decreased

Process for Revision of and Updates to MedDRA

The MedDRA Maintenance and Support Services Organization (MSSO), which is the sole licensee and distributor of MedDRA subscriptions, updates MedDRA twice a year on March 1 and September 1. Core subscribers to MedDRA and Regulators may submit requests for revisions either by submitting the appropriate form or using the WebCR tool. In addition, the MedDRA MSSO staff continually assess MedDRA for adequacy and make changes as appropriate. Every change request must meet at minimum all the following criteria:

- It must be unambiguous.

- It must be within the scope of the terminology.

- It must be medically valid and acceptable by an international panel of medical personnel. (MedDRA MSSO Change Request Information 2008)

Change requests in MedDRA may be both simple and complex. Simple change requests are any changes at the PT level and below in the terminology structure. A simple change request will fall under any of the following categories:

- Add a PT

- Move a PT

- Rename a PT

- Demote a PT to low-level term status

- Swap a PT with a LLT

- Add or delete a PT in a SMQ

- Add or delete a PT link to a HLT

- Add a LLT

- Move a LLT

- Rename a LLT

- Promote a LLT

- Change the status of a LLT

- Reassign the primary SOC of a PT

- Add a new term (MedDRA MSSO Change Request Information 2008)

Complex change requests are any changes involving HLTs, HLGTs, or SOCs because they will affect all underlying terms. The MSSO will consider complex changes based on input from core subscribers or internal analysis. A complex change request can fall under any of the following categories:

- Add a new SOC, HLGT, HLT

- Rename SOC, HLGT, HLT

- Merge HLT

- Merge HLGT

- Link/unlink a HLT

- Link/unlink a HLGT (MedDRA MSSO Change Request Information 2008)

All complex changes to the terminology are made once a year in March.

Subscribers requesting revisions to SMQs must use the specified form posted on the Web site. Updates to the SMQs occur twice a year at the same time as MedDRA.

The MedDRA MSSO accepts change requests from anyone with a valid core subscriber user identification number and change request (CR) identification number. Possession of these identification numbers allows an individual to access the change request information on the MSSO Web site.

Check Your Understanding 14.3

Instructions: Complete the following exercises on a separate piece of paper.

1. The most generic terms in MedDRA are the:
   a. System organ classes
   b. High-level group terms
   c. High-level terms
   d. Low-level terms

2. True or False. The code numbers in MedDRA do not have any meaning themselves but, instead, are assigned alphabetically or sequentially.

3. True or False. A clinical term may be mapped to more than one SOC in MedDRA.

4. Who can request changes to MedDRA?
   a. Anyone
   b. Any pharmaceutical manufacturer
   c. Core subscribers to MedDRA
   d. Any healthcare provider and any pharmaceutical manufacturer

5. Which of the following is not a requirement for a request for a change in MedDRA?
   a. The term must be unambiguous.
   b. The condition must be codeable in ICD-9-CM or ICD-10-CM.
   c. The condition must be within the scope of the terminology.
   d. The condition must be medically valid and internationally accepted.

Introduction to the Systematized Nomenclature of Dentistry

The Systematized Nomenclature of Dentistry (SNODENT) is based on the structure and content of, and is a part of, the Systematized Nomenclature of Medicine (SNOMED) discussed in chapter 7.

Developer of SNODENT

SNODENT was developed by the American Dental Association (ADA). Although SNODENT is not currently in wide use, support is gathering to implement it as the terminology for use in EHRs.

Purpose of SNODENT

SNODENT was developed to provide dentistry with a comprehensive terminology to be used to establish and define dental and oral disease classifications and comorbidities. Dental practitioners recognized that the ICD-9-CM system was inadequate for dental diagnostic coding because it was very general and was not developed in a hierarchical or logical way from a dental standpoint.

According to a written statement by Lapp to the NCVHS Workgroup on Computer-based Patient records, SNODENT was designed to be an integral part of the EHR and thus is composed of diagnoses, signs, symptoms, and complaints (Lapp 1999). It provides the means not only for diagnostic coding, but when collected, compiled, and analyzed, reliable diagnostic treatment outcomes data also can be compiled. Third-party payers can use SNODENT to eliminate the need for narrative descriptions and other attachments. Vendors of dental practice management systems are expected to incorporate SNODENT in their systems to maintain a comprehensive patient health record.

SNODENT code usage was designed to allow for:

- The national collection of data via clearinghouses to analyze treatment outcomes

- Recording of a complete oral risk assessment of the patient

- Use of a single code for synonymous descriptive terms in claim processing to help reduce or eliminate narrative descriptions or other claim attachments

- In-office monitoring of production and treatment (ADA News 2007)

In testimony to the NCVHS Subcommittee on Standards and Security, Schooley (2004) stated the need to include specific diagnosis codes on claims is based on five perceived needs within the dental community:

- *Efficiency:* Diagnostic codes would facilitate operations, improve submission accuracy,

lower administrative costs, and improve claim turnaround times.

- *Fraud detection.* Diagnostic codes would facilitate utilization management activities and monitoring for fraud and abuse. Knowing the specific clinical conditions for treatment allows for more effective disease management programs. Diagnostic codes also will facilitate the process of ensuring that items and services are medically necessary and appropriate.

- *Benefit design:* Diagnostic codes would assist in the development of plan designs. Insurers would have information to structure more qualitative and cost-effective dental benefit plans for employer groups and individuals.

- *Outcomes research:* Diagnostic codes would facilitate more effective outcomes research. Plans would be able to identify treatments that are efficacious and those that are not for a given clinical condition, ultimately improving the public's oral health.

- *Claims attachments:* Diagnostic codes would reduce or eliminate the need for dental claim attachments that discourage dentists from submitting claims electronically.

Content of SNODENT

SNODENT is a comprehensive taxonomy that contains codes for identifying not only diseases and diagnoses, but also anatomy, conditions, morphology, and social factors that may affect health or treatment. It allows dentists to code not only dental conditions, but also concurrent medical conditions and risk behaviors (for example, diabetes, smoking behavior) that might be expected to affect patients' oral health and to influence treatment decisions (Leake 2002).

SNODENT contains approximately 6,000 terms and 4,000 codes. The codes are alphanumeric with seven or eight characters, and are organized according to the etiology of the condition (genetic, infectious, trauma, and so on).

Principles and Guidelines for SNODENT

Because SNODENT is an integral part of SNOMED, it follows the general principles and guidelines of SNOMED. Specifically, SNOMED concept codes should be regarded as entirely meaningless identifiers (keys). The assignment of particular letters and number sequences did originally signify some meaning, but this strategy has been abandoned. Relying on any apparent meaning embedded in the code string will only mislead the user. The category (finding, procedure, topography, morphology, and so on) of a particular concept may be made clear only by examining its position in a hierarchy.

Process for Revision of and Updates to SNODENT

In 2007, the maintenance process for SNODENT became the responsibility of the SNODENT Editorial Panel (ADA News 2007). The Panel is made up of members from the Council on Dental Practice, Council on Dental Benefits Programs, Council on Scientific Affairs, and the Council on Dental Education and Licensure, in addition to a dentist representative (ADA Update 2007). Responsibilities of the Panel include the review, update, and maintenance of the clinical descriptors in SNODENT.

Check Your Understanding 14.4

Instructions: Complete the following exercises on a separate piece of paper.

1. Which of the following are *not* included in the SNODENT coding system?
   a. Dental diagnoses
   b. Medical diagnoses
   c. Dental procedures
   d. Signs and symptoms

2. True or False. SNODENT is an integral part of ICD-10-CM and follows the same principles and guidelines.

3. Who is responsible for maintaining SNODENT?
   a. IHTSDO Editorial Board
   b. NCVHS Subcommittee on Standards
   c. SNOMED Editorial Panel
   d. SNODENT Editorial Panel

Introduction to ABC Codes

ABC codes are a registered vocabulary of HL7 and were incorporated into the NLM's Unified Medical Language System (UMLS) in 1998.

Developer of ABC Codes

ABC Coding Solutions, formally Alternative Link started the development process of the ABC codes in 1996 via interviews, informal surveys, and case studies. This process was followed by systematic research using formal data collection tools and input from individuals such as those from practitioner associations and experts in the field. The final groups involved were subject matter experts from various backgrounds (for example, coding, claims management, and credentialing). The outcome was more than 4,000 five-character alphabetic codes that describe a wide assortment of integrative healthcare practices, two-character alphanumeric practitioner identifiers, **relative value units** (RVUs), and legal practice guidelines.

Purpose of ABC Codes

ABC codes were created to describe the procedures, treatments, and services provided during an encounter with a **complementary and alternative medicine** (CAM), nursing, or other integrative healthcare provider. This area of healthcare is not identified specifically in other codes sets in use today. Figure 14.1 (see page 230) shows the gaps in the national HIPAA code sets addressed by ABC codes.

Molina (2004) states: "Fully deployed and used in conjunction with CPT, HCPCS II, and CDT codes, ABC codes will capture data on an estimated 1.4 billion annual visits to unconventional and nonphysician caregivers and allow for comparisons of the outcomes of these visits to the estimated 1.1 billion visits made to doctors' offices."

Content of ABC Codes

More than 4,000 five-character alphabetic ABC codes describe a wide assortment of integrative

Figure 14.1.   Gaps in the national HIPAA code sets addressed by ABC codes

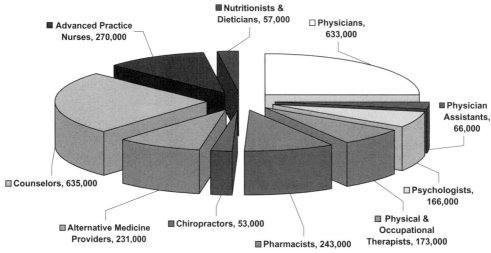

Note: Colored areas indicate gaps in coding targeted by ABC Codes.

healthcare practices, including what is said, done, ordered, prescribed, or distributed by providers of alternative medicine. Figure 14.2 (see page 231) illustrates the coding hierarchy of an ABC code.

In addition, two-character alphanumeric modifiers are available to identify the type of practitioner who rendered the service. (See table 14.1 on page 233.) Modifiers follow the five-character alphabetic ABC code. The two combined into a seven-character code linked with the state-specific scope of practice guidelines available from ABC Coding Solutions can assist in ensuring that practitioners are legally authorized to deliver a specific service.

ABC Coding Solutions also offers RVUs through a license agreement with Relative Value Studies, Inc. (RVSI) that indicate the financial worth of the procedure, treatment, or service. RVUs are established by RVSI by gathering information from the integrative healthcare practitioners. (http://www.abccodes.com/ali/FAQs/general_faq.asp#ALT4).

Principles and Guidelines for ABC Codes

In 2003, the Secretary of the Department of Health and Human Services (HHS) authorized use of ABC codes under an exception to HIPAA. The initial reason for not naming it as a standard was because ABC codes were considered relatively new and evaluation of the system was necessary.

This resulted in a two-year nationwide demonstration project whereby use of the ABC codes to describe the products and services delivered by complementary and alternative medicine and nursing practitioners was tested. HHS approval meant that HIPAA-covered entities (healthcare providers, health plans, and healthcare clearinghouses) used ABC codes to describe products and services in HIPAA transactions. The two-year time period allowed HHS to obtain data on the cost-benefit of ABC codes in HIPAA transactions and assisted in the completion of this code set's evaluation. Although the testing did not guarantee that ABC codes will be named as a HIPAA code set standard, it was seen as

Figure 14.2.   Coding hierarchy of ABC code

Example:
The following description illustrates the coding hierarchy of ABC code NAAGN—Pain management and/or control initial 60 minutes, Managing and/or controlling a patient's pain levels. For additional time, use NAAGO. Service is billed in 60-minute increments.

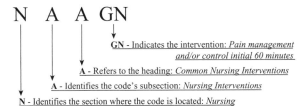

GN - Indicates the intervention: *Pain management and/or control initial 60 minutes*
A - Refers to the heading: *Common Nursing Interventions*
A - Identifies the code's subsection: *Nursing Interventions*
N - Identifies the section where the code is located: *Nursing*

The hierarchal meaning of the first three letters of each ABC code is shown in the following code tree:

A - Clinical practice management
  A - Client evaluation
    A - *New client in-office with ICD diagnosis*
    B - *Existing client in-office with ICD diagnosis*
    C - *New client home-visit with ICD diagnosis*
    D - *Existing client home-visit with ICD diagnosis*
    E - *New client in-facility with ICD diagnosis*
    F - *Existing client in-facility with ICD diagnosis*
  B - Client health maintenance
    A - *New client wellness visit with or without ICD diagnosis*
    B - *Existing client wellness visit with or without ICD diagnosis*
  C - Client assessment
    A - *New client in-office without ICD diagnosis*
    B - *Existing client in-office without ICD diagnosis*
    C - *Remote location, new client without ICD diagnosis*
    D - *Remote location, existing client without ICD diagnosis*
    E - *New client in-office with nursing diagnosis*
    F - *Existing client in-office with nursing diagnosis*
    G - *New client home-visit with nursing diagnosis*
    H - *Existing client home-visit with nursing diagnosis*
    I - *New client in-facility with nursing diagnosis*
    J - *Existing client in-facility with nursing diagnosis*
    K - *New client in-facility with or without ICD diagnosis*
    L - *Existing client in-facility with or without ICD diagnosis*
  D - General service and referral codes
    A - *Consultation between practitioners with or without ICD diagnosis*
    B - *Extended services with or without ICD diagnosis*
    C - *Phone conversations with or without ICD diagnosis*
    D - *Analysis and/or documentation services with or without ICD diagnosis*
    X - *Recommendation and/or prescription services with or without ICD diagnosis*
    Y - *Adjunct Care Orders and/or referrals with or without ICD diagnosis*

    Z - *Preparing and/or dispensing and/or training services with or without ICD diagnosis*
  H - Reference Mapping
    A - *Tracking code use with or without ICD diagnosis*
B - Multiple specialties
  A - Physical modalities
    A - *Cold*
    B - *Electrical or magnetic*
    C - *Heat*
    D - *Water*
    E - *Light*
    F - *Mechanical*
    G - *Sound*
  B - Movement modalities
    A - *Activity or exercise*
    B - *Joint mobilization*
    C - *Traction*
    E - *Aquatic activity*
  C - Rehabilitation and Training Modalities
    A - *Rehabilitative treatments and/or training*
    B - *Work conditioning*
    C - *Ergonomics*
    D - *Taping Services*
  D - Physical Test and/or Measurement Modalities
    A - *Miscellaneous tests and/or measurements*
    B - *Body composition testing*
    C - *Electronic muscle testing*
    D - *Manual muscle testing*
    E - *Physical performance testing*
    F - *Range of motion tests and/or measurements*
  E - Allergy Services
    B - *Allergy Treatments*
  F - Nutrition Services
    A - *Nutritional education*
    B - *Nutritional Management*
C - Practice specialties
  A - Oriental Medicine Services
    B - *General Oriental procedures*
    C - *Oriental Modalities*
    D - *Oriental Therapies*
    E - *Oriental Anesthesia*
  B - Somatic and/or Massage Practices
    A - *Body-Mind*
    B - *Bodywork*
    C - *Energy work*
    E - *Massage*
    G - *Oriental massage*
    H - *Somatic education*
  C - Chiropractic Services
    A - *Spinal adjustments*
    B - *Nonspinal adjustments*
    C - *Miscellaneous chiropractic services*
  D - Mental health services
    A - *Mental Health Counseling*
    B - *Mental Health Testing and/or interpretation*
    C - *Hypnotherapy and/or meditation*
    D - *Psychotherapy*
  E - Reproductive and/or Childbirth services
    A - *Miscellaneous reproductive services*

Figure 14.2.   (Continued)

<table>
<tr><td>

B - *Prenatal*
C - *Labor and Delivery*
D - *Postpartum*
E - *Newborn*
F - *Family planning and/or genetic counseling*
G - *Reproductive system exams and/or treatments*
F - Naturopathic Services
    A - *Osseous manipulations*
    B - *Visceral manipulations*
    C - *Miscellaneous naturopathy*
G - Osteopathic Services
    A - *Miscellaneous osteopathy*
H - Indigenous Healing Practices
    A - *Ayurvedic medicine*
    B - *Native American healing*
    C - *Curandera*
    D - *Shamanism*
I - Spiritual care Services
    A - *Christian Science care*
    B - *Spiritual nursing care*
    C - *Multi-denominational care*
J - Other Specialty Services
    A - *Naprapathic manipulations*
    B - *Parenting education and/or skills training*
    C - *Public health services*
D - Laboratory and/or office procedures
  A - Heart and Vascular Services
    F - *Other Miscellaneous heart or vascular services*
  B - Neurological Services
    B - *Nerve conduction*
  D - Substance administration Services
    A - *Miscellaneous substance administration*
    B - *Injections*
    C - *Substance administration management*
  E - Laboratory Services
    A - *General blood analysis*
    B - *Mineral analysis*
    C - *Nutritional analysis*
    D - *Metabolic analysis*
    E - *Blood vitamin analysis*
    F - *Saliva analysis*

</td><td>

G - *Stool analysis*
I - *Urinalysis*
J - *General laboratory tests*
L - *Chemical screening*
M - *Male-specific tests*
O - *Female-specific tests*
P - *Allergy tests*
Z - *Sample collection*
F - Radiology Services
    A - *Computer-enhanced radiology*
H - Miscellaneous Laboratory and/or Office procedures and
    services
    A - *Spectroscopy*
    C - *Thermography*
E - Physical Resources
  A - Materials and/or Supplies
    A - *Miscellaneous materials and/or supplies*
  B - Applicants
    A - *Miscellaneous applicants*
  C - Solutions
    A - *Allergen solutions*
    B - *Miscellaneous solutions*
G - Herbs and natural substances
  A - Oriental Herbs and Natural Substances
    A to Z - *Oriental herbs and natural substances, letter A - Z*
  B - Western Herbs and Natural Substances
    A to Z - *Western herbs and natural substances, letter A - Z*
  C - Miscellaneous substances
    A - *Flower essences*
    B - *Nutraceuticals*
    C - *Essential oils*
H - Remedies
  A - Homeopathic remedies
    A to Z - *Homeopathic remedies, letter A - Z*
N - Nursing
  A - Nursing Interventions
    A - *Common nursing interventions*
    B - *Common nursing interventions II*
  B - Nursing-facilitated Education
    A - *Patient education and/or counseling*
  C - Speech therapy

</td></tr>
</table>

Source: ABC Coding Manual for Integrated Healthcare 2008.

a step toward either a modification to the HCPCS code set (which already incorporates codes developed by outside entities) or as a separate HIPAA code set for healthcare transactions.

ABC Coding Solutions has included on its Web site (http://www.abccodes.com/ali/etransactions/transactions.asp) companion documents that offer guidelines for using ABC codes in the following HIPAA transactions:

- 270/271 Health Care Eligibility Benefit Inquiry and Response

- 276/277 Health Care Claim Status Request and Response

- 278 Health Care Services Review: Request for Review and Response

- 834 Benefit Enrollment and Maintenance

- 835 Health Care Claim Payment/Advice

- 837 Health Care Claim: Institutional

- 837 Health Care Claim: Professional

Table 14.1.   Disciplines, credential abbreviations, and practitioner specialties

Practitioner Modifier	State-specific Abbreviation	Practitioner Specialty
1A	DC DC	Doctor of Chiropractic Chiropractic Doctor
1B	MT CMT LMP LMT LMT MP n/a n/a n/a n/a	Massage Therapist Certified Massage Therapist Licensed Massage Practitioner Licensed Massage Therapist Licensed Massage Technician Massage Practitioner Master Massage Therapist Massage and Bodywork Therapist Massage and Bodywork Technician Masseur or Masseuse
1C	DOM OMD AcT AP CA DAc LAc DiplAc	Doctor of Oriental Medicine Oriental Medical Doctor Acupuncture Therapist Acupuncture Physician Certified Acupuncturist Doctor of Acupuncture Licensed Acupuncturist Diplomate of Acupuncture
1D	RM CM CPM DEM GM LLM LM LM LTM LDM LMP	Registered Midwife Certified Midwife Certified Professional Midwife Direct Entry Midwife Granny Midwife Licensed Lay Midwife Lay Midwife Licensed Midwife Licensed Traditional Midwife Licensed Direct-Entry Midwife Licensed Midwife Practitioner
1E	ND ND DN NMD	Naturopathic Doctor Naturopathic Physician Doctor of Naturopathy Doctor of Naturopathic Medicine
1F	CNS NS CRNS	Clinical Nurse Specialist Nurse Specialist Clinical Registered Nurse Specialist
1G	CNM NM CRNM	Certified Nurse Midwife Licensed Nurse Midwife Certified Registered Nurse Midwife
1H	ANP APN APRN ARNP CNP CRNP NP RN, NP, C RNP	Advanced Nurse Practitioner Advanced Practice Nurse Advanced Practice Registered Nurse Advanced Registered Nurse Practitioner Certified Nurse Practitioner Certified Registered Nurse Practitioner Nurse Practitioner Registered Nurse, Nurse Practitioner, Certified Registered Nurse Practitioner

(Continued on next page)

Table 14.1.   (Continued)

Practitioner Modifier	State-specific Abbreviation	Practitioner Specialty
1J	LPN LVN	Licensed Practical Nurse Licensed Vocational Nurse

1K	RN
	n/a
	n/a
		Registered Nurse
		   Professional Nurse
		   Professional Registered Nurse

1L	DO DO	Doctor of Osteopathy Osteopathic Doctor

1M	MD
	MD
	MD
	DABMA
		Medical Doctor
		   Allopathic Physician
		   Doctor of Allopathic Medicine
		   Diplomate of the American Board of Medical Acupuncture

1N	PA PA-C	Physician Assistant Physician Assistant, Certified
N/A	HO DHt	Homeopath (for example, secondary license for physicians) Diplomate of Homeotherapeutics
1P	MSW ACSW DSW LCSW QCSW DCSW LICSW LSW MSSW LMSW BSW LiSW	Clinical Social Worker
1Q	MFCC	Marriage and Family Therapist
1R	PhD/EdD PsyD	Psychologist, Doctorate
1S	CS CSB	Christian Science Practitioner Christian Science Practitioner
1T	n/a	Christian Science Nurse
1U	LR RCR	Licensed Reflexologist Registered Certified Reflexologist

1V	DN
	DN
	DN
		Doctor of Naprapathy
		   Naprapathic Doctor
		   Naprapathic Physician

1W	CPC	Licensed Professional Counselor
1X	RD	Registered Dietician
1Y	MH BSW	Nonlicensed Practitioner type
1Z	CNS CN CCN	Certified Nutrition Specialist Certified Nutritionist Certified Clinical Nutritionist

(Continued on next page)

Table 14.1.   (Continued)

Practitioner Modifier	State-specific Abbreviation	Practitioner Specialty
To be assigned	MH	Mental Health Professional (other than Psychiatrist)
	CPC	Certified Professional Counselor
	MFCC	Marriage and Family Counselor
	MSW	Master of Social Work
	ACSW	Academy of Clinical Social Worker
	DSW	Doctorate in Social Work
	LCSW	Licensed Clinical Social Worker
	QCSW	Qualified Clinical Social Worker
	DCSW	Diplomate in Clinical Social Work
	LICSW	Licensed Independent Clinical Social Worker
	LSW	Licensed Social Worker
	MSSW	Master of Science in Social Work
	LMSW	Licensed Master Social Worker
	BSW	Bachelor of Social Work
	LiSW	Licensed Social Worker
	PhD/EdD	Psychologist
	PsyD	Psychologist
	LCP	Psychologist
	MFCC	Psychologist
	MA	Psychologist
To be assigned	HD	Holistic Dentist
	DDS	Doctor of Dental Surgery
To be assigned	OT	Occupational Therapist
To be assigned	PT	Physical Therapist
To be assigned	PharmD	Pharmacist

Source: Alternative Link 2008.

As the guidelines indicate, ABC codes are used in the same insurance forms (CMS-1500 and CMS-1450), data fields, software applications, databases, information systems, and business processes as other HIPAA code sets. Figure 14.3 (see page 235) shows a sample superbill to be used by a practitioner to identify an encounter.

ABC codes are not intended to replace any of the named HIPAA medical code set standards but, rather, to be used alongside them. Consider that, initially, HCPCS was a trilevel coding system with CPT as Level I and national and local code sets as Levels II and III. Although eliminated on December 31, 2003, to comply with HIPAA, state Medicaid agencies, Medicare contractors, and private insurers developed HCPCS Level III codes for use in their specific programs or local areas of jurisdiction. An option under consideration is to name ABC codes as HCPCS Level IV. If HHS chooses to do so, it would close a gap that now exists in the ability to identify services provided during an encounter with a complementary, alternative, nursing, or other integrative healthcare provider. According to information on ABC Coding Solutions' Web site, "The codes fill the gaps left by the existing standard HIPAA code sets and provide for comprehensive and seamless coding. With ABC codes, you gain a superior understanding of the economic and health outcomes of alternative medicine, nursing and other integrative healthcare interventions—the kind of understanding that supports health-promoting, cost-effective and evidence-based healthcare." (Alternative Link 2008).

Figure 14.3.   Superbill

Superbills for Super-Efficiency
Create a personalized list of coded services on your own form to save time and simplify coding.
Call us at 1-877-621-5465 for a price quote.

Sample Group Practice for Oriental Medicine, Refelexology and Massage Therapy
860 Main Street

(505) 875-0001 Office	Anytown, USA 93420	Tax ID # 99- 999999
(505) 875-0002 Fax	mail@ABCcodes.com	State License # 00000

Last Name: _____   First Name: _____
SS#: _____   Referred by: _____
Address: _____   City: _____   State: _____   Zip Code: _____
Home Phone: _____   Work Phone: _____   Cell Phone: _____
E-mail: _____   Miscellaneous: _____
Diagnosis / Complaint: _____

ABC/CPT Code	DESCRIPTION	# / $	ABC/CPT Code	DESCRIPTION	# / $	ABC/CPT Code	DESCRIPTION	# / $
New Wellness Visit w/o ICD Diagnosis			**Multiple Specialties**			**Herbs and Natural Substances**		
ABAAB 99402	Welness 30 minutes		BAAAF 97039	Cold friction each 20 minutes		GAGAG	Ginseng / ren shen / xi yan she	
ABAAC 99403	Wellness 45 minutes		BABAE 97039	Magnet therapy each 15 minutes		GBAAR	Arctostaphylos uva ursi / uva ursi leaf	
Existing client in-office with ICD diagnosis			BAEAC 97039	Cold laser therapy each treatment		GBHAJ	Hydrastis canadensis / goldenseal	
ACAAG 99203	30 minutes in-office Oriental medicine intake		BBAAH 97110	Postural exercise individual each 15 minutes		GCACQ	Five flower formula / rescue remedy	
ACAAH 99499	10 minutes in-office reflexology intake		BBABY 97139	PNF individual each 15 minutes		GCCBQ	Eucalyptus globulus	
ACAAJ 99215	20 minutes in-office massage therapy intake		BCAAS 97110	Range-of-motion therapeutic exercise individual each 15 min.		GCCCA	Jasminum officinalis	
Existing Client Visit w/o Diagnosis			BDCAD 95999	Electronic muscle testing one region each test		GCCCF	Lavendula officinalis	
ACBAF 99212	20 minutes in-office Oriental medicine intake		BDDAB 95831	Extremity or trunk manual testing each 15 minutes		**Substance Administration**		
ACBAI 99499	20 minutes in-office reflexology intake		**Oriental Medicine Services**			DDADV 97139	Essential oil inhalation each 15 minutes	
ACBAD 99212	10 minutes in-office massage therapy intake		CABAB 97810	Auricular acupuncture each 15 minutes		DDADW 97139	Essential oil compress each 15 minutes	
General Services			CABAE 97810	Acupuncture initial 15 minutes		**Common Interventions**		
ADBAA 99050	After-hours care until 10 p.m. narrative required		CABAG 97810	Trigger-point acupuncture each 15 minutes		ADYAB	Laboratory procedure order no charge	
ADYAL	Specialist referral		CACAB 17999	Cupping each 15 minutes		NAAHI 99199	Body pressure management	
ADYAN	Practitioner referral		CACAC	Ear seeds or pellets each 15 minutes		NAANG 97799	Mobility therapy	
ADZAM	Compounding Oriental herbs each 5 minutes		CACAE 97810	Moxibustion each 15 minutes		CBAAA 99199	Core energetics each 15 minutes	
ADZAX	Therapeutic grade essential oil dispensing		CABAH 97810	Auricular therapy each 15 minutes		CBBBM 97140	Reflexology hand each 15 minutes	
Practice Specialties								
CBBAY 97124	Touch for health™ each 15 minutes		CBCAF 99199	Reiki each 15 minutes		CBECB 97124	Swedish massage each 15 minutes	
CBBBC 97124	Zero balancing™ each 30 minutes		CBEAB 97124	Craniosacral therapy each 15 minutes		CBEBH 97124	Trigger-point therapy each 15 minutes	
CBBBN 97140	Reflexology foot each 15 minutes		CBEAG 97124	Infant massage each 15 minutes		CBEBW 97039	Hot stone therapy each 15 minutes	
CBBBQ 87112	Neuromuscular therapy each 15 minutes		CBEAT 97124	Prenatal massage each 15 minutes		CBGAB 97139	Amma therapy each 15 minutes	
CBCAC 99199	Polarity therapy each 15 minutes		CBEBB 97124	Sports massage each 15 minutes		CBGAK 97139	Tuina each 15 minutes	
Client Self-Care Notes:								

SAMPLE

 # / $ Represents Number of Units or Fee Charged

Nutritional Items		Supply Items		Charges	
				Services	
				Nutritional/Supply Items	
				Adjustments	
				TOTAL CHARGES	
				AMOUNT PAID	

Practitioner Signature: _____   Date: _____

Patient Signature: _____   Date: _____

CPT® is a registered trademark of the American Medical Association

The sample Superbill above is based on three separate licenses for one practitioner.
To avoid fraudulent billing, be advised not to copy information from this sample.

Source: Alternative Link 2008.

Process for Revision of and Updates to ABC Codes

ABC Coding Solutions has the primary responsibility for updating ABC codes on an annual basis. Updating is accomplished through an open and impartial process. New codes can be added, obsolete codes retired, and terminology associated with an existing code modified. Anyone can suggest changes to the ABC codes by submitting an ABC Terminology and Code Request Form to ABC Coding Solutions. The form can be downloaded from the Internet at http://www.abccodes.com/ali/abc_codes/code_request.asp.

According to the ABC Coding Solutions' Web site, requests for updates are checked by the Research Department. Once the information is verified, subject matter experts review the proposals and recommendations are made. This process helps to ensure that the ABC codes remain complete and accurate as changes in healthcare practices occur.

Check Your Understanding 14.5

Instructions: Complete the following exercises on a separate piece of paper.

1. True or false. The characters in ABC codes do not have any meaning themselves, but are assigned alphabetically or sequentially.

2. Who can request changes to ABC codes?
    a. Anyone
    b. Only a constituent from a member association
    c. Employees of the Foundation for Integrative Healthcare
    d. Only CAM practitioners

3. The practitioner modifier 1G is used to identify a:
    a. Certified acupuncturist
    b. Certified professional midwife
    c. Certified nurse midwife
    d. Certified midwife

4. True or false. At the conclusion of the two-year testing project, ABC codes were named as a HIPAA code set.

5. Two-character alphanumeric modifiers identify:
    a. Multispecialty interventions
    b. Laboratory and office procedures
    c. The type of practitioner who rendered the service
    d. Homeopathic preparations

Introduction to the International Classification of Functioning, Disability and Health

Released in 2001, the International Classification of Functioning, Disability and Health (ICF) describes how people live with their health conditions. It is a classification of health and health-related domains describing body functions and structures, activities, and participation. The domains are classified from body, individual, and societal perspectives. Because an individual's functioning and disability occur in a context, ICF also includes a list of environmental factors. ICF has been accepted by many countries as the international standard for describing and measuring health and disability.

Developer of ICF

The developer of ICF is the World Health Organization. ICF is a revision of the first version, the **International Classification of Impairments, Disabilities and Handicaps** (ICIDH), published in 1980. Some of the literature refers to the updated version as ICIDH-2, but the current and adopted name is ICF. ICF was developed over a decade with the active participation of sixty-five countries. The 191 member states of the World Health Assembly approved it in May 2001.

Purpose of ICF

According to WHO (2008e), "The International Classification of Functioning, Disability and Health, known more commonly as ICF, provides a unified and standard language and framework for the description of health and health-related states." ICF is a tool for measuring functioning in society, no matter what the reason for the impairment, and there has been a radical shift from emphasizing a person's disability to focusing on the individual's level of health. ICF provides the framework and standard language needed to describe all health and health-related conditions and is intended for use in various sectors such as public health and health planning.

Population health has traditionally been measured by **mortality** based on statistics reported by the International Classification of Diseases (ICD) system. This information proved useful in identifying life expectancy and causes of death, but the data collected gave no further indication of the health status of the living population. As the importance of other health outcomes was identified (for example, functioning and disability in different areas of life), it became clear that additional information on population health was needed. As a result, WHO published the trial supplementary classification of impairments and handicaps in 1980 known as ICIDH. This classification was field-tested and a revision process set in place in 1995 involving several countries, which led to the present ICF.

ICD provides the codes for mortality and **morbidity,** and ICF provides the codes for health status; thus, the two systems are complementary. Users are encouraged to use both tools, wherever applicable, to obtain a broad and meaningful picture of the health status of people or populations.

ICF systematically groups different health and health-related domains for individuals with given health conditions. That is, it categorizes what people can do when they have a certain disease or disorder into different components. The body component defines functions and structures of the body system. The activity and participation component covers a range of life domains people engage in (for example, learning, self-care, moving around, work, and so on). Also listed are environmental factors that interact with all these domains. Thus, ICF encompasses health and health-related outcomes, including nonfatal health outcomes. Because ICF measures how people live with their health conditions and how those conditions can be improved to achieve a productive, fulfilling life, this classification system has implications for the practice of medicine, for the establishment of law and social policy to improve access and treatment, and for the protection of the rights of individuals and groups.

Check Your Understanding 14.6

Instructions: Complete the following exercises on a separate piece of paper.

1. True or False. ICD-10 is used mainly to classify causes of death whereas ICF classifies health.

2. True or False. ICD-10 and ICF complement each other.

3. What organization developed ICF?

Applications of ICF

Because of its flexibility, ICF is believed to offer various applications for use. Besides the service applications indicated in table 14.2, ICF has uses in policy development, economic analyses, research, intervention studies, and environmental factors. (WHO 2008e)

Table 14.2.   ICF applications

ICF Application	Purpose
At the individual level:	• For the assessment of individuals • For individual treatment planning • For the evaluation of treatment and other interventions • For communication among physicians, nurses, physiotherapists, occupational therapists, and other health workers, social service workers, and community agencies • For self-evaluation by consumers
At the institutional level:	• For educational and training purposes • For resource planning and development • For quality improvement • For management and outcome evaluation • For managed-care models of healthcare delivery
At the social level:	• For eligibility criteria for state entitlements such as Social Security benefits, disability pensions, workers' compensation, and insurance • For social policy development, including legislative review, model legislation, regulations and guidelines, and definitions for antidiscrimination legislation • For needs assessments • For environmental assessment for universal design, implementation of mandated accessibility, identification of environmental facilitators and barriers, and changes to social policy

Source: World Health Organization. 2008e. ICF Training Beginner's Guide.

Content/Format of ICF

The following is taken from the introduction to ICF (WHO 2008e):

ICF has two parts and each part has two components.
Part 1. Health Condition
    (a) Body Functions and Structures
    (b) Activities and Participation
Part 2. Contextual Factors
    (c) Environmental Factors
    (d) Personal Factors

Each component consists of various domains composed of categories that are the units of classification. After the appropriate category code is selected, qualifiers are added. These qualifiers are numeric codes that specify the extent or magnitude of the functioning or disability in that category or the extent to which an environmental factor is a facilitator or barrier.

This format is different from ICIDH, which had the following three different parts or classifications:

• Impairments (I code)

• Disabilities (D code)

• Handicaps (H code)

Figure 14.4 illustrates the differences between ICF and ICIDH.

ICF disability and functioning are viewed as outcomes of interactions between health conditions (diseases, disorders, and injuries) and contextual factors (environmental and personal factors). (See figure 14.5.) ICF has provided formal definitions of the components of the system, which are shown in table 14.3.

Figure 14.4.   Differences between ICF and ICIDH

ICF		ICIDH
Body Functions Body Structures	vs.	Impairments
Activities	vs.	Activity limitation 1980 Disability
Participation	vs.	Handicap

Source: World Health Organization. 2008e. ICF Training Beginner's Guide.

Figure 14.5.   Interaction between ICF components

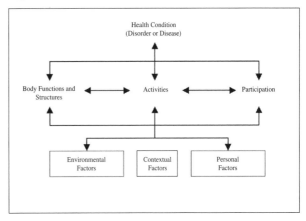

Source: World Health Organization. 2008e. ICF Training Beginner's Guide.

Table 14.3.   Components of the ICF system

Component	Definition
Body functions	Physiological functions of body systems (including psychological functions)
Body structures	Anatomical parts of the body such as organs, limbs, and their components
Impairments	Problems in body function or structure such as a significant deviation or loss
Activity	Execution of a task or action by an individual
Participation	Involvement in a life situation
Activity limitations	Difficulties an individual may have in executing activities
Participation restrictions	Problems an individual may experience in involvement in life situations
Environmental factors	The physical, social, and attitudinal environment in which people live and conduct their lives

Source: World Health Organization. 2008e. ICF Training Beginner's Guide.

Check Your Understanding 14.7

Instructions: Complete the following exercises on a separate piece of paper.

1. True or False. ICF can be used in performing research.

2. True or False. ICF consists of three parts.

3. Was the classification of handicaps part of ICIDH or ICF?

4. True or False. Environmental factors consist only of the physical environment in which people live.

Table 14.4.   Domains of ICF (body functions)

Level	Example	Coding
Chapter	Chapter 5: Functions of the digestive, metabolic and endocrine systems	b5
Second level	Ingestion functions	b510
Third level	Swallowing	b5105
Fourth level	Oral swallowing	b51050

Source: World Health Organization. 2008e. ICF Training Beginner's Guide.

Structure of ICF

The domains of ICF are arranged in a hierarchy that includes:

- A chapter
- A second level
- A third level
- A fourth level

Each of these domains is reflected in the coding as shown in table 14.4. To review the structure and codes online, go to http://www.who.int/classification/icf and select ICF Online.

Table 14.5 shows the list of chapters available in ICF.

The list of domains becomes a classification when qualifiers are added. The qualifiers identify the presence and severity of a problem in functioning. They vary depending on the components involved.

The qualifiers available for impairments of body functions are identified on a five point scale ranging from no impairment through mild, moderate, and severe, to complete impairment, as listed below:

0 No impairment
1 Mild impairment
2 Moderate impairment
3 Severe impairment
4 Complete impairment
8 Not specified
9 Not applicable

Table 14.6 (see page 242) lists the qualifiers applicable for impairments of body structures.

The next component, activity limitations and participation restrictions, has two types of qualifiers: the performance qualifier and the capacity qualifier. The performance qualifier describes what an individual does in his or her current environment; the capacity qualifier describes the individual's ability to execute a task or an action. Table 14.7 (see page 242) lists the qualifiers available within the activity limitations and participation restriction component.

As previously mentioned, the final component is that of environmental factors. Environmental factors make up the physical, social, and attitudinal environment in which people lead their lives. The qualifiers in this component draw a distinction between environmental barriers and facilitators. (See table 14.8 on page 242.)

A checklist, available on the WHO Web site, is a practical tool that can be used to elicit and record information on the functioning and disability of a particular individual. This checklist assists in information gathering and identification of the applicable qualifier. It is not intended to be used to assign the complete code because it does not go into each of the domains; rather, it provides an outline of the chapter and second-level domains. It should be used in conjunction with ICF full version or the ICF pocket version.

Principles and Guidelines for ICF

The essential principles of universality, parity, neutrality, and environmental factors are components of the ICF model and guide the revision process. These principles are listed in table 14.9 (see page 242).

Process for Revision of and Updates to ICF

The process for periodically updating ICF is similar to the process used for updating ICD. Three successive versions have been field-tested, and the results from international field tests have shown that ICF is a useful and meaningful framework for health reporting and decision making. The World Health Assembly will revise ICF at intervals that ensure the stability of the classification system and the incorporation of new knowledge.

Revision activities for ICF in the United States and Canada have been under the auspices of the

Table 14.5.   ICF chapters

Body	
Function	**Structure**
Mental functions	Structure of the nervous system
Sensory functions and pain	The eye, ear, and related structures
Voice and speech functions	Structures involved in voice and speech
Functions of the cardiovascular, haematological, immunological, and respiratory systems	Structures of the cardiovascular, immunological, and respiratory systems
Functions of the digestive, metabolic, and endocrine systems	Structures related to the digestive, metabolic, and endocrine systems
Genitourinary and reproductive functions	Structures related to genitourinary and reproductive systems
Neuromusculoskeletal and movement-related functions	Structures related to movement
Functions of the skin and related structures	Skin and related structures
Activities and Participation	
Learning and applying knowledge General tasks and demands Communication Mobility Self-care Domestic life Interpersonal interactions and relationships Major life areas Community, social, and civic life	
Environmental Factors	
Products and technology Natural environment and human-made changes to environment Support and relationships Attitudes Services, systems, and policies	

Source: World Health Organization. 2008e. ICF Training Beginner's Guide.

Table 14.6.   Qualifiers applicable for impairments of body structures

First Qualifier: Extent of Impairment	Second Qualifier: Nature of the Change

0 No impairment
1 Mild impairment
2 Moderate impairment
3 Severe impairment
4 Complete impairment
8 Not specified
9 Not applicable
	0 No change in structure
	1 Total absence
	2 Partial absence
	3 Additional part
	4 Aberrant dimensions
	5 Discontinuity
	6 Deviating position
	7 Qualitative changes
	   in structure, including
	   accumulation of fluid
	8 Not specified
	9 Not applicable

Source: World Health Organization. 2008e. ICF Training Beginner's Guide

WHO Collaborating Center for the Classification of Diseases for North America since 1993, renamed the WHO Collaborating Center for the Family of International Classifications for North America. The North American Collaborating Center (NACC), is housed at the **National Center for Health Statistics** (NCHS). According to the NCHS, decisions on the first updates are expected in 2009 (NCHS 2008a).

Check Your Understanding 14.8

Instructions: Complete the following exercises on a separate piece of paper.

1.   True or False. The domains of ICF are arranged in a hierarchy.

2.   True or False. Each component of ICF has the same qualifiers.

3.   True or False. Qualifiers are added to provide the presence and severity of a problem.

4.   True or False. An ICF checklist assists in information gathering and the identification of appropriate qualifiers.

Table 14.7.   Qualifiers for activity limitations and participation restriction

First Qualifier: Performance Extent of Participation Restriction	Second Qualifier: Capacity (Without Assistance) Extent of Activity Limitation
0 No difficulty	0 No difficulty
1 Mild difficulty	1 Mild difficulty
2 Moderate difficulty	2 Moderate difficulty
3 Severe difficulty	3 Severe difficulty
4 Complete difficulty	4 Complete difficulty
8 Not specified	8 Not specified
9 Not applicable	9 Not applicable

Source: World Health Organization. 2008e. ICF Training Beginner's Guide.

Table 14.8.   Qualifiers for environmental factors

Barrier	Facilitator
0 No barriers	0 No facilitator
1 Mild barriers	+1 Mild facilitator
2 Moderate barriers	+2 Moderate facilitator
3 Severe barriers	+3 Substantial facilitator
4 Complete barriers	+4 Complete facilitator

Source: World Health Organization. 2008e. ICF Training Beginner's Guide.

Table 14.9.   Component principles of the ICF model that guide the revision process

Component	Guiding Principles
Universality	A classification of functioning and disability should be applicable to all people regardless of their health condition. ICF is about all people. Persons with disabilities should not be labeled as a separate group.
Parity	There should be no distinction between mental and physical conditions. Disability should not be differentiated by etiology.
Neutrality	Domain names should be worded in neutral language so that the classification can express both positive and negative aspects of functioning and disability.
Environmental factors	ICF includes contextual factors, in which environmental factors are listed. The factors range from physical factors such as climate to social attitudes, institutions, and laws. Interaction with environmental factors is a key aspect of understanding functioning and disability.

Source: World Health Organization. 2008e. ICF Training Beginner's Guide.

Introduction to the International Classification of Health Interventions

The International Classification of Health Interventions (ICHI) is under development to fill a need to classify interventions. This need was identified in 1971 and was limited initially to surgical procedures. A preliminary system, the International Classification of Procedures in Medicine (ICPM) was published in 1978, but stopped in 1989 because of difficulties in keeping the system updated due to the rapid and extensive changes in the healthcare field. Several countries then worked on individual systems for national purposes, but those classifications did not provide adequate tools for use at the international level. It has again been recognized that an international classification is needed for interventions. In the interim, the Network of WHO Collaborating Centres for the Family of International Classifications promoted developing a short list of health interventions to use internationally. This list is based on the Australian Modification of the International Classification of Diseases, 10th revision (ICD-10-AM). This would be utilized by those countries without their own classification of interventions.

Developer of ICHI

The International Classification of Health Interventions (ICHI) will be part of the WHO-FIC family of reference classifications (along with ICD and ICF). ICHI is currently under development. It can be a lengthy and complex process to develop a new classification. A process has been established for developing and nominating classifications to be brought into the WHO-FIC. Table 14.10 lists the steps to bring a classification into the WHO-FIC.

Purpose of ICHI

According to WHO, "the purpose of this classification is to provide Member States, health care service providers and organizers, and researchers with a common tool for reporting and analyzing the distribution and evolution of health interventions for statistical purposes (WHO 2007)."

Content of ICHI

WHO anticipates that the ICHI will cover a wide range of measures taken for curative and preventive purposes by medical, surgical, and other health-related care services (WHO 2007). WHO states that this classification should be a multiaxial capture of the underlying knowledge.

Principles and Guidelines for ICHI

ICHI is structured with various degrees of specificity to be used at different levels of health systems. And like all WHO reference classifications, ICHI uses common, accepted terminology to permit comparison of data between countries and services, and ICHI must conform to those standards. To review the principles for including classifications in the WHO Family of International Classifications, see Attachment 1 in the World Health Organization Family of International Classifications: definition, scope and purpose document at: http://www.who.int/classifications/en/FamilyDocument2007.pdf

Current Status/Process for Revision of and Updates to ICHI

An initial ICHI version is being adapted to meet present day needs. Because of rapid change in science and technology, it is expected that frequent up-dates will be required. Therefore, adequate technical solutions must be developed. WHO states, "The Family Development Committee of the Network of WHO Collaborating Centers for the Family of International Classifications is actively developing plans and canvassing support to that end (WHO 2008h)."

After the classification is implemented, a revision and update procedure will be established according to WHO-FIC guidelines.

Check Your Understanding 14.9

1. ICHI is a:
    a. Derived classification
    b. Related classification
    c. Reference classification
    d. All of the above.

2. ICHI is being developed to classify:
    a. Diagnoses
    b. Disabilities
    c. Causes of injury
    d. Interventions

3. True or False. ICHI will be part of the WHO-FIC family of classifications.

Summary

The Universal Medical Device Nomenclature System (UMDNS), the Global Medical Device Nomenclature (GMDN), the Medical Dictionary for Regulatory Activities (MedDRA), the Systematized Nomenclature of Dentistry (SNODENT), the ABC codes, the International Classification of Functioning, Disability and Health (ICF), and the International Classification of Health Interventions (ICHI) represent specialized vocabularies, terminologies, or classifications with relatively narrow applications. For example, ABC codes have specific applications to complementary and alternative medicine, nursing, and other integrative healthcare providers.

The maintenance of UMDNS, GMDN, MedDRA, and SNODENT is the responsibility of a specific regulatory body, and each requires a license for use. ABC codes and ICF are copyrighted by their

Table 14.10.   Steps to bring a classification into the WHO-FIC

Step 1	The network is informed of the intention to either: • Develop a new classification, a derived, or related classification. Alpha status nominated. OR • Bring an existing classification for consideration for inclusion in the family. Beta status nominated.
Step 2 Alpha phase	Development and conceptual testing. Beta status nominated.
Step 3 Beta phase	Establishment of validity and reliability through testing in the field.
Step 4	Review of testing and full endorsement in the WHO-FIC.

Source: International Classifications: Definition, scope and purpose.

founding organizations, and each requires a license for use. Alternative Link, original developer of the ABC codes, also maintains, and updates, these classifications. WHO has plans to implement an update process for ICF in 2009; and ICHI is under development to classify interventions in order to provide a common tool to report and analyze healthcare interventions for statistical purposes.

These terminologies represent only some of the many alternate vocabularies in use in both the United States and internationally.

References

ADA News. 2007. Creating the dental piece of the EHR. American Dental Association. http://www.ada.org/prof/resources/pubs/adanews/adanewsarticle.asp?articleid=2642.

ADA Update: Dentistry and the Electronic Health Record. 2007. American Dental Association. http://www.ada.org/prof/resources/topics/nhii_ehr_update01.pdf.

ADA Washington Weekly Update. 2006. Health Information Technology Issues Common Questions and Answers. http://www.ada.org/prof/resources/topics/healthtech_questions.pdf.

Alternative Link. 2008. *ABC Coding Manual for Integrative Healthcare*. Albuquerque: Alternative Link.

Alternative Link. 2008. ABC coding solutions. http://www.alternativelink.com/ali/home/.

Alternative Link. 2004. The commercial use and cost-benefit of ABC codes in HIPAA transactions and the NHII. Report submitted on October 11, 2004, to the Office of the Secretary, U.S. Department of Health and Human Services. 45 CFR 162.940.

Bowman, Sue. 2004. ICD-10: All in the family. *Journal of the American Health Information Management Association* 75(10):62–63.

ECRI. 2006. http://www.ecri.org/Documents/UMDNS_2006flyer.pdf.

ECRI. 1997. Comments on coding and classification issues in connection with the requirements of the Health Insurance Portability and Accountability Act of 1996, National Committee on Vital and Health Statistics, Subcommittee on Health Data Needs, Standards and Security, April 11, 1997. http://www.ncvhs.hhs.gov/97041620.htm.

Giannini, Melinna. 2003 (October). ABC codes and improvements in US healthcare. *Proceedings of AHIMA's 75th Anniversary National Convention and Exhibit*. Chicago: American Health Information Management Association.

Global Medical Device Nomenclature. 2005. http://www.gmdnagency.com/.

GMDN Nomenclature structure, 2005, GMDN Agency. http://www.gmdnagency.com/?id=userinfo.

GMDN User Guidance, Version 2008.1, (2008) GMDN Agency. http://www.gmdnagency.com/.

Greenberg, Marjorie S., and Judith M. Jones. 1997. Toward standardization of health information. *Journal of the American Health Information Management Association* 68(2):22–28.

Introductory Guide for Standardised MedDRA Queries (SMQs) Version 11.1. 2008. International Federation of Pharmaceutical Manufacturers and Associations.

Lapp, Robert. Written statement for the NCVHS Workgroup on Computer-based Patient Records. May 17-18, 1999. http://www.ncvhs.hhs.gov/990517t3.htm.

Leake, James L. 2002. Diagnostic codes in dentistry: Definition, utility, and developments to date. *Journal of the Canadian Dental Association* 68(7):403–406.

MedDRA. 2008. http://www.meddramsso.com/MSSOWeb/index.htm.

MedDRA. MSSO Change Request Information. 2008a. Northrop Grumman Corporation

MedDRA. Introductory Guide Version 11.1. 2008b. International Federation of Pharmaceutical Manufacturers and Associations.

Molina, Synthia. 2004a. ABC codes: An essential tool for health benefit cost management and consumer-driven health plans. *ABC Coding Solutions Compensation and Benefits Review* (September/October). http://www.alternativelink.com/ali/ARTabout_link/ARTCompBenReview-Aug04.asp.

Molina, Synthia. 2004b. ABC codes: A new opportunity to capture CNS contributions to U.S. healthcare. *Clinical Nurse Specialist: The Journal for Advanced Nursing Practice* 18(5):238–45. http://www.nursingcenter.com/prodev/ce_article.asp?tid=527528.

National Center for Complementary and Alternative Medicine. 2005. http://nccam.nih.gov/health/.

National Center for Health Statistics. 2008a. International Classification of Functioning, Disability and Health (ICF). http://www.cdc.gov/nchs/about/otheract/icd9/icfhome.htm

National Center for Health Statistics. 2008b. WHO Collaborating Center for the Family of International Classifications for North America. http://www.cdc.gov/nchs/about/otheract/icd9/nacc.htm

Norwegian Centre for Informatics in Health and Social Care. 2007. ICPC-2e download. http://www.kith.no/templates/kith_WebPage____1111.aspx.

Norwegian Nomenclature. 2005. Information on GMDN maintenance. http://www.haukeland.no/nkkn/gmdn/intro.htm.

O'Mahony, Brian. 1997. International classification of primary care (ICPC): Comments and comparisons. Unpublished paper posted on personal Web site. http://homepages.iol.ie/~bom/ICPC.htm.

Prophet, Sue. 1999. Alternative medicine: Growing trend for the new millennium, part II. *Journal of the American Health Information Management Association* 70(5):65–70.

PSI International. 2003. http://www.meddrahelp.com/qaforum_cod_a.htm#_I_am_coding

Rulon, Vera. 2000. A global language for pharmaceutical regulation. *Journal of the American Health Information Management Association* 71(1):58–60.

Schooley, Ed. 2004. Testimony before the NCVHS Subcommittee on Standards and Security. http://www.ncvhs.hhs.gov/040128p3.htm.

Wonca International Classification Committee. 2005. http://www.ulb .ac.be/esp/wicc/.

WONCANews. 2008. Wonca. http://www.globalfamilydoctor.com/ publications/woncanews/WN%20Aug%2008/index.htm.

World Health Organization. 2008a. ICF Application and Training Tools. http://www.who.int/classifications/icf/icfapptraining/en/index.html.

World Health Organization. 2008b. ICF Application Areas. http:// www.who.int/classifications/icf/appareas/en/index.html.

World Health Organization. 2008c. ICF Browser. http://www.who.int/ classifications/icfbrowser/.

World Health Organization. 2008d. ICF Checklist. http://www.who.int/ classifications/icf/training/icfchecklist.pdf.

World Health Organization. 2008e. ICF Training Beginner's Guide. http://www.who.int/classifications/icf/training/icfbeginnersguide.pdf.

World Health Organization. 2008f. ICF training materials. http://www .who.int/classifications/icf/en/.

World Health Organization. 2008g. WHO-FIC Strategic Documents. http://www.who.int/classifications/docs/en/index.html.

World Health Organization. 2008h. The WHO Family of International Classifications. http://www.who.int/classifications/en/.

World Health Organization. 2007. World Health Organization Family of International Classifications: Definition, scope and purpose. http:// www.who.int/classifications/en/FamilyDocument2007.pdf.

World Organization of Family Doctors. 2005. http://www .globalfamilydoctor.com/wicc/icpcstory.html.

Application Exercises

1. The MedDRA Term Selection Points to Consider is the current standard for application of MedDRA terms. Go to the MedDRA MSSO Web site at http:// www.meddramsso.com. Select Documentation Library and MedDRA Term Selection: Points to Consider Document. Review this document and answer the following questions:

    How should diagnoses reported with signs and symptoms be coded?
    How are provisional diagnoses reported?
    For reporting purposes, is death considered an outcome, an adverse effect, or an adverse drug reaction?
    How are abnormal laboratory results reported?
    How does the coding of poisonings and adverse effects differ from ICD-9-CM?

2. Research the status of the two-year ABC codes testing project and write a report on the government's decision regarding naming it as a HIPAA code set.

3. Visit the WHO Web site for ICF http://www.who .int/classification/icf and select ICF Online. Review a chapter and then proceed through the various domains and levels to find a code at the fourth level.

4. Visit the WHO Web site and open the World Health Organization Family of International Classifications: definition, scope and purpose. Identify the Principles for including classifications in the WHO Family of International Classifications and prepare a report of this criteria.

Review Quiz

1. Which of the following are not described by UMDNS codes?
    a. Medical devices and materials
    b. Adverse effects of medical devices
    c. Clinical laboratory equipment
    d. Hospital furniture

2. True or False. Embedded within UMDNS are all diagnosis and procedure codes included in ICD-9-CM.

3. In UMDNS, entry terms are followed by:
    a. A direction to see another term
    b. A five-digit code
    c. Either a see direction or a code
    d. A six-digit code

4. Who can suggest changes to UMDNS?
    a. Licensed users of UMDNS
    b. Employees of ECRI
    c. Anyone
    d. Any device manufacturer

5. GMDN was developed by:
    a. ECRI
    b. Food and Drug Administration
    c. European Committee for Standardization
    d. International Standards Organization

6. Which of the following are not included in GMDN?
    a. Implantable devices
    b. Hospital forms
    c. Diagnostic and therapeutic radiation equipment
    d. Reusable instruments

7. An equivalent term in GMDN is defined as:
   a. A term used to classify groups of medical devices
   b. A collective term for grouping similar preferred terms
   c. A term having an alternative name to a preferred term
   d. A term that is equal in concept to a preferred term

8. The term "Cardiac, Catheter, balloon <specify>" is an example of a(n) _____ term in GMDN.
   a. Template
   b. Equivalent
   c. Preferred
   d. Invalid

9. True or False. The FDA requires the use of MedDRA to report adverse effects of pharmaceuticals.

10. In the MedDRA hierarchy, preferred terms map to:
    a. Lowest-level terms
    b. High-level terms
    c. A system organ class term
    d. A high-level group term

11. True or False. In MedDRA, the same clinical diagnosis may map to different terms depending on the mapping path followed.x

12. In MedDRA, how are diagnoses qualified as "possible," "probable," and so on coded?
    a. They are not coded.
    b. They are coded as if present.
    c. They are coded with a P modifier.
    d. They are coded with a ? modifier.

13. Which of the following is not a simple change request in MedDRA?
    a. Add a preferred term
    b. Add a lowest-level term
    c. Add a new term
    d. Add a high-level group term

14. Which of the following does SNODENT not contain codes for?
    a. Social conditions
    b. Risk behaviors
    c. Dental procedures
    d. Dental diagnoses

15. SNODENT terms are arranged on the basis of:
    a. Alphabetical order
    b. Etiology of the condition
    c. Part of the mouth involved
    d. Sequence, depending on when they were added

16. SNODENT is a part of, and completely embedded within:
    a. ICD-9-CM
    b. ICD-10-CM
    c. SNOMED
    d. Both ICD-10-CM and SNOMED

17. True or False. When approved, ABC codes will replace HCPCS Level I codes as a HIPAA standard medical code set.

18. What is the meaning of the third character G for Section C, Practice specialties, subsection B, Somatic practices and massage?
    a. Energy work
    b. Oriental massage
    c. Massage
    d. Somatic education

19. True or False. ABC codes are an integral part of HCPCS and follow the same principles and guidelines.

20. Which of the following insurance claim forms may be used to submit ABC codes?
    a. 271
    b. 278
    c. 1500
    d. 270

21. True or False. Codes are retired from the ABC code set when they are found to be obsolete.

22. ICF measures:
    a. Mortality
    b. Morbidity
    c. Death
    d. Life

23. In ICF, _____ are problems in body function or structure, such as a significant deviation or loss.

24. Mobility is part of:
    a. Body function
    b. Body structure
    c. Activities and participation
    d. Environmental factors

25. True or False. ICF has two major parts, and each part has two components.

26. True or False. To be included in WHO-FIC classifications certain guiding principles must be met.

Part III

Data Standards for Healthcare

Chapter 15

Data Set Standards

Kathy Giannangelo, MA, RHIA, CCS, CPHIMS, FAHIMA,
and Judith J. Warren, PhD, RN, BC, FAAN, FACMI

Learning Objectives

- To distinguish between data dictionary, element domain, and data set

- To explain the general purpose of healthcare data sets

- To recognize the relationship between healthcare data sets and vocabularies, terminologies, and classification systems

- To recognize the names and purpose of data set standards including the Uniform Hospital Discharge Data Set, the Minimum Data Set for Long-term Care, the Outcomes and Assessment Information Set, and various nursing data sets, among others

Key Terms

Data dictionary
Data element domain
Data Elements for Emergency Department Systems (DEEDS)
Data set
Essential Medical Data Set (EMDS)
Minimum Data Set for Long-term Care (MDS)
Nursing Management Minimum Data Set (NMMDS)
Nursing Minimum Data Set (NMDS)
Outcomes and Assessment Information Set (OASIS)
Patient Care Data Set (PCDS)
Perioperative Nursing Dataset (PNDS)
Uniform Ambulatory Care Data Set (UACDS)
Uniform Hospital Discharge Data Set (UHDDS)

Introduction

Having standard vocabularies, terminologies, and classifications available enables the numerous bits of data contained in the health record to be coded. However, how does one know which standard should be applied to each specific bit of data to ensure consistency of usage? One must decide what to collect. **Data sets** and their data dictionaries provide the answer.

This chapter briefly explains data sets and data dictionaries and then discusses specific examples of data sets used in certain healthcare settings. Part of the data dictionary for the **Uniform Hospital Discharge Data Set** (UHDDS) is included to illustrate how a data dictionary is an integral part of a data set specification.

Developer

Both **data sets** and **data dictionaries** may be created internally by healthcare providers or produced externally by either standards organizations such as the Health Level Seven (HL7) or government agencies such as the Centers for Medicare and Medicaid Services (CMS). The owner of the data dictionary and data set determines the process for revisions and updates.

Purpose and Content

The terms *data dictionary* and *data set* have been defined as follows (LaTour and Eichenwald 2002, p. 122):

- A data dictionary is a descriptive list of data elements to be collected in an information system or database.

- A data set is a list of recommended data elements with uniform definitions.

Standardized data sets encourage healthcare providers to collect and report data in a standardized manner (Amatayakul 2004). In addition to the list of data elements, a data dictionary provides definitions

for data elements that comprise a data set and includes each data element's principles and guidelines for use. According to Shakir (1999), the data dictionary includes other information such as **data element domain** that is key to data set creation. Shakir defines data element domain as "a specification of the allowable values for each data element."

Data attributes such as length also are a part of a data dictionary. For example, the **Uniform Hospital Discharge Data Set** (UHDDS), which is considered a core data set for hospital reporting, contains a data dictionary where the principal diagnosis, a data element, is defined along with its allowable value, an ICD-9-CM code.

Check Your Understanding 15.1

Instructions: Complete the following exercises on a separate piece of paper.

1. Which of the following is *not* part of a data dictionary?
   a. Allowable values for a data element
   b. Length of a data element
   c. List of standard data to collect
   d. Definition of a data element

2. In the UHDDS, the principal diagnosis data element is defined in the _____.

3. True or False. Data sets and data dictionaries describe and define data elements to be collected.

Uniform Hospital Discharge Data Set

Created more than thirty years ago, the UHDDS is a core set of data elements that are collected by acute care, short-term stay (usually less than thirty days) hospitals to report inpatient data elements in a standardized manner. It was developed through the National Committee on Vital and Health Statistics (NCVHS) and has been required by Department of Health and Human Services (HHS) policy since January 1, 1975. Revisions have taken place twice since 1975, in 1984 and again in 1986. Although

NCVHS recommended and circulated a revision in 1992, with additional recommendations from an Interagency Task Force in 1993, HHS has made no decisions on any of these recommended revisions.

The UHDDS has become a de facto standard in the hospital inpatient area for data collection by federal and state agencies as well as by public and private data-abstracting organizations (Greenburg 1995). It is the basis of the hospital discharge data systems in thirty-four states (AHRQ 2005).

The UHDDS also has had an influence on the UB-92, the claim form on which Medicare and Medicaid data sets are based. In fact, the UB-92 is a major vehicle for collecting UHDDS data elements. When diagnosis-related groups (DRGs) were implemented in 1983, UHDDS definitions were incorporated into the inpatient prospective payment system (PPS) regulations. Other payers also require use of UHDDS.

The purpose of the UHDDS is to specify standard definitions that facilitate collection of uniform and comparable health information from hospitals. An integral part of the UHDDS is the data dictionary, where specific definitions of the core data elements collected on acute inpatient hospitalizations are listed along with each data element's guidelines for use. When UHDDS definitions or principles are ignored, data may be reported inaccurately.

Table 15.1 presents examples from UHDDS's data dictionary.

Uniform Ambulatory Care Data Set

The **Uniform Ambulatory Care Data Set** (UACDS), a core set of data elements for reporting ambulatory data elements in a standardized manner, also was created through the work of NCVHS. Development of a data set for a uniform minimum data set for ambulatory care began in 1972 and was first approved by NCVHS in 1975. This data set was reviewed again in 1987, and a revision was published in 1989. NCHVS reviewed it again in 1993

Table 15.1. Portions of the UHDDS data dictionary

Data Element	Definition
Personal identification	The unique number assigned to each patient within the hospital that distinguishes the patient and his or her hospital record from all others in that institution
Discharge date	Month, day, and year of discharge
Principal diagnosis	The condition, after study, to be chiefly responsible for occasioning the admission of the patient to the hospital for care
Other diagnosis	All conditions that coexist at the time of admission or that develop subsequently or that affect the treatment received and/or length of stay. Diagnoses that relate to an earlier episode and have no bearing on the current hospital stay are to be excluded.

and enhancements were recommended, but the overall conclusion was that the data set was essentially sound. Although the UACDS has been widely disseminated, it has never been officially promulgated.

The purpose of the UACDS is to identify data elements for a uniform minimum data set on ambulatory care. The CMS 1500 is the main method for collecting UACDS data elements.

Table 15.2 shows sixteen data items found in the UACDS.

Table 15.2. UACDS data items

Patient Data Items	1. Personal identification 2. Residence 3. Date of birth 4. Sex 5. Race and ethnic background 6. Living arrangement and marital status
Provider Data Items	7. Provider identification 8. Location or address 9. Profession
Encounter Data Items	10. Date, place, or site and address of encounter, if different from item 8 11. Patient's reason for encounter 12. Problem, diagnosis, or assessment 13. Services 14. Disposition 15. Patient's expected sources of payment 16. Total charges

Check Your Understanding 15.2

Instructions: Complete the following exercises on a separate piece of paper.

1. True or False. UHDDS is considered a data dictionary.

2. UHDDS was developed by which of the following?
   a. NCVHS
   b. DHHS
   c. CMS
   d. The Social Security Act that created Medicare

3. The main method for collecting data elements in the UACDS is:
   a. UB-82 claim form
   b. UB-92 claim form
   c. CMS 1500 form
   d. Hospital abstracting systems

Minimum Data Set for Long-term Care

A long-term care minimum data set was part of the uniform minimum health data set work done by NCVHS in the mid-1970s. Reports on a long-term care minimum data set were published in 1980 and 1987. Then in 1987, the Omnibus Budget Reconciliation Act amended sections of the Social Security Act to include requirements for the secretary of HHS to specify a minimum data set of core elements for use in conducting comprehensive assessments and to designate one or more resident assessment instruments (RAIs) based on the minimum data set. The outcome was the Minimum Data Set (MDS) for Nursing Facility Resident Assessment and Care Screening and the RAI. The RAI is a uniform assessment instrument developed by CMS to standardize the collection of skilled nursing facility patient data. It includes the **Minimum Data Set for Long-term Care** (MDS 2.0), triggers, and resident assessment protocols.

MDS 2.0 is the foundation of the comprehensive assessment for all residents of long-term care facilities certified to participate in Medicare or Medicaid. It is a core set of screening, clinical, and functional status elements, including common definitions and coding categories. MDS provides a way to standard-ize communication about resident problems and conditions within facilities, between facilities, and between facilities and outside agencies. All nursing facilities are required to report the uniform set of elements extracted from the RAI on nursing facility residents.

The MDS was originally intended to serve as an assessment tool in identifying resident care problems addressed in individualized care plans. However, additional reasons for the MDS have developed over time, including the use of data collected from MDS assessments for Medicare and Medicaid reimbursement systems. For example, the MDS is used to collect data used to classify Medicare and Medicaid residents into Resource Utilization Groups (RUG-III). The RUG-III classification system is used in the PPS for nursing facilities, hospital swing-bed programs, and many state Medicaid case-mix payment systems.

Monitoring the quality of care provided to nursing facility residents is another way the MDS is used. Researchers developed a set of twenty-four quality indicators to assist state staff in identifying potential care problems. Providers use the data to assist in their ongoing quality improvement activities. In addition, surveyors find the MDS helpful in identifying potential problem areas that should be addressed during the survey process. Finally, CMS uses it for long-term quality monitoring and program planning.

Contained in the MDS are items that reflect the acuity level of the resident, including diagnoses, treatments, and evaluations of functional status. Figure 15.1 (see page 256) presents the required components of the MDS as specified by Version 2.0 of the MDS user's manual.

CMS is working on MDS 3.0. MDS 3.0 content must conform to Consolidated Health Informatics (CHI) endorsed standards, including Systematized Nomenclature of Medicine Clinical Terms (SNOMED CT), Logical Observation Identifier Names and Codes (LOINC), and HL7 messaging and vocabulary standards using an electronic metathesaurus software program (Dougherty and Mitchell

Figure 15.1.   Components of the MDS

Section AA—The Basic Assessment Tracking Form
This form contains identification information items 1–9, which consist of identifying information needed to uniquely identify each resident, the nursing facility in which he or she resides, the reason(s) for assessment, and item AA9 a-l, signatures of persons completing a portion of the MDS or tracking form.

Sections AB, AC, AD—Background (Face Sheet) Information at Admission Form
This form contains section AB (demographic information), section AC (customary routine), and section AD (face sheet signatures). This information is to be completed at the time of the resident's initial admission to the nursing facility. A new face sheet is also required to be completed, along with an admission assessment, for an individual who returns to the facility after a discharge in which return was not anticipated.

Sections A–Q—Clinical Assessment
Sections A–Q contain the clinical data items used to assess residents in the nursing facility. Section A9 is where staff sign that they have completed portions of the assessment and agree to the attestation statement.

Section R—Signature and Completion Date
Section R contains the signature of the RN coordinating the assessment. This is the section that records participation of the resident, family, and/or significant other in the assessment process.

Section S—State Section
Some states have added items to the core MDS that must be completed for each resident when a comprehensive assessment, full MDS Medicare PPS assessment form (MPAF), or quarterly assessment is required. Thus, while the basic MDS form is the standard foundation for all states, other items may have been added at the end of the form (in section S) for a particular state.

Section T—Supplement
Required for all Medicare assessments. Optional at state discretion for all other types of assessments.

Section U—Medications
Not used by CMS. Can be required by the state.

Section V—Resident Assessment Protocol Summary
Section V contains the form used to document triggered RAPs, the location of documentation describing the resident's clinical status, factors that impact the care planning decision, and whether or not a care plan has been developed for each RAP area. Note that the RAP need not have triggered for a care plan to be developed for that particular area. A RAP summary form must be completed each time a comprehensive RAI is required under the federal schedule. If a care plan is written from a nontriggered RAP, it should be noted on the RAP summary form.

Source: CMS. 2002. User's Manual for the Minimum Data Set (MDS) Version 2.0 (2002).

2004). The draft is available online at http://www.cms.hhs.gov/NursingHomeQualityInits/25_NHQIMDS30.asp#TopOfPage.

In the interim, CMS has published manual updates on its Web site for August 2003, April 2004, June 2004, and May 2005. These updates can be downloaded from http://www.cms.hhs.gov/MinimumDataSets20/025_WhatsNew.asp. CMS also has developed a procedure to review, respond, and distribute clarifications to the MDS coding process. Following are the steps from the CMS Web site:

1. Clinicians who have a question about a particular MDS item should first review the manual and then contact their state RAI coordinator for clarification. If necessary, the state RAI coordinator contacts the appropriate CMS staff if he or she is unable to answer a specific question.

2. CMS determines whether a clarification of an item is needed and posts new clarifications on the CMS Web site. A clarification posted on the official CMS Web site can be considered policy. The MDS 2.0 Web site at http://www.cms.hhs.gov/NursingHomeQualityInits/20_NHQIMDS20.asp can be checked for regular updates.

Outcomes and Assessment Information Set

The **Outcomes and Assessment Information Set** (OASIS) is a core group of data elements that represent items of a comprehensive assessment for an adult home care patient. Most data items in the OASIS were derived in the context of a CMS-funded national research program (cofunded by the Robert Wood Johnson Foundation) to develop a system of outcome measures for home healthcare (CMS 2004). It has been reviewed and refined several times since it was originally developed.

Two regulations relating to the collection and reporting of OASIS data were published in the *Federal*

Register in January 1999. The June 18, 1999 *Federal Register* notice published the effective date for the mandatory use, collection, encoding, and transmission of OASIS data for all Medicare and Medicaid patients receiving skilled services in the home. The regulation specified that the home care agency must use a standard core assessment data set as part of its comprehensive assessment.

OASIS forms the basis for measuring patient outcomes for purposes of outcome-based quality improvement. In addition, OASIS data have three important uses:

- Patient assessment and care planning for individual adult patients

- Agency-level case-mix reports that contain aggregate statistics on various patient characteristics such as demographic, health, or functional status at the start of care

- Internal home health agency performance improvement (CMS 2004)

The OASIS contains items such as those that encompass sociodemographic, environmental, support system, health status, and functional status attributes of adult (nonmaternity) patients. CMS provides an extensive OASIS user's manual that includes data element definitions, principles, and guidelines. Chapter 8 of the manual includes item-by-item tips to assist in the completion. (See figure 15.2 on page 258 for an example from the manual.)

The most recent version of the data set is OASIS-B1 (12/2002). OASIS-related announcements, corrections, and updates are found on the CMS Web site under OASIS: What's New (www.cms.hhs.gov/OASIS/).

Check Your Understanding 15.3

Instructions: Complete the following exercises on a separate piece of paper.

1. True or False. All long-term care nursing facilities are required to report the uniform set of elements extracted from the RAI on nursing facility residents.

2. Which of the following items on the MDS is *not* required by CMS?
   a. Diagnoses
   b. Treatments
   c. Functional status
   d. Medications

3. Which of the following is *not* found in section AA of the MDS?
   a. Patient identification
   b. Reason for the comprehensive assessment
   c. Signature of the RN who coordinated the assessment
   d. Name of the nursing facility

4. What core group of data elements represents items of a comprehensive assessment for an adult home care patient?
   a. MDS
   b. OASIS
   c. UHDDS
   d. UACDS

5. True or False. One use of OASIS data is patient assessment and care planning for individual adult patients.

Data Elements for Emergency Department Systems

The **Data Elements for Emergency Department Systems** (DEEDS) is designed to support the uniform collection of data in a twenty-four-hour, hospital-based emergency department. Although not intended to be a minimum data set, it does provide uniform specifications for data elements that emergency departments may use in their record systems. The uniform specifications encourage greater consistency and integrate existing health data standards, particularly standards for electronic health records. For example, data types and field lengths conform to HL7 specifications.

The Centers for Disease Control and Prevention (CDC) was instrumental in the development of DEEDS. Along with other federal agencies and professional organizations such as the American Health Information Management Association (AHIMA), the CDC formed a group to organize a workshop and to draft data elements. In January 1996, the

Figure 15.2.   Excerpt from the OASIS Manual

OASIS ITEM:

(M0245)   Payment Diagnoses (Optional): If a V code was reported in M0230 in place of a case-mix diagnosis, list the primary diagnosis and ICD-9-CM code, determined in accordance with OASIS requirements in effect before October 1, 2003—no V codes, E codes, or surgical codes allowed. ICD-9-CM sequencing requirements must be followed. Complete both lines (a) and (b) if the case-mix diagnosis is a manifestation code or in other situations where multiple coding is indicated for the primary diagnosis; otherwise complete line (a) only.

        <u>(M0245) Primary Diagnosis</u>   <u>ICD-9-CM</u>

    a. _____   (__ __ __.__ __)

        (M0245 First Secondary Diagnosis   ICD-9-CM

    b. _____   (__ __ __.__ __)

DEFINITION:

A case-mix diagnosis is a primary diagnosis that assigns patients with selected conditions to an orthopedic, diabetes, neurological, or burns/trauma group for Medicare PPS case-mix adjustment. A case-mix diagnosis may involve manifestation coding.

TIME POINTS ITEM(S) COMPLETED:

Start of care
Resumption of care
Follow-up

RESPONSE-SPECIFIC INSTRUCTIONS:

- V codes and E codes may not be entered in M0245 (a) or (b) as these pertain to the Medicare PPS case-mix diagnosis only.
- M0245 is for patients with a payment source of Medicare traditional fee for service (M0150, response 1). M0245 should always be blank for ALL other payer sources (M0150, response 0, 2, 3, 4, 5, 6, 7, 8, 9, 10, 11. UK).
- Complete M0245 only if a V code has been reported in place of a case-mix diagnosis in M0230.
- Do not complete M0245 if a V code has not been reported in M0230 in place of a case-mix diagnosis.

ASSESSMENT STRATEGIES

Select the code(s) that would have been reported as the primary diagnosis under the OASIS-B1 (8/2000) instructions:
1.   No surgical codes—list the underlying diagnosis.
2.   No V codes or E codes—list the relevant medical diagnosis.
3.   If the patient's primary home care diagnosis is coded as a combination of an etiology and a manifestation code, the etiology code should be entered in M0245 (a) and the manifestation code should be entered in M0245 (b).
4.   You can refer to CMS Guidelines for selecting a diagnosis under PPS at: www.cms.hhs.gov/providers/ hhapps/hhdiag.pdf.

(Continued on next page)

Figure 15.2.   (Continued)

OASIS ITEM:

(M0250) Therapies the patient receives <u>at home</u>: **(Mark all that apply.)**
- ☐ 1 - Intravenous or infusion therapy (excludes TPN)
- ☐ 2 - Parenteral nutrition (TPN or lipids)
- ☐ 3 - Enteral nutrition (nasogastric, gastrostomy, jejunostomy, or any other artificial entry into the alimentary canal)
- ☐ 4 - None of the above

DEFINITION:

Identifies whether the patient is receiving intravenous, parenteral nutrition, or enteral nutrition therapy at home.

TIME POINTS ITEM(S) COMPLETED:

Start of care
Resumption of care
Follow-up
Discharge from agency—not to an inpatient facility

RESPONSE-SPECIFIC INSTRUCTIONS:

- Include only such therapies administered at home. Exclude similar therapies administered in outpatient facilities
- If the patient will receive such therapy as a result of this assessment (e.g., the IV will be started at this visit; the physician will be contacted for an enteral nutrition order; etc.), mark the applicable therapy.
- If a patient receives intermittent medications or fluids via an IV line (e.g., heparin or saline flush), mark Response 1. If IV catheter is present, but not active (e.g., site is observed only or dressing changes are provided), do <u>not</u> mark Response 1.
- If any enteral nutrition is provided, mark Response 3. If a feeding tube is in place, but not currently used for nutrition, Response 3 does <u>not</u> apply. A flush of a feeding tube is <u>not</u> considered to provide nutrition.

ASSESSMENT STRATEGIES:

Determine from patient/caregiver interview, nutritional assessment, review of past health history, and referral orders. Assessment of hydration status or nutritional status may result in an order for such therapy (therapies).

National Workshop on Emergency Department Data was held to review and discuss the draft of DEEDS. Based on participant feedback, revisions were made. Release 1.0 was completed in January 1997.

Another data set connected to DEEDS is the **Essential Medical Data Set** (EMDS). The National Information Infrastructure Health Information Network (NII-HIN) created EMDS in 1997. EMDS is a standardized medical history data set containing the data elements for demographics, problem lists, medications, allergies, and previous critical encounters (ACEP 2001). The data definitions in DEEDS are identical to those in EMDS.

Release 1.0 of DEEDS contains 156 data elements organized into eight sections. Following are the eight section titles along with the titles of the thirty-two data elements for section 4:

- Patient Identification Data

- Facility and Practitioner Identification Data

- ED Payment Data

- ED Arrival and First Assessment Data

  —Date/Time First Documented in ED

  —Mode of Transport to ED

  —EMS Unit That Transported ED Patient

  —EMS Agency That Transported ED Patient

  —Source of Referral to ED

  —Chief Complaint

  —Initial Encounter for Current Instance of Chief Complaint

  —First ED Acuity Assessment

  —Date/Time of First ED Acuity Assessment

  —First ED Acuity Assessment Practitioner ID

  —First ED Acuity Assessment Practitioner Type

  —First ED Responsiveness Assessment

  —Date/Time of First ED Responsiveness Assessment

  —First ED Glasgow Eye Opening Component Assessment

  —First ED Glasgow Verbal Component Assessment

  —First ED Glasgow Motor Component Assessment

  —Date/Time of First ED Glasgow Coma Scale Assessment

  —First ED Systolic Blood Pressure

  —Date/Time of First ED Systolic Blood Pressure

  —First ED Diastolic Blood Pressure

  —First ED Heart Rate

  —First ED Heart Rate Method

  —Date/Time of First ED Heart Rate

  —First ED Respiratory Rate

  —Date/Time of First ED Respiratory Rate

  —First ED Temperature Reading

  —First ED Temperature Reading Route

  —Date/Time of First ED Temperature Reading

  —Measured Weight in ED

  —Pregnancy Status Reported in ED

  —Date of Last Tetanus Immunization

  —Medication Allergy Reported in ED

- ED History and Physical Examination Data

- ED Procedure and Result Data

- ED Medication Data

- ED Disposition and Diagnosis Data

Documentation of each data element follows a specific format, as shown in figure 15.3.

Figure 15.3.   Example of DEEDS documentation format

4.06 CHIEF COMPLAINT

PART OF THE CHIEF COMPLAINT GROUP (4.06 AND 4.07)*

Definition

Patient's reason for seeking care or attention, expressed in terms as close as possible to those used by patient or responsible informant.

Uses

Data collected on the patient's chief complaint are pivotal to the clinical process and provide an important resource for measuring and evaluating health care services. The chief complaint figures prominently in triage decision making and is a key determinant of the direction and extent of history taking, physical examination, and diagnostic testing in the ED. When ED data on chief complaint are aggregated and linked with process, diagnosis, and financial data, they take on added value for clinical and epidemiologic research, practitioner training, quality management, and health care administration and finance.

Discussion

Chief complaints encompass more than reports of symptoms or complaints. A chief complaint may also be a request for:
— a diagnostic, screening, or preventive procedure
— treatment or compliance with a practitioner's instructions to seek a specific treatment, procedure, or medication
— test results
— an examination required by a third party
— a referral, such as follow-up initiated from this ED or elsewhere
— intervention for a stated diagnosis or disease

Although data describing the chief complaint are routinely and often repetitively recorded during a single ED visit, the data generally are not classified, coded, and stored in a form that facilitates aggregate analysis. Several established systems are candidates for classifying and coding ED chief complaints, but modifications or adaptations are likely to be needed for routine ED use. Among the candidate systems are the *International Classification of Primary Care (IPCP), Reason for Visit Classification and Coding Manual (RC), Systematized Nomenclature of Human and Veterinary Medicine—SNOMED International, Read Codes Version 3*, and the *International Classification of Diseases, 9th Revision, Clinical Modification (ICD-9-CM)*. In the interim, text descriptions or local codes can be used.

Data Type (and Field Length)

CE—coded element (200).

Repetition

Yes; if there is more than one chief complaint, the Chief Complaint Group repeats.

---

*The Chief Complaint Group includes data elements 4.06 and 4.07. A single iteration of this group is used to report each chief complaint.

(Continued on next page)

Figure 15.3.   (Continued)

Field Values

Component 1 is the chief complaint code.

Component 2 is the chief complaint descriptor.

Component 3 is the coding system identifier.

Components 4–6 can be used for an alternate code, descriptor, and coding system identifier.

For example, to encode headache using the *International Classification of Primary Care* (ICP):

Component 1 = N01

Component 2 = Headache

Component 3 = ICP

Text data also can be entered without an accompanying code, as follows:

Component 1 = ' "

Component 2 = Headache

If the chief complaint is unknown, enter data in the following manner:

Component 1 = Unknown

Data Standards or Guidelines

None

Other References

ICPC (Lamberts and Wood, 1987), *RVC* (National Center for Health Statistics, 1994). *SNOMED International* (Cote et al., 1993), *Read Codes Version 3: A User Led Terminology* (O'Neill et al., 1995), and *ICD-9-CM* (U.S. Department of Health and Human Services, 1995).

Available online at http://www.cdc.gov/ncipc/pub-res/pdf/deeds.pdf.

When published, subsequent revisions will be found on the National Center for Injury Prevention and Control Web site at http://www.cdc.gov/ncipc/pub-res/deedspage.htm.

Check Your Understanding 15.4

Instructions: Complete the following exercises on a separate piece of paper.

1. How does DEEDS encourage electronic health records?
   a. By defining the EHR data set
   b. By requiring an EHR in order to use it
   c. By conforming with HL7 specifications
   d. All of the above

2. What is the difference between DEEDS and EMDS?
   a. The data definitions are different.
   b. They are designed for different types of facilities.
   c. DEEDS must be used in an EHR; EMDS can be used in a hospital information system.
   d. DEEDS supports collection of data in an emergency department system whereas EMDS contains only the emergency department data related to medical history.

3. Release 1.0 of DEEDS contains how many data elements?
   a. 8
   b. 32
   c. 156
   d. 256

Nursing Minimum Data Set

The **Nursing Minimum Data Set** (NMDS) was created to standardize the collection of nursing data. It is a minimum set of elements with uniform definitions and categories concerning the specific dimensions of nursing. Included in NMDS are the label and conceptual definition of elements that are used on a regular basis by most nurses across all settings.

The broad categories of elements are:

- Nursing care
- Patient or client demographics
- Service elements

The specific elements for these categories are shown below. Elements that also are included in the UHDDS are indicated with an asterisk.

Nursing Care Elements
1. Nursing Diagnosis
2. Nursing Intervention
3. Nursing Outcome
4. Intensity of Nursing Care

Patient or Client Demographic Elements
*5. Personal Identification
*6. Date of Birth
*7. Sex
*8. Race and Ethnicity
*9. Residence

Service Elements
*10. Unique Facility or Service Agency Number
*11. Unique Health Record Number of Patient or Client
12. Unique Number of Principle Registered Nurse Provider
*13. Episode Admission or Encounter Date
*14. Discharge or Termination Date
*15. Disposition of Patient or Client
*16. Expected Payer for Most of This Bill (Anticipated Financial Guarantor for Services) (University of Minnesota 2009)

It is possible to use NMDS for manual documentation and data collection, but computerization is required to optimize the system. The USA Nursing Minimum Data Set Consortium is charged with the maintenance and ongoing implementation and evaluation of NMDS.

The NMDS Web site is found at http://www.nursing.umn.edu/ICNP/USANMDS/home.html.

Check Your Understanding 15.5

Instructions: Complete the following exercises on a separate piece of paper.

1. Which of the following elements is included in the broad categories of this terminology?
   a. Occupational hazards
   b. Physician orders
   c. Pharmaceuticals
   d. Service

2. Disposition of the Patient or Client belongs in which element?
   a. Demographics
   b. Nursing Intervention
   c. Service
   d. Nursing Outcome

Nursing Management Minimum Data Set

The **Nursing Management Minimum Data Set** (NMMDS) addresses the contextual covariates of patient outcomes derived from the setting in which nursing care is delivered. NMMDS provides the data needed by nurse managers and administrators in making decisions about care management. It supports the description, analysis, and comparison of nursing care and nursing care resources with greater precision regarding the effects of context on complex healthcare outcomes. NMMDS is designed to complement the clinical patient-oriented data designated in the **Nursing Minimum Data Set** (NMDS) (University of Minnesota 2009)

NMMDS is registered with the HL7 standards organization. Relevant mapping has occurred within SNOMED CT, and experiments have been conducted to determine the usefulness of the LOINC structure for data reporting.

The Nursing Information and Data Set Evaluation Center (NIDSEC) has acknowledged the contribution of NMMDS as essential to support nursing practice. Moreover, NMDS and NMMDS are core to the advancement of the International Nursing Minimum Data Set (I-NMDS), cosponsored by the International Council of Nurses (ICN) and the International Medical Informatics Association Nursing Informatics Special Interest Group (IMIA NI-SIG).

NMMDS work is significant in that it:

- Identifies the core nursing management variables to measure the context of nursing care and improve outcomes

- Provides standardized definitions and measures for the collection of contextual data

- Is research based

- Is compatible with clinical data sets (for example, NMDS)

- Is integrated into national and international standards (for example, HL7, SNOMED CT)

- Is applicable across the care continuum

- Provides nurse manager and administrator database decision support

- Facilitates benchmarking and adoption of best practices

- Supports the integration of nursing data into clinical and administrative information applications

- Supports outcome measure validation required by accreditation bodies (University of Iowa 2005).

Check Your Understanding 15.6

Instructions: Complete the following exercises on a separate piece of paper.

1. Which of the following statements is true?
   a. NMMDS is designed to complement NMDS.
   b. NMMDS is designed to replace NMDS.
   c. NMDS was created by HL7 as part of the EHR functional model.
   d. NMDS was designed to create a unique method of expressing nursing data distinct from other clinical data sets.

2. True or False. NMMDS is mapped to SNOMED CT, LOINC, NMDS, and HL7.

Perioperative Nursing Data Set

The Association of PeriOperative Registered Nurses (AORN) developed the **Perioperative Nursing Data Set** (PNDS) to identify the perioperative experience of the patient from preadmission to discharge. PNDS can be used in any surgical setting and at any time during the perioperative experience. It includes 74 nursing diagnoses, 133 nursing interventions, and 28 nurse-sensitive patient outcomes.

There are a number of reasons for using PNDS. As a universal language for perioperative nursing practice, for example, it can serve as a framework for standardizing documentation. In addition, PNDS contributes data that can be used to measure and evaluate patient outcomes in the perioperative arena or for perioperative nursing research. Other uses include communication among clinicians, benchmarking activities, orientation programs and competency evaluation, effectiveness research, and activity-based costing (AORN 2005).

The American Nursing Association (ANA) has recognized PNDS as a data set useful for perioperative nursing practice.

PNDS is available for purchase from AORN from its Web site at http://www.aorn.org and has been incorporated into a number of clinical information software systems involving surgical care data management.

Patient Care Data Set

The **Patient Care Data Set** (PCDS) originates from work by Judy Ozbolt at the University of Virginia in collaboration with member institutions of the University Health System Consortium. Ozbolt has continued her work on PCDS at Vanderbilt University Medical Center where future versions will be maintained. PCDS is intended to provide standard terms for representing and capturing clinical data for patient care information systems.

Version 4.0 of PCDS includes a data dictionary along with sets of terms and codes. PCDS is organized into twenty-two components. Examples of components include activity, cognition, metabolism, and nutrition. Each component has three axes (problems, goals, and orders), and each axis contains atomic-level elements such as status, method, or laterality.

Check Your Understanding 15.7

Instructions: Complete the following exercises on a separate piece of paper.

1. True or False. PCDS is a vocabulary that will never be revised in order to serve as a reference vocabulary for other terminologies used in nursing.

2. Which of the following aspects of the Perioperative Nursing Data Set is correct?
   a. PNDS provides a universal language for perioperative nursing practice.
   b. Surgeons use PNDS as a framework for creating operative reports.
   c. AORN does not yet recognize PNDS as a standardized nursing vocabulary.
   d. PNDS is used to calculate surgical reimbursement for hospital inpatients.

Summary

As health information management (HIM) professionals know, not everyone requires exactly the same set of data. Thus, it is not surprising that a number of data set standards and their corresponding data dictionaries exist. Nonetheless, data sets and their data dictionaries are important to ensuring consistent data collection and data reporting for internal and external uses.

As the transition from a paper-based record to an electronic health record occurs, data set standards will need to be revised and updated. To keep abreast of changes, HIM professionals should monitor the various Web sites of the data set developers referenced in this chapter for continuing work in this area.

References

American College of Emergency Physicians. 2001. Patient safety in the emergency department environment. Report of the Patient Safety Task Force. http://www.acep.org/WorkArea/downloadasset.aspx?id=8970.

Agency for Healthcare Research and Quality. 2005. Healthcare informatics standards. http://www.ahrq.gov/data/infostd2.htm.

Amatayakul, Margret K. 2004. *Electronic Health Records: A Practical Guide for Professionals and Organizations*. Chicago: American Health Information Management Association.

Association of PeriOperative Registered Nurses. 2005. Perioperative nursing data set. http://www.aorn.org/research/pnds.htm.

Brandt, Mary. 2000. Health informatics standards: A user's guide. *Journal of the American Health Information Management Association* 71(4):39–43.

Brandt, Mary D., and Daniel A. Pollock. 2000. Initiative supports standardized data for emergency departments. *Journal of the American Health Information Management Association* 71(10):70–71.

Carpenter, Jennifer E. 1999. OASIS cracks down on home care. *Journal of the American Health Information Management Association* 70(5):56–57.

Centers for Medicare and Medicaid Services. 2002. *Revised Long-Term Care Resident Assessment Instrument (RAI) User's Manual for the Minimum Data Set (MDS), Version 2.0*. http://www.cms.hhs.gov/nursinghomequalityinits/20_NHQIMDS20.asp/.

Centers for Medicare and Medicaid Services. 2004. OASIS User's Manual. http://www.cms.hhs.gov/OASIS/05_UserManual.asp.

Dougherty, Michelle, and Sue Mitchell. 2004. Getting better data from the MDS: Improving diagnostic data reporting in long-term care facilities. *Journal of the American Health Information Management Association* 75(10):28–33.

Fletcher, Donna M. 1997. Outcome Assessment Information Set (OASIS) for home care. *Journal of the American Health Information Management Association* 68(8):46,48.

Greenberg Majorie. 1995. History of health care core data set development. Attachment 1 to Common Core Health Data Sets, 1/31/95 (unpublished).

LaTour, Kathleen, and Shirley Eichenwald, eds. 2002. *Health Information Management: Concepts, Principles, and Practice*. Chicago: American Health Information Management Association.

Manny, Barbara. 1991. Implementing the minimum data set in nursing facilities. *Journal of AMRA* 62(2):6.

National Center for Injury Prevention and Control. 1997. *Data Elements for Emergency Department Systems* (DEEDS Release 1.0). Atlanta: Centers for Disease Control and Prevention.

National Committee on Vital and Health Statistics. 2005. National Committee on Vital and Health Statistics 1949–1999: A History. http://www.ncvhs.hhs.gov/50history.htm.

National Committee on Vital and Health Statistics. 2005. The Patient Care Data Set. http://www.ncvhs.hhs.gov/990518t3.pdf.

National Committee on Vital and Health Statistics. 1996 (August). Core health data elements. Report of the National Committee on Vital and Health Statistics, U.S. Department of Health and Human Services. http://www.ncvhs.hhs.gov/ncvhsr1.htm.

Shakir, Abdul-Malik. 1999. Tools for defining data. *Journal of the American Health Information Management Association* 70(8):48–53.

University of Minnesota. 2009. http://www.nursing.umn.edu/ICNP/home.html.

USA Nursing Minimum Data Set Consortium. 2003. Brief synopsis of the Nursing Minimum Data Set (NMDS). http://www.nursing.umn.edu/ICNP/USANMDS/home.html
.

Application Exercises

1. Research your state's data-reporting requirements. Determine whether your state is one of the thirty-four states that use UHDDS as the basis for the hospital discharge data system.

2. Review MDS 3.0 at http://www.cms.hhs.gov/NursingHomeQualityInits/25_NHQIMDS30.asp#TopOfPage and prepare a report that identifies how it is different from MDS 2.0.

3. Visit http://www.cdc.gov/ncipc/pub-res/pdf/deeds.pdf. Search the report and identify where ICD-9-CM is mentioned. Create a report based on your findings.

Review Quiz

1. OASIS forms the basis for measuring patient _____.

2. True or False. DEEDS allows for entering more than one chief complaint on a single patient's visit to the emergency department.

3. Which of the following is defined as a specification of the allowable values for each data element?
    a. Data set
    b. Data element domain
    c. Data definition
    d. Data field

4. Which of the following statements is true?
    a. Data dictionaries limit how aggregate data can be viewed.
    b. Data sets and data dictionaries communicate data standards so that data can be collected and used consistently.
    c. Hospitals have been unable to agree on a uniform data set for reporting inpatient data.
    d. UACDS is the official, mandated data set for ambulatory care.

5. The principal diagnosis for inpatient acute care hospital inpatients is defined in which of the following data sets?
    a. UHDDS
    b. EMDS
    c. OASIS
    d. UACDS

6. The purpose of the _____ is to specify standard definitions that facilitate collection of uniform and comparable health information on hospital inpatients.

7. How is the MDS used?
    a. As an assessment tool to identify problems to be addressed in an individualized care plan
    b. To collect data for Medicare and Medicaid reimbursement systems
    c. To classify residents into resource utilization groups
    d. To monitor the quality of care provided to nursing facility residents
    e. For long-term quality monitoring and program planning by CMS
    f. All of the above
    g. a and b only

8. True or False. Data items collected on the MDS may vary from state to state.

9. The RAI is part of which of the following data sets?
    a. EMDS
    b. MDS
    c. NMDS
    d. PNDS

10. Which of the following data sets defines the payment diagnosis for home care patients?
    a. MDS
    b. UHDDS
    c. UACDS
    d. OASIS

11. Which of the following is not intended to be a minimum data set?
    a. DEEDS
    b. MDS
    c. UACDS
    d. UHDDS

12. Which of the following systems specifically integrates standards for electronic health records, for example, by conforming to HL7 specifications?
    a. DEEDS
    b. MDS 2.0
    c. UHDDS
    d. OASIS

13. True or False. The data definitions in DEEDS are identical to those in EMDS.

14. Data elements specified in UHDDS are collected for which type of patient?
    a. Ambulatory care patients
    b. Long-term care patients
    c. Home care patients
    d. Acute care inpatients

15. True or False. Some of the elements included in NMDS also are included in UHDDS.

16. True or False. NMMDS provides the data needed by nurse managers and administrators to make decisions about care management.

17. Which of the following is not an axis of PCDS?
    a. Problems
    b. Orders
    c. Nutrition
    d. Goals

18. Which organization developed the Perioperative Nursing Data Set?
    a. Association of PeriOperative Registered Nurses
    b. International Council of Nurses
    c. USA Nursing Minimum Data Set Consortium
    d. American Nurses Association

Chapter 16

Data Interchange Standards

Kathy Giannangelo, MA, RHIA, CCS, CPHIMS, FAHIMA,
and Judith J. Warren, PhD, RN, BC FAAN, FACMI

Learning Objectives

- To discuss standards development organizations and transmission standards

- To explain the general purpose of healthcare data interchange standards

- To understand the relationship between healthcare data interchange standards and vocabularies, terminologies, and classification systems

- To recognize the names and purpose of the major healthcare data interchange standards

Key Terms

Accredited Standards Committee (ASC) X12N
American National Standards Institute (ANSI)
Consolidated Health Informatics (CHI)
Designated standards maintenance organization (DSMO)
Digital Imaging and Communications in Medicine (DICOM)
Electronic data interchange (EDI)
Health Level Seven (HL7)
Institute of Electrical and Electronics Engineers Standards Association (IEEE-SA)
National Council for Prescription Drug Programs (NCPDP)
Semantic interoperability
Standards development organizations (SDOs)
Transmission standards

Introduction

To manage healthcare data and information resources, health information management professionals must be knowledgeable not only in the various types of vocabulary, terminology, and classification systems and data sets, but also in the standards used in the exchange of data. There are many varieties of healthcare data interchange standards. Some are suitable for a paper-based environment; others are created expressly for use in an electronic world. For example, the five categories of healthcare informatics standards are information standards including structure and content of the electronic health record and message format standards; clinical data representation standards including vocabularies, clinical classification systems, and terminologies; technical standards such as electronic data interchange; medication standards; and data privacy and security standards (LaTour 2006, 160).

This chapter focuses on the messaging standards for patient medical record information (PMRI) recommended by the National Committee on Vital and Health Statistics (NCVHS) to the Department of Health and Human Services (HHS). These include HL7 as the core PMRI standard and DICOM, NCP-DP SCRIPT, and IEEE 1073 as standards for specific PMRI market segments. According to NCVHS, PMRI standards are important "because they will facilitate significant improvements in the quality of patient care, promote patient safety, control rising healthcare costs, enhance the productivity of clinical research, and strengthen the nation's ability to identify and respond to healthcare emergencies" (NCVHS 2002).

Other transaction standards, ASC X12 Version 5010 and the NCPDP's Telecommunication Standard Version D0, and equivalent NCPDP Batch Standard, also are discussed. Finally, the chapter includes illustrations of the relationship of vocabularies, terminologies, and classification systems to healthcare data interchange standards.

Developer

Private-sector **standards development organizations** (SDOs) accredited by the **American National Standards Institute** (ANSI) are the primary developers of data exchange standards. Other SDOs include federal agencies, professional societies, and trade associations. ANSI coordinates the development of voluntary standards to increase global competitiveness in a variety of industries, including healthcare. Its Healthcare Information Technology Standards Panel (ANSI HITSP) provides an open, public forum for the voluntary coordination of healthcare informatics standards among all U.S. SDOs.

According to the Institute of Medicine (IOM) report titled *Patient Safety: Achieving a New Standard for Care,* data exchange standards are established in the following three ways:

- Federal mandate by legislation or regulation,

- Voluntary consensus through balloting of an industry professional group or sector, or

- *De facto* as the result of dominance in the commercial marketplace (IOM 2004).

Figure 16.1 (see page 272) presents an overview of processes used to set standards for the exchange of healthcare data in the United States.

Purpose and Content

Data exchange standards are necessary to access, combine, manipulate, and share data for various purposes. Healthcare data exchange standards supply specifications for the format and content of data exchanges, thereby providing the ability to send and receive medical and administrative data in an understandable and usable manner across information systems. **Transmission standards**, also referred to as communication, messaging, and transaction standards,

Figure 16.1.   Overview of processes used to set standards for the exchange of healthcare data in the United States

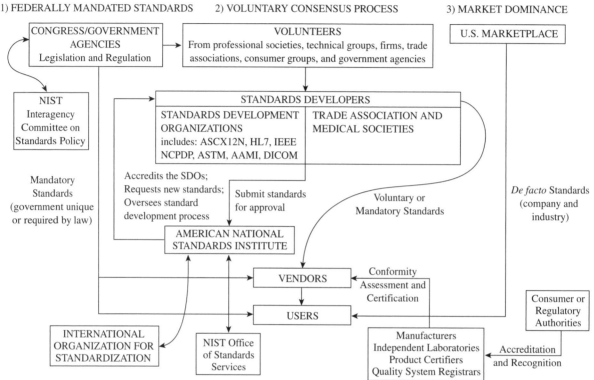

Reprinted with permission from *Patient Safety: Achieving a New Standard for Care*. ©2004 by the National Academy of Sciences, courtesy of the National Academies Press, Washington, D.C.

support the uniform format and sequence of data during transmission from one healthcare entity to another. **Electronic data interchange** (EDI) is a standard transmission format using strings of data for business information communicated among the computer systems of independent organizations.

The most recognized data exchange standards are the electronic transaction standards adopted under the Health Insurance Portability and Accountability Act (HIPAA). These standards apply to health plans, healthcare clearinghouses, and healthcare providers that transmit any health information in electronic form in connection with the following transactions:

- Health claims or equivalent encounter information

- Healthcare payment and remittance advice

- Health claim inquiry and response

- Eligibility inquiry and response

- Enrollment and disenrollment in a health plan

- Health plan premium payments

- Referral certification and authorization inquiry and response

- Coordination of benefits

- Health claims attachments

- First report of injury

In addition to mandating specific transaction standards, the HIPAA provisions established a new category of organization to maintain the standards adopted and criteria for the process to be used in such maintenance. This category of organization is the **designated standards maintenance organization** (DSMO). DSMOs include the following:

- **Accredited Standards Committee X12** (ASC X12)

- The Dental Content Committee

- **Health Level Seven** (HL7)

- **National Council for Prescription Drug Programs** (NCPDP)

- National Uniform Billing Committee (NUBC)

- National Uniform Claim Committee (NUCC)

The secretary of HHS is required to consult with the DSMOs before adopting any standard for electronic healthcare transactions. The DSMOs are responsible for maintaining standards for healthcare transactions adopted by the secretary and receiving and processing requests for adopting a new standard or modifying an adopted standard. When the secretary decides that a new code set should be adopted, the DSMOs oversee the various standards modifications needed to accommodate the new code set (for example, a move from a five-character numeric to a seven-character alphanumeric code). A DSMO also might be called on during the hearing process to explain how the proposed change would affect different transaction standards. Finally, DSMOs coordinate the updating of transaction guides for inclusion of the new standard. Additional information about DSMOs is available online at www.hipaa-dsmo.org.

Consolidated Health Informatics Initiative

A driver of healthcare data exchange standard adoption is the **Consolidated Health Informatics** (CHI) initiative. A government initiative that includes the departments of HHS and Defense and the Veterans Administration (VA), CHI adopts standards for domains related to health information for federal health data systems, enabling all agencies in the federal health enterprise to "speak the same language." CHI standards work in conjunction with the HIPAA transaction records and code sets provisions. NCVHS serves as a vehicle for CHI to receive comments from the private sector on data exchange standards under review.

The following standards have been approved for adoption to allow for the electronic exchange of health information across the federal government:

- HL7 messaging standards to ensure that each federal agency can share information that will improve coordinated care for patients such as entries of orders, scheduling appointments and tests, and better coordination of the admittance, discharge, and transfer of patients.

- NCPDP standards for ordering drugs from retail pharmacies to standardize information between healthcare providers and pharmacies. These standards already have been adopted under HIPAA.

- The IEEE 1073 series of standards that enables healthcare providers to plug medical devices into information and computer systems in order to monitor information from an intensive care unit or through telehealth services on Indian reservations, and in other circumstances.

- **Digital Imaging Communications in Medicine** (DICOM) standards that enable images and associated diagnostic information to be retrieved and transferred from various manufacturers' devices as well as from medical staff workstations.

- Laboratory Logical Observation Identifier Name Codes (LOINC) to standardize the electronic exchange of clinical laboratory results.

- The International Health Terminology Standards Development Organisation's Systematized Nomenclature of Medicine Clinical Terms (SNOMED CT) for laboratory result contents, nonlaboratory interventions and procedures, anatomy, diagnosis and problems, and nursing. HHS is making SNOMED CT available for use in the United States at no charge to users.

- HL7 vocabulary standards for demographic information, units of measure, immunizations, and clinical encounters, and HL7's Clinical Document Architecture standard for text-based reports.

- LOINC to standardize the electronic exchange of laboratory test orders and drug label section headers.

- The HIPAA transactions and code sets for the electronic exchange of health-related information to perform billing or administrative functions. These are the same standards now required under HIPAA for health plans, healthcare clearinghouses, and those healthcare providers who engage in certain electronic transactions.

- A set of federal terminologies related to medications, including the Food and Drug Administration's names and codes for ingredients, manufactured dosage forms, drug products, and medication packages; the National Library of Medicine's RxNORM for describing clinical drugs; and the VA's National Drug File Reference Terminology (NDF-RT) for specific drug classifications.

- The Human Gene Nomenclature (HUGN) for exchanging information on the role of genes in biomedical research in the federal health sector.

- The Environmental Protection Agency's Substance Registry System for nonmedicinal chemicals of importance to healthcare.

- The National Cancer Institute's Anatomy component of the NCI Thesaurus, which extends present anatomy terminologies into subcellular structures required for research and internationally-based clinical trials. Ad-

ditionally, the remaining anatomy terminology may serve as an alternate for SNOMED CT. It is recommended that the two terminologies be related through mapping (CHI 2009).

The CHI has completed its charge of identifying the standards need for federal healthcare use (HHS 2008). The ongoing work of this initiative is subsumed under the Federal Health Architecture (FHA) program, available online at http://www.hhs.gov/healthit/initiatives. The FHA is responsible for a federal healthcare information technology (IT) infrastructure that can support national health IT efforts and ensure the exchange of federal health data between and among federal agencies, with state and local governments, and with private healthcare organizations.

Check Your Understanding 16.1

Instructions: Complete the following exercises on a separate piece of paper.

1. Which of the following is *not* a CHI standard?
   a. IEEE 1073
   b. DICOM
   c. NUBC
   d. HL7

2. True or False. DICOM is a designated standards maintenance organization.

3. Which of the following supports the uniform format and sequence of data during transmission from one healthcare entity to another?
   a. Code set standards
   b. Transmission standards
   c. Vocabulary standards
   d. Electronic data interchange

Health Level Seven

Health Level Seven (HL7) is a not-for-profit, ANSI-accredited SDO founded in 1987 that produces standards for clinical data exchange (for example, transmission of patient and patient stay information, clinical orders, and clinical results), vocabulary, and document architecture. It aims to identify and support the needs of users, vendors, and consultants. Its mission is to provide a comprehensive framework and related standards for the exchange, integration, sharing, and retrieval of electronic health information that supports clinical practice and the management, delivery, and evaluation of healthcare services. The HL7 messaging standard is the accepted messaging standard for communicating clinical data and is the most widely implemented standard for healthcare information in the world.

The HL7 messaging standards support electronic communication between applications within the facility as well as exchanges outside the facility. They enable the exchange of data and information, regardless of the clinical system. The focus is on **semantic interoperability,** or agreement on the meaning of the exchanged information, enabling one system not only to receive data from another system, but also to understand them. HL7 does not develop terminology per se but, rather, defines the role of registered terminologies for encoding in its messaging formats.

Technical Committees and Special Interest Groups within HL7

Within HL7 are a number of technical committees (TCs) and special interest groups (SIGs). These volunteer-led groups are responsible for defining the HL7 standard protocol. For example, the goal of the Vocabulary TC is to "provide an organization and repository for maintaining a coded vocabulary that, when used in conjunction with HL7 and related standards, will enable the exchange of clinical data and information so that sending and receiving systems have a shared, well defined, and unambiguous knowledge of the meaning of the data transferred" (HL7 2009).

Another group within HL7 that has responsibility tied to vocabularies is the Attachments SIG (ASIG). This group is involved in the development of the HIPAA claims attachment standard, which uses LOINC codes. In addition, ASIG represents HL7 in HIPAA DSMO efforts.

Versions of HL7

HL7 messaging standards exist in various versions and in various stages of development. For example, Version 2.6 was approved as an ANSI standard in June 2007 and is the latest published update in the HL7 Version 2.x series. The introduction to Version 2.6 states: "The Standard currently addresses the interfaces among various healthcare IT systems that send or receive patient admissions/registration, discharge or transfer (ADT) data, queries, resource and patient scheduling, orders, results, clinical observations, billing, master file update information, medical records, scheduling, patient referral, patient care, clinical laboratory automation, application management and personnel management messages." (HL7 2007).

Version 3 differs from the 2.x series in that it is being built on a single-object model, the Reference Information Model, and is more focused on specific contexts, terminology, models, and conceptual definitions and relationships. However, both the V2.x series and V3 require a controlled terminology specified at the data element level to support interoperability (IOM 2004). The third normative edition of Version 3.0 standard consists of a suite of specifications. According to an HL7 Press Release, "HL7 Version 3 Normative Edition 2008 is a comprehensive assembly of the HL7 Version 3 specifications that have reached normative status—as either a Normative Standard or a Draft Standard for Trial Use (DSTU)—since 2004."

Guidelines for Determining Which Terminologies to Use

HL7 is an important forum for defining the role of vocabularies in the context of clinical data interchange. According to Rose et al. (2001), the following set of guidelines was developed by the Vocabulary TC to help organizations using HL7 decide which terminology to use:

- The terminology must be compliant with the HL7 message structure.

- The terminology provider must be willing to participate in HL7 efforts.

- The healthcare organization needs to take responsibility for maintaining and updating the terminology.

- License fees should be reasonable and proportional to their use.

- The terminology should be comprehensive.

- Certain terminologies may be mandated by regulatory agencies.

Check Your Understanding 16.2

Instructions: Complete the following exercises on a separate piece of paper.

1. The HL7 messaging standard is the accepted messaging standard for communicating:
   a. Administrative data
   b. Medical device data
   c. Clinical data
   d. Prescription data

2. True or False. The HL7 Vocabulary TC is responsible for developing vocabularies used in HL7 messages.

3. Which version was approved as an ANSI standard in June 2007 and is the latest published update to the HL7 standard?
   a. 2.3
   b. 2.6
   c. 3.0
   d. 2.5

Accredited Standards Committee, Insurance Subcommittee X12N

In 1979, ANSI chartered the **Accredited Standards Committee** (ASC) X12 to develop standards for EDI. ASC X12N, the subcommittee for insurance and insurance-related business processes, develops and maintains X12 EDI and Extensible Markup Language (XML) standards, standards interpretations, and standards guidelines. Within X12N are a number of task groups and workgroups. (See figure 16.2.) These groups develop data standards (both national

Figure 16.2.   Structure of ASC X12N

X12N	Insurance
	includes the following task groups:
TG01	Property and Casualty
	includes the following workgroups:
	WG1 Policy Administration
	WG2 Claims
	WG5 Subrogation
TG02	Healthcare
	includes the following workgroups:
	WG1 Healthcare Eligibility
	WG2 Healthcare Claims
	WG3 Claim Payments
	WG4 Enrollments
	WG5 Claims Status
	WG9 Patient Information
	WG10 Healthcare Services Review
	WG12 Interactive Healthcare Claims
	WG15 Provider Information
	WG20 Insurance Transaction Acknowledgement
TG03	Transaction Coordination and Modeling
	includes the following workgroup:
	WG3 HIPAA Implementation and Coordination
TG04	Implementation Guides
TG08	Architecture Review
TG11	Education

and international) and implementation guides (IGs) for the exchange of administrative data within the healthcare community.

Use of Implementation Guides

X12 standards are commonly used within the healthcare industry for reimbursement and insurance-related messaging. With the implementation of HIPAA, use of X12 specifications has increased. By mandating specific electronic transaction standards, the burden of administrative costs on the healthcare system is reduced. Healthcare organizations that use HIPAA-defined transactions must use the ANSI ASC X12N standard formats.

The X12N IGs explain the proper use of a standard for a specific business purpose. For example, an IG provides details on how each transaction is to be implemented, including field sizes, data definitions, and conditions (whether specific fields are mandatory or situational). IGs also are the primary reference documents used by businesses implementing the associated transactions and are incorporated into the HIPAA regulations by reference.

Figure 16.3. Element summary

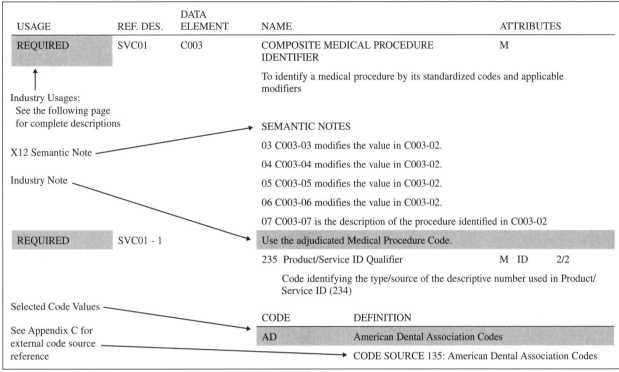

Source: Washington Public Co. 2003.

Use of HIPAA Transaction Sets

Often a number is used to refer to the message format standards. Following is a list of the HIPAA transaction sets and their corresponding number:

- Health Care Eligibility Benefit Inquiry and Response (270/271)

- Health Care Services Review: Request for Review and Response (278)

- Payroll Deducted and Other Group Premium Payment for Insurance Products (820)

- Benefit Enrollment and Maintenance (834)

- Health Care Claim Payment/Advice (835)

- Health Care Claim and Coordination and Benefits (837) (The 837 includes HIPAA X12N 837 institutional, professional, and dental healthcare transactions.)

Other transaction sets that have been developed by the X12N include:

- Health Care Provider Information (274)

- Patient Information (275)

- Health Care Claim Status Request and Response (276/277)

An X12 message is defined by reference to a grouping of data or a transaction set. The transaction set contains groups of segments, each of which can consist of several data elements. A data element dictionary defines each data element and specifies the format for it. All coded elements have their allowable code values listed within the data dictionary or have a reference to the external source for the codes. (See figure 16.3)

The new version of the standard for electronic healthcare transactions (Version 5010 of the X12 standard) was approved in 2009 for implementation by

2012. This new version is essential to the use of ICD-10 codes because the current X12 standard (Version 4010/4010A1) cannot accommodate the use of the greatly expanded ICD-10 code sets. Accordingly, HHS closely coordinated the development of the final rules, and the rules are being announced simultaneously.

Other terminologies and classifications used in X12N messaging include ICD-9-CM, CPT, and HCPCS. A message format for health claim attachments is in development and proposes to use LOINC. In January 2009, ICD-10-CM was approved for implementation by 2013. The expanded ICD-10 code sets will support quality reporting, pay-for-performance, bio-surveillance, and other critical activities. Conversion to ICD-10 is essential to development of a nationwide electronic health information environment.

Data Interchange Standards Association

The Data Interchange Standards Association (DISA), ASC X12's secretariat, publishes X12's standards documents. The X12N's IGs are published by the Washington Publishing Company and can be downloaded from its Web site at http://www.wpc-edi.com/products/publications. According to the Web site, each of the X12N IGs originally published for use under HIPAA have had addenda created for them. In January 2009, HHS adopted the updated X12 standard, Version 5010, and the National Council for Prescription Drug Programs standard, Version D.0, for electronic transactions, such as healthcare claims. Version 5010 is essential to use of the ICD-10 codes.

Check Your Understanding 16.3

Instructions: Complete the following exercises on a separate piece of paper.

1. True or False. The focus of the X12N subcommittee is insurance.

2. Which of the following transaction sets was *not* developed by the X12N?
   a. Benefit Enrollment and Maintenance (834)
   b. Health Care Payer Information (836)
   c. Health Care Claim and Coordination and Benefits (837)
   d. Health Care Claim Payment/Advice (835)

3. True or False. Instructional guides provide details on how to implement each transaction.

Digital Imaging and Communications in Medicine

The first (1985) and second (1988) versions of a standard for transferring images and associated information between devices were developed by the American College of Radiology (ACR) and the National Electrical Manufacturers Association (NEMA). These same two organizations created a joint committee and developed the **Digital Imaging and Communications in Medicine** (DICOM) standard. First available in 1994, DICOM is a standard for the interchange of computerized biomedical images and image-related information within and between healthcare providers.

The DICOM standard contains the following parts:

- PS 3.1: Introduction and Overview
- PS 3.2: Conformance
- PS 3.3: Information Object Definitions
- PS 3.4: Service Class Specifications
- PS 3.5: Data Structure and Encoding
- PS 3.6: Data Dictionary
- PS 3.7: Message Exchange
- PS 3.8: Network Communication Support for Message Exchange
- PS 3.9: Retired
- PS 3.10: Media Storage and File Format for Media Interchange
- PS 3.11: Media Storage Application Profiles
- PS 3.12: Storage Functions and Media Formats for Data Interchange
- PS 3.13: Retired
- PS 3.14: Grayscale Standard Display Function

- PS 3.15: Security and System Management Profiles

- PS 3.16: Content Mapping Resource

- PS 3.17: Explanatory Information

- PS 3.18: Web Access to DICOM Persistent Objects (WADO)

The DICOM standard has been incorporated into the product designs of many diagnostic medical imaging vendors. Its application is rapidly spreading to every medical profession that uses images, including cardiology, dentistry, endoscopy, mammography, ophthalmology, pathology, radiation therapy, radiology, surgery, and so on. Using DICOM can result in the transfer of medical images in a multivendor environment, can ease the development and expansion of picture archiving and communication systems, and can interface with clinical information systems.

According to PS 3.1 above, the DICOM standard results in interoperability of medical imaging equipment by indicating (NEMA 2004):

- A set of protocols to be followed by devices claiming conformance to the standard (for network communications)

- The syntax and semantics of commands and associated information, which can be exchanged using these protocols

- A set of media storage services to be followed by devices claiming conformance to the standard, as well as a file format and a medical directory structure to facilitate access to the images and related information stored on interchange media (for media communication)

- Information that must be supplied with an implementation for which conformance to the standard is claimed

Updates occur according to the procedures of the DICOM Standards Committee. Working groups of the committee perform most of the maintenance through subject matter groups, such as angiography or nuclear medicine, and end users of the standard.

Check Your Understanding 16.4

Instructions: Complete the following exercises on a separate piece of paper.

1. The DICOM messaging standard is the accepted messaging standard for communicating:
   a. Medical imaging data
   b. Medical device data
   c. Prescription data
   d. Administrative data

2. Which of the following organizations developed the DICOM standard?
   a. Royal College of Radiologists
   b. American Board of Radiology
   c. Radiological Society of North America
   d. American College of Radiology

3. True or False. Conformance to the DICOM standard is key to interoperability of medical imaging equipment.

National Council for Prescription Drug Programs

The **National Council for Prescription Drug Programs** (NCPDP) is a not-for-profit, ANSI-accredited SDO founded in 1977. It produces standards, IGs, and a data dictionary for data interchange and processing standards for pharmacy transactions. According to the NCPDP Web site,

The standard comprises technical rules and guidance for the format and usually the data layout or format of transaction(s).

The IG usually provides more information about the transaction(s), such as business rules, guidance for usage, matrices of usage, and examples. An IG is designed to go together with a standard.

The data dictionary has the field identifiers, format, values, descriptions, and reject codes for the data elements supported in the various standards. It is also designed for use with a standard and implementation guide (NCPDP 2009).

For example, the telecommunication standard and IG address the data format and content, the transmission protocol, and other appropriate telecommunication requirements for the electronic communication of transactions among pharmacy providers, payers, and other responsible parties (NCPDP 2009).

Impact of HIPAA Implementation on NCPDP Standards

NCPDP standards are used within the healthcare industry for pharmacy reimbursement and insurance-related messaging. The implementation of HIPAA has meant an increased use of NCPDP specifications because those entities that use HIPAA-defined transactions must use the NCPDP standard formats.

Regulations published as a result of HIPAA designate the NCPDP's Telecommunication Standard Implementation Guide Version D Release Ø and Equivalent Batch Standard Batch Implementation Guide, Version 1 Release 2 (1.2) for Retail Pharmacy Transactions include:

- Health claims and equivalent encounter information, retail pharmacy claims

- Healthcare eligibility benefit inquiry and response, retail pharmacy eligibility

- Coordination of benefits, retail pharmacy claims

- Healthcare services, referral certification and authorization, retail pharmacy claims

The HIPAA standard for the healthcare claim payment and remittance advice, retail pharmacy drug claims and remittance advice, is the ASC X12N 835 Health Care Claim Payment/Advice.

The NCPDP Telecommunication Standard Version D.Ø is an online, real-time conversation of a request from the pharmacy to the health plan AND a response from the health plan to the pharmacy. The NCPDP Batch Standard works in the same manner as a request and response, but is submitted via batch means instead of real-time. The pharmacy submits the NCPDP Standard for the billing of a claim and receives the NCPDP Standard response from the health plan.

Changes to the National Drug Code Set

The sole HIPAA medical code standard for claims from all sectors originally was the National Drug Code (NDC). However, after the initial EDI transaction standards were adopted, a significant number of change requests were submitted through the DSMO process. As required by Congress as a part of HIPAA, HHS worked with the DSMOs to revise the proposed changes to the standards. Those changes deemed essential for initial implementation by the DSMOs were presented to NCVHS. Public hearings were held, and NCVHS recommended that the secretary of HHS adopt all the changes proposed by the DSMOs as modifications to the national standards. One significant change concerned the NDC set.

In the May 31, 2002 *Federal Register*, a proposed rule was published to repeal the NDC as the standard medical data code set for reporting drugs and biologics in institutional, professional, and dental claims (that is, nonretail pharmacy drug claims). HHS solicited comments on an alternative standard for reporting drugs and biologics on nonretail pharmacy transactions. In that same rule, HHS proposed that the HCPCS code set be the alternative standard.

HHS received approximately 200 comments regarding a standard code set for reporting drugs and biologics. The comments fell into the following three major categories:

- Repeal the NDC as the standard medical data code set for professional, institutional, and dental claims and have no standard code set

- Repeal the NDC but adopt HCPCS as the standard code set

- Retain the NDC as the sole standard code set for claims from all sectors

The Centers for Medicare and Medicaid Services (CMS) considered comments from the public, comments from others such as the National Uniform Billing Committee, and information received from the Subcommittee on Standards and Security of the NCVHS public hearings regarding HIPAA implementation issues and the NDC. In the February 20, 2003 *Federal Register*, HHS published the Final Rule on Health Insurance Reform: Modifications to Electronic Data Transaction Standards and Code

Sets (HHS 2003). In it, the medical code set standards from the August 2000 final rule were retained with one exception: the final rule repealed adoption of the NDC for institutional and professional claims. No identified standard medical data code set was named for reporting drugs and biologics on nonretail pharmacy transactions. However, the final rule did state that the NDC remains the standard medical data code set for reporting drugs and biologics for retail pharmacy claims.

Another NCPDP standard, SCRIPT, was recommended as a PMRI standard for a specific market segment. This standard communicates prescription information between prescribers and pharmacies. The transactions included are new prescriptions, prescription refill requests, prescription fill status notifications, and cancellation notifications (NCVHS 2002).

Development of and Modifications to NCPDP Standards

NCPDP workgroups (WGs) are charged with development of and modification to the NCPDP standards. Meetings of the joint technical WGs occur four times a year in March, May, August, and November. Task groups are created to assist with WG projects and are open to non-NCPDP members. Task groups work virtually (via conference calls, e-mails). Suggested changes or modifications to existing standards also may be submitted via documents and forms posted on the NCPDP Web site. Proposals are reviewed at the joint technical WG meetings.

Institute of Electrical and Electronics Engineers Standards Organization

The **Institute of Electrical and Electronics Engineers Standards Association** (IEEE-SA) is a nonprofit standards-setting body that has been in existence for over a century. One set of standards developed by IEEE-SA is the 1073 Point of Care Medical Device Communication Standards, which pertain to communication of patient data from medical devices (patient monitors, ventilators, infusion pumps, and so on). This medical device communications standards series (IEEE 1073 [1.1.1, 1.2.1, 1.3, 2.1.1, 3.2]) was identified by NCVHS as an emerging PMRI market segment message format standard.

With more than 850 standards and more in development, IEEE-SA has an established open standards development process. Working groups and sponsors are key to the process as is the Project Authorization Request (PAR).

A number of manuals and documents that explain the procedures can be found online at http://www.standards.ieee.org/resources. One such publication is the *IEEE Standards Companion*. According to this manual, a standard is valid for five years from its publication date (IEEE 2003). Revisions or extensions to the standard can occur within the five-year time period. At the end of the five years, the standard will be reaffirmed, revised, or withdrawn. When approved by the standards board, the standard remains in force for another five years. When an approved standard no longer requires maintenance, it can be labeled as "stabilized." More information on the update process is available online at http://www.standards.ieee.org/guides/companion/part1.html#PAR.

In July 2004, IEEE-SA approved four standards in the IEEE 1073 series involving communications for point-of-care medical devices. According to the press release, the new standards provide a data dictionary and a domain information model for medical device communications, message syntax and encoding for device profiles, and a protocol for short-range infrared communication with medical devices (IEEE 2004).

Check Your Understanding 16.5

Instructions: Complete the following exercises on a separate piece of paper.

1. Which transaction is *not* included in the NCPDP's Telecommunication Standard Implementation Guide Version D Release Ø and Equivalent Batch Standard Batch

Implementation Guide, Version 1 Release 2 (1.2) for Retail Pharmacy Transactions mandated under HIPAA?

   a. Health claims and equivalent encounter information, retail pharmacy claims
   b. Health care services, referral certification and authorization, retail pharmacy claims
   c. Health care eligibility benefit inquiry and response, retail pharmacy eligibility
   d. Health care claim payment and remittance advice, retail pharmacy drug claims and remittance advice

2. The NCPDP messaging standard is the accepted messaging standard for communicating:
   a. Administrative data
   b. Medical imaging data
   c. Clinical data
   d. Prescription data

3. True or False. IEEE standards are revised every other year.

Summary

Being informed of data interchange and transmission standards is an important part of understanding how data can be shared or exchanged among individuals, organizations, and clinical information systems. Today, healthcare information technology (HIT) standards organizations, such as HL7, NCPDP, and ASC X12, are collaborating to advance standardization efforts, avoid redundancy in standards development, and facilitate the harmonization of standards relevant to healthcare. Doing so has the potential to reduce the costs of reaching interoperability.

The healthcare data exchange standards developed by the HIT standards-development organizations may cover a number of domains, such as the HL7 for clinical data, ASC X12N for administrative data, DICOM for medical images, NCPDP for prescription data, and IEEE for medical device data. Because of their purpose, many of these transmission standards also are tied to vocabularies, terminologies, and classification systems.

References

AHIMA Workgroup on Core Data Sets as Standards for the EHR. 2004. E-HIM strategic initiative: core data sets. Appendix A: Core data sets as standards for the EHR, part. 2: Healthcare standards organizations. *Journal of the American Health Information Management Association* 75(8): Web extra.

Brandt, Mary. 2000. Health informatics standards: A user's guide. *Journal of the American Health Information Management Association* 71(4):39–43.

Cassidy, Bonnie. 2000. HIPAA: Understanding the requirements. *Journal of the American Health Information Management Association* 71(4):16A–D.

Consolidated Health Informatics. 2009. http://www.hhs.gov/healthit/chi.html.

Department of Health and Human Services. 2002 (May 31). Proposed Rule on health insurance reform: Modifications to transactions and code set standards for electronic transactions. Federal Register. 67(105). http://www.frwebgate.access.gpo.gov/cgi-bin/getdoc.cgi?dbname=2002_register&docid=02-13615-filed.pdf.

Department of Health and Human Services. 2003 (February 20). Final Rule on health insurance reform: Modifications to electronic data transaction standards and code sets. Federal Register. http://www.aspe.hhs.gov/admnsimp/FINAL/FR03-8381.pdf.

Department of Health and Human Services. 2008. http://www.hhs.gov/healthit/standards/other.

Department of Health and Human Services. 2009. Health insurance reform: Standards for electronic transactions. 2000 (August 17). 45 CFR Parts 160 and 162. Federal Register 65(160). http://frwebgate.access.gpo.gov/cgi-bin/getdoc.cgi?dbname=2000_register&docid=00-20820-filed.pdf.

Federal Health Architecture (FHA) Program. http://www.hhs.gov/healthit/initiatives.

Health Level 7. 2007. Messaging Standard Version 2.6. Application protocol for electronic data exchange in healthcare environments. Chapter 1, p. 3. Ann Arbor: Health Level 7.

Health Level 7. 2008. Health Level Seven announces release of Version 3 Normative Edition 2008. http:www.hl7.org/documentcenter/public/pressreleases/HL7_PRESS_20080814.pdf.

Health Level 7. 2009. Vocabulary. http://www.hl7.org/about/.

Institute of Electrical and Electronics Engineers Standards Association. 2003. IEEE Standards Companion, second edition. http://www.standards.ieee.org/guides/companion/index.html.

Institute of Electrical and Electronics Engineers Standards Association. 2004 (July 6). IEEE okays four point-of-care medical device communication standards. Press Release. http://www.standards.ieee.org/announcements/pr_1073.html.

Institute of Electrical and Electronics Engineers Standards Association. 2005. http://www.standards.ieee.org.

Institute of Medicine. 2004. Patient Safety: Achieving a New Standard for Care. http://www.nap.edu/openbook.php?record_id=10863.

LaTour, Kathleen. 2006. Healthcare information standards. In *Health Information Management: Concepts, Principles, and Practice*, edited by Kathleen LaTour and Shirley Eichenwald, p. 160. Chicago: American Health Information Management Association.

National Cancer Institute. 2004. External data standards review. http://www.cabig.nci.nih.gov/workspaces/VCDE/Documents/NCI_ExtStdsReviewAppend.pdf.

National Council for Prescription Drug Programs. 2004 (September). HIPAA Final Rule Information on Electronic Transactions as it relates to the pharmacy industry. http://www.ncpdp.org/PDF/finalrule.pdf.

National Council for Prescription Drug Programs. 2009. Basic guide to standards. http://www.ncpdp.org/PDF/basic_guide_to_standards.pdf.

National Council for Prescription Drug Programs. 2009a. E-prescribing incentive program. http://www.cms.hhs.gov/PQRI/03_EPrescribingIncentiveProgram.asp#TopOfPage.

National Committee on Vital and Health Statistics. 2002 (February 27). Letter to the Secretary, U.S. Department of Health and Human Services. http://www.ncvhs.hhs.gov/020227lt.htm.

National Committee on Vital and Health Statistics. 2007 (September 26). Letter to the Secretary, U.S. Department of Health and Human Services. http://www.ncvhs.hhs.gov/070926lt.pdf.

National Electrical Manufacturers Association. 2004. Digital Imaging and Communications in Medicine (DICOM). Part 1: Introduction and overview. http://www.medical.nema.org/dicom/2004/04_01PU.pdf.

National Electrical Manufacturers Association. 2005. DICOM. http://www.medical.nema.org/.

Radiology Society of North America. 2005. Practice resources, DICOM: The value and importance of an imaging standard. http://www.rsna.org/Technology/DICOM/index.cfm.

Rose, J., B. Fisch, W, Hogan, et al. 2001. Common medical terminology comes of age, part two: Current code sets—strengths and weaknesses. *Journal of Healthcare Information Management* 15(3).

Scichilone, Rita A. 2002. DSMOs shed light on future coding systems, data sets. *Journal of the American Health Information Management Association* 73(7):74–77.

Washington Publishing Company. 2003. X12N 837 Implementation Guide. http://www.wpc-edi.com/products/publications.

Application Exercises

1. Go to DSMO Web site at http://www.hipaa-dsmo.org. Review the changes that have been requested in transaction standards. Click on one of the active change requests. Review the details and determine which HIPAA transaction standard is affected by the request and which DSMO has expressed interest.

2. Visit the HL7 Web site (http://www.hl7.org) and locate information on Version 3. Write a brief report on the reference information model and the requirements for vocabularies.

3. Visit the Washington Publishing Company's Web site at http://www.wpc-edi.com/products/publications. Access and review the implementation guide for X12N 837

Institutional. Create a report that identifies the coded elements that have a reference to the ICD-9-CM codes.

Review Quiz

1. Which of the following is *not* an SDO?
   a. ASC X12N
   b. HL7
   c. IEEE-SA
   d. ANSI

2. Which of the following organizations developed a data interchange standard for medical devices?
   a. DICOM
   b. IEEE-SA
   c. ASC X12N
   d. NCPDP

3. ____ is a standard transmission format using strings of data for business information communicated among the computer systems of independent organizations.
   a. Electronic data interchange
   b. Semantic interoperability
   c. Extensible Markup Language
   d. Data interchange standards

4. Which HL7 volunteer-led group represents HL7 in the HIPAA DSMO efforts?
   a. Vocabulary TC
   b. RIM SIG
   c. EHR TC
   d. Attachments SIG

5. True or False. Healthcare organizations that use HIPAA-defined transactions must use the HL7 standard formats.

6. The X12N messaging standard is the accepted messaging standard for communicating:
   a. Clinical data
   b. Medical device data
   c. Administrative data
   d. Medical imaging data

7. ____ is a standard for the interchange of computerized biomedical images and image-related information within and between healthcare providers.
   a. DICOM
   b. NCPDP
   c. IEEE
   d. X12N 270

8. Which of the following developed a data interchange standard for reimbursement and insurance-related messaging?
    a. HIPAA
    b. IEEE-SA
    c. ASC X12N
    d. ANSI

9. ____ produces standards, IGs, and a data dictionary for data interchange and processing standards for pharmacy transactions.
    a. HL7
    b. NCPDP
    c. IEEE-SA
    d. NDC

10. Which NCPDP standard was recommended as a PMRI standard?
    a. BS V1.1
    b. IEEE 1073
    c. TS V5.1
    d. SCRIPT

Part IV

Application of Vocabulary, Terminology, and Classification Systems in Healthcare

Chapter 17

Database of Vocabulary, Terminology, and Classification Systems

Kathy Giannangelo, MA, RHIA, CCS, CPHIMS, FAHIMA

Learning Objectives

- To review the development and purpose of the Unified Medical Language System (UMLS)

- To examine the component parts of the UMLS

- To review the process for updating the UMLS

Key Terms

Concept unique identifier (CUI)

Healthcare Information Technology Standards Panel (HITSP)

MetamorphoSys

Metathesaurus

Semantic Network

SPECIALIST Lexicon

UMLS Knowledge Source Server (UMLSKS)

Unified Medical Language System (UMLS)

Introduction

The number of vocabulary, terminology, and classification systems in healthcare has grown substantially over the past twenty or so years, and systems that have been around for several years have undergone revisions and updates expanding their size. Although consolidation in some instances may occur in the future, multiple systems are required for interoperable healthcare information. The National Committee on Vital and Health Statistics (NCVHS) study titled *Recommendations for Patient Medical Record Information (PMRI) Terminology Standards* (NCVHS 2000) and the U.S. government-wide standards by the Consolidated Health Informatics (CHI) eGov initiative support this. In addition, the work of the **Healthcare Information Technology Standards Panel** (HITSP) in standards harmonization has resulted in the identification of not one but a suite of terminology standards. These standards are needed for the electronic exchange of clinical health information and as a requirement for interoperability.

With so many systems available and some of them being quite large, a centralized location is needed to maintain consistent terminology use. This chapter examines one such centralized database: the Unified Medical Language System (UMLS).

Unified Medical Language System

The **Unified Medical Language System** (UMLS) (http://www.nlm.nih.gov/research/umls) is a tool that links existing computer-based clinical terminologies together as well as with biomedical literature and knowledge bases (Watzlaf 2002).

Developer

UMLS was initiated by the National Library of Medicine (NLM) to build an intelligent, automated system that can understand biomedical concepts, words, and expressions and their interrelationships. It contains a set of Knowledge Resources: **Metathe-saurus, Semantic Network,** and **SPECIALIST Lexicon** and Lexical Tools.

Begun in 1986 as an NLM research and development project, UMLS continues to evolve through the inclusion of new vocabulary, terminology, and classification systems, and redesigns of its resources and tools based on available information technology. For example, Version 6.0 of the **UMLS Knowledge Source Server** (UMLSKS) added a new Web-services-based application programming interface (API), a new Web interface based on portal technology, two new UMLS browsing capabilities, Tree Browser which allows for viewing, expanding, and collapsing Metathesaurus source hierarchies, and UMLS and Source View where the user can view concept data in source and Metathesaurus (NLM 2008).

Although the UMLS Knowledge Sources are provided by the NLM free of charge, a license agreement must be signed to allow access to them. The Semantic Network and Lexical Tools both have terms of use and the Metathesaurus requires a license agreement due to the different restrictions placed on each vocabulary or terminology by its creator. Each Metathesaurus licensee must submit a brief annual report describing how it is being used.

Access to the Knowledge Resources is through the Knowledge Source Server Web interface or DVD and via download. The full data may be downloaded from the UMLSKS.

Purpose

According to the NLM, the purpose of UMLS is to make it simple for health professionals and researchers to retrieve and integrate information from a variety of sources and for users to link disparate information systems, including EHRs, bibliographic databases, factual databases, and expert systems. UMLS includes more than a hundred vocabularies, terminologies, and classifications, some in multiple languages.

The UMLS Knowledge Sources make a wide variety of applications programs possible to overcome retrieval problems caused by differences in terminology and the scattering of relevant information across many databases. The NLM Web site lists the following applications where the UMLS could be used:

- Information retrieval
- Creation of patient and research data
- Natural language processing
- Automated indexing
- Development of enterprise-wide vocabulary services

NLM's own applications include PubMed, the NLM Gateway, ClinicalTrials.gov, and the Indexing Initiative.

Results from an analysis of the 2004 UMLS user annual reports show the main activities to be research, software development, healthcare provision, and education (Fung et al. 2006). This same study reported the UMLS uses were terminology research, mapping between terminologies, the creation of a local terminology, information indexing/retrieval, and natural language processing.

In addition, a survey distributed to the UMLS user mailing list reported 119 uses with the top three being terminology research, information retrieval, and terminology translation (Chen et al. 2007).

Content

UMLS is a multipurpose resource that includes concepts and terms from many different source vocabularies developed for very different purposes. All segments and disciplines of the healthcare process are covered in UMLS, but the total scope is controlled by the combined scope of its source vocabularies.

The Metathesaurus, a very large, multipurpose, and multilingual vocabulary database, is the central vocabulary component of UMLS. Its structure is concept oriented and does not include an overarching hierarchy. Although the Metathesaurus does not supply a universal hierarchy, it does contain the individual hierarchies of the source vocabularies. When the same concept appears in different hierar-

chical contexts in different source vocabularies, the Metathesaurus includes all the hierarchies. The Metathesaurus preserves the meanings, concept names, and relationships from its source vocabularies, but also certain synonymous relationships, concept attributes, and some concept names have been added (NLM 2008).

Other parts of the UMLS include the following (NLM 2008):

- The SPECIALIST Lexicon and Lexical Tools supplies the lexical information and programs needed for the SPECIALIST natural language processing system.
- Semantic Network represents a consistent categorization of all concepts represented in the UMLS Metathesaurus.
- UMLS Knowledge Source Server provides Internet access to the Knowledge Sources and other related resources made available by developers using UMLS.
- **MetamorphoSys** is the installation wizard and customization program included in each release of UMLS.

The source vocabularies found in the Metathesaurus include terminologies designed for use in patient-record systems (for example, SNOMED CT used to capture clinical data, and large disease and procedure classifications used for statistical reporting and billing, such as ICD-9-CM and CPT). The Department of Health and Human Services (HHS) signed a licensing agreement in 2003 with the College of American Pathologists (CAP) allowing users to have access to SNOMED CT at no charge through UMLS by obtaining a UMLS license. In 2007, the International Health Terminology Standards Development Organisation (IHTSDO) became the owner of SNOMED CT and, as a result, an Affiliate Licence Agreement was signed by the United States. With this change, new license terms became a part of the License for Use of the UMLS Metathesaurus and licensees had available SNOMED CT in multiple formats (NLM 2008). SNOMED CT remains free of charge to those with a UMLS license. The SNOMED CT to ICD-9-CM cross map is a part of the SNOMED CT International Release. Additional information on mapping is found in chapter 18 of this book.

NLM plans to include all the code sets required for administrative transactions under the Health Insurance Portability and Accountability Act (HIPAA) and all terminologies recommended as U.S. government-wide standards by the CHI eGov initiative and/or as core terminology standards by NCVHS.

Principles and Guidelines

The Metathesaurus is organized by concept. It reflects and preserves the meanings, concept names, and relationships from its source vocabularies. Each concept or meaning in the Metathesaurus has a permanent **concept unique identifier** (CUI). The CUI has no intrinsic meaning and never changes, regardless of changes over time in the names that are attached to it in the Metathesaurus or in the source vocabularies. However, a CUI is removed from the Metathesaurus when it is discovered that two CUIs actually name the same concept. In such cases, the process is to retain one of the two CUIs, link all relevant information in the Metathesaurus to it, and retire the other CUI. Retired CUIs are never reused. According to the NLM, "CUIs also serve as permanent, publicly available identifiers for biomedical concepts or meanings to which many individual source vocabularies are linked" (NLM 2008a).

The Metathesaurus includes many relationships among different concepts in addition to the synonymous relationships, most of which come from the individual source vocabularies. The Semantic Network includes data on the categories to which all Metathesaurus concepts have been assigned and the permissible relationships among these types.

Metathesaurus construction involves understanding the intended meaning of each name in each source vocabulary and linking all the names from all the source vocabularies that mean the same thing (the synonyms). Although its editors decide what view of synonymy to represent in the Metathesaurus concept structure, each source vocabulary's view of synonymy is also present, whether or not it agrees with the Metathesaurus view.

Process for Revision and Updates

UMLS is directed by a multidisciplinary team of NLM staff and maintained by public funding. The Knowledge Sources are iteratively refined and expanded based on feedback from those applying each successive version. Each edition of the Metathesaurus includes files that detail any changes from the previous edition.

A formal methodology for expanding content involves four major steps (UMLS 2008b):

1. Analysis and inversion. The semantics and structure of the vocabulary are analyzed and then "inverted" into a standard Metathesaurus input format.

2. Insertion. The terminology is inserted into the Metathesaurus maintenance system.

3. Human editing. Experts with the requisite expertise review and edit the Metathesaurus entries affected by the automated insertion routines.

4. Quality assurance. Standard and source-specific quality assurance queries are run to identify potential errors of commission and omission.

Part of the procedure includes eight general evaluation criteria that must be addressed with all requests for a source vocabulary addition to the UMLS.

There are no restrictions as to who can suggest a vocabulary for inclusion in the UMLS Metathesaurus. However, NLM may not be able to include additions, which would consume large amounts of effort in analysis, processing, or editing. NLM encourages broad use of the UMLS products by distributing semiannual updates in April and November free of charge.

Summary

Having access to vocabulary, terminology, and classification systems from a single source is being made possible through the efforts of the unified language systems. The Unified Medical Language System (UMLS) is a multipurpose resource that includes concepts and terms from many different source vocabularies developed. The UMLS Knowledge Sources and associated software tools go a long way toward providing health information systems developers with what they need to build or improve applications for health information systems used in an electronic patient record system.

References

Chen, V., Y. Perl, J. Geller, and J. Cimino. 2007. Analysis of a study of the users, uses, and future agenda of the UMLS. *Journal of the American Medical Informatics Association* 14(2): 221–231.

Fenton, Susan. 2005. Introduction to the Unified Medical Language System. *Journal of the American Health Information Management Association* 76(5):60–62.

Fung, K. W., W. T. Hole, and S. Srinivasan. 2006. Who is using the UMLS and how—Insights from the UMLS user annual reports. AMIA 2006 Symposium Proceedings. 274-278.

Halamka, J. 2008. Standardizing How We Share Information in Healthcare. Healthcare Information Technology Standards Panel. Webinar 1. http://www.hitsp.org/webinars.aspx.

Humphreys, B. L., D. Lindberg, H. M. Schoolman, and G. O. Barnett. 1998. The Unified Medical Language System: An informatics research collaboration. *Journal of the American Medical Informatics Association* 5(1):1–11.

National Committee on Vital and Health Statistics. 2000. Recommendations for Patient Medical Record Information (PMRI) Terminology Standards. Washington, DC: NCVHS.

National Library of Medicine, National Institutes of Health. 2006. Fact sheet: UMLS Metathesaurus. Available online at http://www.nlm.gov/pubs/factsheets/umlsmeta.html.

National Library of Medicine, National Institutes of Health. 2006. Fact sheet: UMLS Semantic Network. http://www.nlm.nih.gov/pubs/factsheets/umlssemn.html.

National Library of Medicine, National Institutes of Health. 2008. About the UMLS resources. http://www.nlm.nih.gov/research/umls/about_umls.html.

National Library of Medicine, National Institutes of Health. 2008a. UMLS release: 2008AA documentation. http://www.nlm.nih.gov/research/umls/documentation.html.

National Library of Medicine, National Institutes of Health. 2008b. UMLS Metathesaurus Source Vocabularies FAQs. http://www.nlm.nih.gov/research/umls/faq_main.html.

National Library of Medicine, National Institutes of Health. 2008c. Unified Medical Language System Basics. http://www.nlm.nih.gov/research/umls/online%20learning/index.htm

National Library of Medicine, National Institutes of Health, 2008d. Unified Medical Language System SNOMED Clinical Terms. http://www.nlm.nih.gov/research/umls/Snomed/snomed_main.html.

Watzlaf, Valerie. 2002. The impact of clinical terminologies and structured vocabularies. Presentation given at the 2002 Annual HIMSS Conference and Exhibition, San Diego, January 29.

Application Exercise

1. Access the NLM Web site at http://www.nlm.nih.gov/research/umls/umlsdoc.html and locate the information on UMLS Metathesaurus source vocabularies. Develop a table or grid that identifies the code sets required for administrative transactions under HIPAA, the terminologies recommended as U.S. government-wide standards by the CHI eGov initiative, and as core terminology standards by NCVHS.

Review Quiz

1. Which of the following is *not* one of the steps in NLM's methodology for expanding UMLS content?
    a. Quality assurance
    b. Analysis and inversion
    c. Human editing
    d. Public hearings

2. True or False. MetamorphoSys is a very large, multi-purpose, and multilingual vocabulary database found in ULMS.

3. The Metathesaurus is organized by:
    a. Concept
    b. Relationships
    c. Diagnosis
    d. Disease

4. True or False. A licensing agreement was signed by HHS with IHTSDO that allows U.S. users access to SNOMED CT at no charge through UMLS.

5. Which one of the following is *not* one of the UMLS's Knowledge Resources?
    a. SPECIALIST Lexicon
    b. Semantic Network
    c. MetamorphoSys
    d. Metathesaurus

Chapter 18

Use of Vocabulary, Terminology, and Classification Systems

Kathy Giannangelo, MA, RHIA, CCS, CPHIMS, FAHIMA

Learning Objectives

- To review the use of vocabulary, terminology, and classification systems in electronic health record systems

- To examine the use of vocabulary, terminology, and classification systems in administrative applications

- To explain how vocabularies, terminologies, and classification systems work together in an electronic healthcare environment

- To identify implementation issues surrounding the use of vocabulary, terminology, and classification systems in healthcare

- To explain the terminology connection to semantic interoperability

Key Terms

Coding
Electronic health record (EHR)
EHR system (EHR-S)
Information model
Interoperability
Mapping
Semantic interoperability

Introduction

Envision the entry of data such as drug allergies that are encoded at the point of care using a standard clinical terminology. By using various applications, the data are linked to knowledge resources whereby an alert regarding possible drug interactions is produced that assists the physician in determining the proper care for the patient. Using these same data, automated cross-maps are employed, resulting in the assignment of administrative code sets for claim submission. Or visualize the encoding of data such as diagnostic studies, patient vital signs, nursing diagnoses, and interventions using a standard clinical terminology. These data are stored via a terminology management system in a data mart and later mined to analyze how patient outcomes were affected by clinical decisions and to determine the effectiveness of specific interventions.

These are just two examples of the extent of options available when **interoperability** has been achieved. However, the promises of interoperability and its desired outcomes (cost reduction, increased efficiency, and improved quality of data exchange) will not be possible without the use of vocabularies, terminologies, and classification systems working together in an electronic healthcare environment that involves an information model. This chapter discusses how those promises might be achieved.

Electronic Health Record Applications

In order to try and obtain a consensus on health information technology (HIT) terms, a project was funded by the Office of the National Coordinator for Health Information Technology. As a result, NAHIT produced a report containing definitions for six HIT terms, one of which was EHR.

An **electronic health record** (EHR) is defined as an electronic record of health-related information on an individual that conforms to nationally recognized interoperability standards and that can be created, managed, and consulted by authorized clinicians and staff across more than one healthcare organization (NAHIT 2008).

A report by the Institute of Medicine (IOM) titled *Key Capabilities of an Electronic Health Record System* states that an **EHR system** (EHR-S) includes (IOM 2003):

- Longitudinal collection of electronic health information for and about persons, where health information is defined as information pertaining to the health of an individual or healthcare provided to an individual

- Immediate electronic access to person- and population-level information by authorized, and only authorized, users

- Provision of knowledge and decision support that enhance the quality, safety, and efficiency of patient care

- Support of efficient processes for healthcare delivery. Critical building blocks of an EHR system are the electronic health records (EHRs) maintained by providers (hospitals, nursing homes, ambulatory settings, and so on) and by individuals (also called personal health records).

The IOM report also points out the need to clearly define a functional model of key capabilities for an EHR-S. Health Level Seven (HL7) has taken the lead in the development of an EHR functional model. In 2007, the EHR-S Functional Model Normative Standard (ANSI-approved) was published. Divided into three sections, Direct Care, Supportive, and Information Infrastructure, it contains over 140 functional characteristics of EHR systems.

For those functions of an EHR-S related to data capture, data should be captured using standardized code sets or terminology, depending on the nature of the data. All the uses of an EHR-S identified in the IOM report require data in order to deliver the results; therefore, encoded data in the form of a standard terminology are required to accomplish the things an EHR-S is expected to do. Bottom line, the healthcare operations where a clinical terminology would be used relate directly to the functionality and capabilities of the EHR-S.

Because terminologies form the basis of all coded data sets and provide the data structure required for a fully functional EHR-S, which terminology system will meet EHR-S needs? The answer is that more than one system will be required. This is supported by a National Committee on Vital and Health Statistics (NCVHS) study that concluded that multiple vocabularies, terminologies, and classification systems were needed (NCVHS 2003). Multiple systems also have been recommended as U.S. government-wide standards by the Consolidated Health Informatics (CHI) eGov initiative.

For example, after a lengthy analysis of forty-six candidate terminologies based on specific criteria, NCVHS narrowed the pool of candidate terminologies to ten in its Patient Medical Record Information Terminology Analysis Reports. The general criteria used by NCVHS to make its recommendations for the PMRI terminology standards were (NCVHS 2002):

- The extent to which the standard enables interoperability between information systems

- The ability of the standard to facilitate the comparability of data

- The aspects of the standard that support data quality, accountability, and integrity

- The degree of market acceptance of the standard

After additional testimony, NCVHS recommended a core set of PMRI terminology standards. The core set includes:

- Systematized Nomenclature of Medicine Clinical Terms (SNOMED CT)

- Logical Observation Identifiers Names and Codes (LOINC)

- Federal Drug Terminologies: A set of controlled terminologies and code sets developed and maintained as part of a collaboration between the Food and Drug Administration, National Library of Medicine, Veterans Health Administration, National Cancer Institute, and Agency for Healthcare Research and Quality related to medications, including medication proprietary and nonproprietary names, clinical drug code (RxNorm); ingredient names and Unique Ingredient Identifiers (UNII); routes of administration, dosage forms, and units of presentation from the NCI Thesaurus (NCIt); and certain pharmacological drug classes from the National Drug File Reference Terminology (NDF-RT).

The NCVHS report also revealed that messaging format standards include their own vocabulary, terminology, and classification systems. These systems are used to represent information needed for standard messaging exchanges. As the NCVHS report mentions, the "lack of coordination between messaging and terminology standards allows redundant representations, which render data exchange more difficult and error prone" (NCVHS 2002).

In addition to NCVHS, the work of the Healthcare Information Technology Standards Panel (HITSP) in standards harmonization has resulted in the identification of not one but a suite of terminology standards. These standards are needed for the electronic exchange of clinical health information and as a requirement for interoperability. The major terminology standards named thus far are:

- ICD-9-CM

- CPT

- HCPCS

- LOINC

- SNOMED CT

- NDF–RT

- RxNorm

Check Your Understanding 18.1

Instructions: Complete the following exercises on a separate piece of paper.

1. True or false. Interoperability and its desired outcomes are possible without the use of vocabularies, terminologies, and classification systems.

2. Which of the following terminologies was named by NCVHS as part of the core set of PMRI terminology standards?
   a. LOINC
   b. ICD-10-CM
   c. ICD-9-CM
   d. CPT

Administrative Applications

In addition to naming a core set of PMRI terminology standards, NCVHS recommended that "important related terminologies" (for example, ICD-9-CM, CPT, CDT) be recognized and that **mappings** among those terminologies and the core set be created and maintained. NCVHS recognized the continued use of related terminologies in administrative applications; thus, compatibility with the recommended core set of PMRI standards was necessary.

Several vocabularies, terminologies, and classification systems are required for administrative applications. Those most recognized are the Health Insurance Portability and Accountability Act (HIPAA) of 1996 standard medical code sets. These include the *International Classification of Diseases, Ninth Revision, Clinical Modification (ICD-9-CM), Volumes 1–3*, Current Procedural Terminology, Fourth Edition (CPT), Code on Dental Procedures and Nomenclature (CDT), National Drug Codes (NDC), and the Centers for Medicare and Medicaid Services (CMS) Healthcare Common Procedure Coding System (HCPCS). In addition, in 1999, the United States implemented International Statistical Classification of Diseases and Related Health Problems, Tenth Revision (ICD-10), for reporting mortality statistics.

Vocabularies, Terminologies, and Classification Systems Working Together to Achieve Interoperability

The National Alliance for Health Information Technology (NAHIT) has defined interoperability as "the ability of different information technology systems, software applications and networks to communicate, to exchange data accurately, effectively and consistently, and to use the information that has been exchanged" (NAHIT 2005). NAHIT is a partnership of groups that include the American Health Information Management Association, the American Hospital Association, the Federation of American Hospitals, and the Joint Commission.

In 2006, an Executive Order mandating the Federal Government use interoperable standards stated the following:

> "Interoperability" means the ability to communicate and exchange data accurately, effectively, securely, and consistently with different information technology systems, software applications, and networks in various settings, and exchange data such that clinical or operational purpose and meaning of the data are preserved and unaltered (Bush 2006).

Three types of interoperability—technical, semantic, and process—were defined by the HL7 EHR Interoperability Work Group. The Work Group's definition of **semantic interoperability** stated in their paper is:

> The ability of information shared by systems to be understood…so that non-numeric data can be processed by the receiving system.

What is the terminology connection to semantic interoperability? Recognizing all three types of interoperability as important, it is semantic interoperability which gives meaning to the data. Thus, common standard terminologies are a fundamental part of semantic interoperability.

The practicality of vocabulary, terminology, and classification system usage within healthcare is tied to the applications that employ these systems. Such applications have specific purposes or "use cases" and specific users. Thus, just as certain vocabulary, terminology, and classification systems are more appropriate for the collection of clinical data at the point of care, so are specific systems suitable for administrative applications.

For instance, although classifications are limited with regard to their usability in clinical decision making at the time of care, they do allow granular clinical concepts captured by a terminology to be aggregated into manageable categories for secondary data purposes. Examples of applications where aggregate data are necessary include:

- Reporting basic health statistics

- Reporting medical diagnoses, procedures, and services on healthcare claims in order to receive third-party payment

- Performing epidemiological studies and clinical trials

- Conducting medical education and research by providing a useful basis for local, regional, and national utilization comparisons

- Setting health policy

- Designing healthcare delivery and payment systems

- Monitoring resource utilization

- Developing guidelines for medical care review

- Improving clinical, financial, and administrative performance

- Identifying fraudulent or abusive practices

- Tracking public health and risks

- Processing healthcare claims to determine the correct payment for healthcare services

On the other hand, terminologies are very granular and comprehensive and thus able to codify the clinical content of a health record and support patient care processes. For example, a standard clinical terminology interacting within an EHR system enables:

- Access to complete and legible clinical data with links to medical knowledge for real-time clinical decision support

- Information exchange between providers, thereby speeding care delivery and reducing duplicate testing and duplicate prescribing

- Information retrieval to produce practitioner alerts (for example, allergy alerts, reminders for preventive medicine screening tests, notifications of potential drug interactions or abnormal test results)

- Access to standards of care for benchmarking, measuring, and interpreting effectiveness and quality improvement

Given the various use cases and users, vocabularies, terminologies, and classifications should be utilized according to their purpose(s) and design to accomplish interoperability.

Implementation Issues

Although multiple vocabularies, terminologies, and classification systems are clearly needed, they do present various implementation opportunities and challenges. Consider the capture of clinical data at the point of care for efficient and effective administrative application through mapping. At its simplest, mapping is linking content from one terminology or classification scheme to another. It requires deciding how they match or, in some instances, how they are similar or do not match at all. Mapping considers different purposes, levels of detail, and coding guidelines of source and target. The mapping process uses a standard method in which the terminology concept or classification description are interpreted between systems. With the use of a mapping, the terminology used to capture the clinical data in an EHR can be chosen by the documenter and data reuse is still possible (Foley et al. 2007). However, while mappings exist, there are no nationally recognized standards for map development and validation, and the lack of coordination among terminology development organizations inhibits the development of maps (AHIMA and AMIA 2006).

The National Library of Medicine (NLM) was recommended as the body to coordinate and/or develop and disseminate mappings between standard clinical terminologies and other important terminologies within the UMLS Metathesaurus. In October, 2006, the NLM published nine basic mapping project assumptions to assist with existing and new mapping projects.

Coding is translating descriptions of diseases, injuries, and procedures into numeric or alphanumeric designations. It involves using a health record as the source for determining code assignment. Automated maps are efficient because they minimize duplicative data entry and patient data integration across a wide variety of applications. In essence, they provide the opportunity to implement the "code once, use many times" functionality. Essential to the success of data reuse is the representation of the information using controlled terms (Cimino 2007).

Although coordinating terminologies is essential to the development of a unified EHR-S, this step alone will not result in interoperability. An **information model** needs to be implemented. The process of data or information representation begins with information models, not just terms and codes alone (AHIMA and AMIA 2006). In its Patient Medical Record Information Terminology Analysis Reports, NCVHS acknowledges that standard representation of the full meaning of patient medical data requires integrating terminology models with models of context and other structural relationships. Together, the terminology model and the additional elements necessary to fully represent the meaning of clinical information constitute a complete information model.

NCVHS also concluded that if PMRI standards do not include both a comprehensive information model and a terminology model, mapping between the core set of terminologies and the important related terminologies will require information about the specific (nonstandard) medical record structures of each provider. This would result in an increased cost of such mappings and would restrict the benefits of standardizing PMRI data. Although integration of the two models is best, NCVHS notes that no clinically-specific information models yet exist. In the interim, NCVHS recommends coordination with messaging standards such as HL7 to minimize ambiguities and redundancies demonstrated in information exchanges using both messaging standards and the core terminology standard. HL7's work on a clinical information model is also showing potential in achieving the integration of the two models.

The IOM report titled *Key Capabilities of an Electronic Health Record System* also notes the importance of information models. According to this report, reference information models for defining relationships among data elements, clinical templates for structuring data as they are exchanged, and clinical document architectures support semantic interoperability among the heterogeneous computer-based systems that form an integrated information system.

Check Your Understanding 18.2

Instructions: Complete the following exercises on a separate piece of paper.

1. Which of the following is best used in applications where aggregate data are necessary?
   a. Vocabulary
   b. Terminology
   c. Classification system
   d. Nomenclature

2. True or false. Mapping involves using a health record as the source for determining code assignment.

3. True or false. To accomplish interoperability, terminologies and classifications should be utilized according to their purpose(s) and design.

Summary

According to the American Health Information Management Association's Vision of the eHIM™

Future report, the future state of health information is electronic, patient-centered, comprehensive, longitudinal, accessible, and credible. Collectively, vocabularies, terminologies, and classification systems provide the common medical language necessary for this future state. Standard clinical terminologies are necessary for semantic interoperability.

Depending on the "use case," certain vocabulary, terminology, and classification systems are appropriate for chosen applications. For example, by definition, classification systems group together similar diseases and procedures and organize related entities for easy retrieval. However, they are inadequate for primary documentation of clinical care. In the same vein, because of their size, significant granularity, intricate hierarchies, and lack of reporting rules, many vocabularies and terminologies are insufficient for serving the purposes for which classification systems are used.

While clinical terminologies form the basis of all coded data sets and provide the data structure required for a fully functional EHR-S, significant implementation issues for standard vocabulary, terminology, and classification systems include the use of maps and an information model. Reducing duplicative data entry via "code once, use many times" is minimized via automated maps. In addition, there is no standard model to date, although the National Committee on Vital and Health Statistics has pointed out that implementation of an information model is needed to attain interoperability. In the meantime, standards for both data structure within electronic health records and communications among them are required in order to share and aggregate data.

References

AHIMA and AMIAA. 2006. Healthcare Terminologies and Classifications: An Action Agenda for the United States. http://library.ahima.org/xpedio/groups/public/documents/ahima/bok1_032401.html.

Bowman, Sue. 2005. Coordinating SNOMED-CT and ICD-10: Getting the most out of electronic health record systems. *Journal of the American Health Information Management Association* 76(7):60–61.

Brouch, Kathy. 2003. AHIMA project offers insights into SNOMED, ICD-9-CM mapping process. *Journal of the American Health Information Management Association* 74(7):52–55.

Bush, George W. 2006. Executive Order: Promoting Quality and Efficient Health Care in Federal Government Administered or Sponsored Health Care Programs. http://www.whitehouse.gov/news/releases/2006/08/20060822-2.html.

Cimino, James J. 2007. Collect Once, Use Many: Enabling the reuse of clinical data through controlled terminologies. *Journal of the American Health Information Management Association* 78(2):24–29.

Consolidated Health Informatics. http://www.whitehouse.gov/omb/egov/c-3-chi.html.

e-HIM Task Force. 2003. *A Vision of the eHIM™ Future.* Chicago: American Health Information Management Association. http://www.ahima.org.

Foley, Margaret, Candace Hall, Kathryn Perron, and Rachael D'Andrea. 2007. Translation, please. *Journal of the American Health Information Management Association* 78(2):24–38.

Giannangelo, Kathy. 2004. Clinical vocabulary basics. AHIMA audio seminar, August 26.

Health Level Seven. 2007. Health Level Seven EHR-S Functional Model Normative Standard (ANSI-approved). http://www.hl7.org/ehr/downloads/index_2007.asp.

Health Level Seven EHR Interoperability Work Group. 2007. Coming to Terms: Scoping Interoperability for Health Care. http://www.hln.com/assets/pdf/Coming-to-Terms-February-2007.pdf.

Institute of Medicine. 2003. *Key Capabilities of an Electronic Health Record System. Letter Report of the Committee on Data Standards for Patient Safety, Board on Health Care Services, Institute of Medicine.* Washington, D.C.: National Academies Press.

Johns, Merida. 2000. A crystal ball for coding. *Journal of the American Health Information Management Association* 71(1):26–33.

National Alliance for Health Information Technology. 2005. The National Alliance for Health Information Technology stakes out definition for healthcare interoperability, calls for input. Press release, March 8. http://www.nahit.org:9006/alliance2/index.do.

National Alliance for Health Information Technology. 2008. NAHIT releases HIT definition. Press release, May 20. http://www.nahit.org./pandc/press/pr5_20_2008_1_33_49.asp.

National Committee on Vital and Health Statistics. 2002. Patient medical record information terminology analysis reports. http://www.ncvhs.hhs.gov/031105rpt.pdf.

National Committee on Vital and Health Statistics. 2003. Reports and recommendations. http://www.ncvhs.hhs.gov/reptrecs.htm.

Smith, Paul. 2004. Electronic health records and the national health information infrastructure. http://library.findlaw.com/2004/Oct/27/133614.html.

Application Exercise

Review the white paper, *Healthcare Terminologies and Classifications: An Action Agenda for the United States*, found here: http://library.ahima.org/xpedio/groups/public/documents/ahima/bok1_032401.htm

1. The Task Force identified four recommendations. Choose the recommendation you believe will be the most difficult to accomplish. Write up a report explaining your rationale.

Appendix A

Answer Key for
"Check Your Understanding" Exercises

Chapter 2

Check Your Understanding 2.1

1. c
2. c
3. d

Check Your Understanding 2.2

1. a
2. False
3. True

Check Your Understanding 2.3

1. True
2. True
3. False
4. a. D
   b. D
   c. P
   d. D
   e. P
   f. D
   g. P

Check Your Understanding 2.4

1. False
2. True
3. False

Check Your Understanding 2.5

1. Blocks
2. d
3. True

Check Your Understanding 2.6

1. False
2. True
3. True

Check Your Understanding 2.7

1. True
2. False

Check Your Understanding 2.8

1. False
2. True
3. True
4. b
5. False
6. Body part

Check Your Understanding 2.9

1. d
2. True
3. False

Check Your Understanding 2.10

1. a. Completeness
   b. Expandability
   c. Multi-axial
   d. Standard terminology

Note: These may be listed in any order.

2. False

3. b

Check Your Understanding 2.11

1. True
2. False
3. d

Check Your Understanding 2.12

1. Bypass
2. a. Transplantation
   b. Resection or excision (depending on whether all or part of the appendix was removed)
   c. Inspection
   d. Fragmentation
3. True

Chapter 3

Check Your Understanding 3.1

1. True
2. b

Check Your Understanding 3.2

1. b
2. c
3. a

Check Your Understanding 3.3

1. True
2. a
3. b
4. d

Check Your Understanding 3.4

1. c
2. False
3. c
4. c

Chapter 4

Check Your Understanding 4.1

1. The primary purpose of HCPCS is to meet the operational needs of Medicare and Medicaid reimbursement programs.

2. Centers for Medicare and Medicaid Services
3. True

Check Your Understanding 4.2

1. HCPCS level I is a CPT numeric coding system maintained by AMA. The codes have five characters and two-digit modifiers. HCPCS level II codes, or national codes, are maintained by CMS. These codes were established to submit claims for items that are not identified by CPT.

2. Temporary codes allow insurers the flexibility to establish codes that are needed before the next January 1 annual update and can be changed quarterly. Usually, temporary codes are implemented within 90 days to allow for preparation and implementation.

3. Maintained by the HCPCS National Panel, permanent national codes represent a standardized coding system that is managed jointly by private and public insurers. The system is updated annually. The CMS HCPCS Workgroup is responsible for any changes to the permanent national alphabetic numeric codes.

4. Miscellaneous codes are used when a supplier submits a bill for an item or service that no existing national code adequately describes. These codes can be used during the period of time a request for a new code is being considered under the HCPCS review process.

Check Your Understanding 4.3

1. a. Dental procedures
   b. Durable medical equipment
   c. Medical services
   d. Hearing services and Vision services
2. True

Chapter 5

Check Your Understanding 5.1

1. NDCs serve as universal product identifiers for prescription drugs.

2. True

3. The Drug Listing Act dictated the expansion of the NDC to include human over-the-counter drugs and veterinary drugs in addition to prescription

drugs. Also, the *NDC Directory* was suspended until provisions could be limited.

4. True

Check Your Understanding 5.2

1. True
2. The components of National Drug Codes are the labeler code, the product code, and the package code. The labeler code is assigned by the FDA and is the first part of the three-part code; the product code is assigned by the firm and is the second part of the three-part code; and the package code is assigned by the firm and is the third part of the three-part code.
3. The product and package code are assigned by the firm.
4. NDC Search Results on 62856
   Firm Name: EISAI INC
   Address Header: ATTN CHARLES J CAL-
                     LAHGAN REG AFFAIRS
   Street: 55 CHALLANGER RD 6TH FLOOR
   PO Box:
   Foreign Address:
   City, State, Zip: RIDGEFIELD PARK, NJ
                       07660
   Country Name: UNITED STATES

Chapter 6

Check Your Understanding 6.1

1. The Code
2. ADA
3. b
4. d
5. False

Check Your Understanding 6.2

1. CDT procedure code and nomenclature
2. True
3. a
4. d
5. The code manual suggests providing a narrative description when the nomenclature of a code includes "by report."

Check Your Understanding 6.3

1. False
2. The Code voting membership includes one representative from each payer sector and six representatives from the ADA Council on Dental Benefit Programs. The additional representatives from the ADA Council on Dental Benefit Programs provide an equal voting balance between the payer sector and the dental community.
3. True
4. b
5. False

Chapter 7

Check Your Understanding 7.1

1. b
2. False. Even the earlier versions were intended to be used in the background of electronic health records.
3. c
4. b

Check Your Understanding 7.2

1. a
2. b
3. c
4. False. SNOMED International included mapping to LOINC codes.
5. Both are concept-based controlled reference terminologies. The biggest difference is that SNOMED CT reflects the combination of SNOMED RT and the National Health Service's Clinical Terms Version 3 (CTV3). SNOMED RT contains approximately 120,000 concepts, whereas SNOMED CT contains an estimated 300,000 concepts.

Check Your Understanding 7.3

1. a
2. False. SNOMED is designed to fulfill this function, but it is not a characteristic of a classification.
3. Classifications, by nature, are designed to classify or group like things together. In contrast, SNOMED is designed to uniquely identify clinical information

in great detail. Classifications are used to aggregate data for administrative purposes. A controlled terminology is used to capture data at its most granular level. Controlled terminologies are designed to be used as a data input mechanism whereas classifications are most useful for data output.

Check Your Understanding 7.4

1. True
2. c
3. a

Check Your Understanding 7.5

1. Concept
2. a
3. False. It is the least granular concept.
4. c
5. Concepts, descriptions, and relationships

Check Your Understanding 7.6

1. False. SNOMED CT codes are without embedded meaning and without digit restrictions.
2. c
3. True
4. The SNOMED Terminology Solutions performs the development and maintenance tasks.

Chapter 8

Check Your Understanding 8.1

1. False
2. d
3. b

Check Your Understanding 8.2

1. True
2. c
3. a

Chapter 9

Check Your Understanding 9.1

1. b
2. True

3. c
4. False
5. d

Check Your Understanding 9.2

1. True
2. a
3. a
4. True

Check Your Understanding 9.3

1. True
2. False
3. a
4. False
5. False
6. c

Chapter 10

Check Your Understanding 10.1

1. Documentation resources available to learn more about LOINC include the User's Guides and Manuals, answers to Frequently Asked Questions, Other Resources, Issues, Debate, and Discussion Documents, Background Information, and LOINC Community Resources.
2. A LOINC Workshop is often offered with the Laboratory Committee Meetings.

Check Your Understanding 10.2

1. The word *niche* has many definitions. Used in this context, it refers to a specialized market or something of which an activity or thing is best fitted. LOINC is a vocabulary specifically designed for reporting clinical observations.
2. b
3. Clinical LOINC
4. The Consolidated Health Informatics initiative (CHI)

Check Your Understanding 10.4

1. Parts 2, 3, 5 and 6 (type of property, timing, scale, and method) correspond exactly in meaning between laboratory and clinical LOINC codes.

2. The advantage is the ability to deal with all of the unique kinds of circumferences which have not yet been defined as a pre-coordinated term

Chapter 11

Check Your Understanding 11.1

1. c
2. False
3. c
4. b
5. a. Route: Continuous IV infusion
   b. Form: Enteric-coated tablet

Check Your Understanding 11.2

1. d
   a
   e
   c
   b
2. e
   d
   a
   c
   b

Check Your Understanding 11.3

1. a, c, d
2. a, b, c, d, e
3. d
4. True
5. c

Check Your Understanding 11.4

1. f
   c
   g
   a
   e
   d
   b
2. a
3. a

Check Your Understanding 11.5

1. True
2. True
3. False
4. True
5. True
6. False
7. True
8. False
9. True

Chapter 12

Check Your Understanding 12.1

1. b
2. c

Check Your Understanding 12.2

1. b. NIC is used for intervention classification, and NOC is used to classify outcomes.
2. d

Check Your Understanding 12.3

1. d
2. c

Check Your Understanding 12.4

1. True
2. d
3. a

Chapter 13

Check Your Understanding 13.1

1. The site of origin of the neoplasm
2. True
3. False

Check Your Understanding 13.2

1. False
2. a.   Malignant, primary site
   b.   Uncertain whether benign or malignant
   c.   Malignant, metastatic site

d.   Carcinoma in situ
e.   Malignant, primary site
f.   Benign

3.   C21.1

Check Your Understanding 13.3

1.   Histologic grading or differentiation
2.   5
3.   False

Check Your Understanding 13.4

1.   True
2.   False
3.   d

Check Your Understanding 13.5

1.   a
2.   False
3.   c
4.   b
5.   True

Chapter 14

Check Your Understanding 14.1

1.   b
2.   False
3.   b
4.   False
5.   b

Check Your Understanding 14.2

1.   a
2.   True
3.   b
4.   False

Check Your Understanding 14.3

1.   a
2.   True
3.   True
4.   c
5.   b

Check Your Understanding 14.4

1.   c
2.   False
3.   d

Check Your Understanding 14.5

1.   False
2.   a
3.   c
4.   False
5.   c

Check Your Understanding 14.6

1.   True
2.   True
3.   World Health Organization

Check Your Understanding 14.7

1.   True
2.   False
3.   ICDIH
4.   False. Environmental factors also include social and attitudinal environmental factors.

Check Your Understanding 14.8

1.   True
2.   False
3.   True
4.   True

Check Your Understanding 14.9

1.   c
2.   d
3.   True

Chapter 15

Check Your Understanding 15.1

1.   c
2.   Data dictionary
3.   True

Check Your Understanding 15.2

1. False
2. a
3. c

Check Your Understanding 15.3

1. True
2. d
3. c
4. b
5. True

Check Your Understanding 15.4

1. c
2. d
3. c

Check Your Understanding 15.5

1. d
2. c

Check Your Understanding 15.6

1. a
2. False

Check Your Understanding 15.7

1. False
2. a

Chapter 16

Check Your Understanding 16.1

1. c
2. False
3. b

Check Your Understanding 16.2

1. c
2. False
3. b

Check Your Understanding 16.3

1. True
2. b
3. False

Check Your Understanding 16.4

1. a
2. d
3. True

Check Your Understanding 16.5

1. d
2. d
3. False

Chapter 17

Check Your Understanding 17.1

1. d
2. False
3. False

Chapter 18

Check Your Understanding 18.1

1. False
2. a

Check Your Understanding 18.2

1. c
2. False
3. True

Appendix B
Glossary

ABC codes: A registered vocabulary of HL7 incorporated into the National Library of Medicine's Unified Medical Language System in 1998, which describes the procedures, treatments, and services provided during encounters with complementary and alternative medicine, nursing, and other integrative healthcare providers

Accredited Standards Committee (ASC) X12N: The subcommittee for insurance and insurance-related business processes that develops and maintains X12 EDI and Extensible Markup Language (XML) standards, standards interpretations, and standards guidelines

Alternative Link: The original developer of the ABC codes

American Dental Association (ADA): A professional dental association dedicated to the public's oral health, ethics, science, and professional advancement

American Medical Association (AMA): The national professional membership organization for physicians that distributes scientific information to its members and the public, informs members of legislation related to health and medicine, and represents the medical profession's interests in national legislative matters

American National Standards Institute (ANSI): The agency that coordinates the development of voluntary standards to increase global competitiveness in a variety of industries, including healthcare

American Psychiatric Association (APA): A medical specialty society with more than 35,000 member physicians in the United States and abroad who work together to ensure humane care and effective treatment for all persons with mental disorders

America's Health Insurance Plans (AHIP): A national trade association representing companies providing health benefits to Americans; formerly known as the Health Insurance Association of America (HIAA)

Attributes: Properties or characteristics of concepts; used in SNOMED CT to characterize and define concepts

Blue Cross/Blue Shield Association (BCBSA): The national association of state and local Blue Cross and Blue Shield healthcare insurance plans

Carriers (Medicare Part B): Financial agents that serve under contract with the Centers for Medicare and Medicaid Services to work with providers and the federal government to locally administer Medicare Part B claims. See also Medicare Administrative Contractors

Catalog name: *See* product trade name

Centers for Medicare and Medicaid Services (CMS): The division of the Department of Health and Human Services that is responsible for developing healthcare policy in the U.S. and for administering the Medicare program and the federal portion of the Medicaid program; called the Health Care Financing Administration (HCFA) prior to 2001

Classification: A system that arranges or organizes like or related entities; also, a system for assigning numeric or alphanumeric code to represent specific diseases and/or procedures

Clinical Data Abstraction Centers (CDACs): Independent review firms contracted by the Centers for Medicare and Medicaid Services to perform data collection

Clinical drug: A pharmaceutical product given to, or taken by, a patient with a therapeutic or diagnostic intent

Clinical Hierarchy: In MEDCIN, the structure that leads clinicians to document from less detail to more precision

Clinical proposition: According to the developer of the MEDCIN system, "a phrase containing a unique intellectual clinical content" (Goltra 1997)

Clinical terminology: A set of standardized terms and their synonyms that record patient findings, circumstances, events, and interventions with sufficient detail to support clinical care, decision support, outcomes research, and quality improvement

Clinical Terms Version 3 (CTV3): A crown copyright work of the National Health Service in the United Kingdom that comprises a coded terminology designed to facilitate the exchange, retrieval, and analysis of key data in the medical record; formerly known as the Read Codes

Code Revision Committee: The entity responsible for updating Current Dental Terminology

Code Set: Under HIPAA, any set of codes used to encode data elements, such as tables of terms, medical concepts, medical diagnostic codes, or medical procedure codes; includes both the codes and their descriptions

Coding: The process of translating descriptions of diseases, injuries, and procedures into numeric or alphanumeric designations

Coding Clinic for ICD-9-CM: A publication issued quarterly by the American Hospital Association and approved by the Centers for Medicare and Medicaid Services to give coding advice and direction

College of American Pathologists (CAP): A medical specialty organization of board-certified pathologists that was until April 2007 the owner of SNOMED CT

Comité Européen de Normalisation (CEN), or European Committee for Standardization: Consisting of the national standards bodies in Europe as well as associates representing broad industrial sectors and social and economic partners, they adopt European Standards and other formal documents that promote free trade, the safety of workers and consumers, interoperability of networks, environmental protection, exploitation of research and development programs, and public procurement

Complementary and alternative medicine (CAM): A group of diverse medical and healthcare systems, practices, and products that are not presently considered to be part of conventional medicine (National Center for Complementary and Alternative Medicine 2009)

Computer-based Patient Record Institute (CPRI): A private organization founded in 1992 to develop a strategy to support the development and adoption of computer-based patient records; incorporated into an operating unit within HIMSS in 1992

Concept: A unique unit of knowledge or thought created by a unique combination of characteristics

Concept orientation: Term referring to the fact that concepts in a controlled medical terminology are based on meanings, not words

Concept permanence: Term referring to the fact that a code representing a concept in a controlled medical terminology is not reused and thus meanings do not change

Concept unique identifier (CUI): An identifier that serves to preserve the meanings, concept names, and relationships in the UMLS Metathesaurus

Consolidated Health Informatics (CHI): A government initiative that adopts standards for domains related to health information for federal health data systems, facilitating communication among all federal health agencies

Controlled medical terminology: A coded vocabulary of medical concepts and expressions used in healthcare

Controlled vocabulary: A restricted set of phrases, generally enumerated in a list and perhaps arranged into a hierarchy (Hardiker and Casey 2000)

Cooperating Parties for ICD-9-CM: A group of four organizations (the American Health Information Management Association, the American Hospital Association, the Centers for Medicare and Medicaid Services, and the National Center for Health Statistics) that collaborates in the development and maintenance of ICD-9-CM coding guidelines

CPT Editorial Panel: The 17-member group that has oversight responsibility for the update and revision of Category I and II CPT codes

Council on Dental Benefit Programs: The group responsible for developing a standard set of codes describing dental procedures, which led to CDT-1

Counseling: A discussion by the physician of one or more of the following topics: diagnostic results and impressions, prognosis, risks and benefits of management, instruction for management, importance of compliance, risk factor reduction, and patient and family education

Current Dental Terminology (CDT): A coding system developed to report services performed by the dental profession; formerly called the Uniform Code on Dental Procedures and Nomenclature

Current Procedural Terminology® (CPT®): A comprehensive list of descriptive terms and codes published by the American Medical Association and used for reporting diagnostic and therapeutic procedures and other medical services performed by physicians

Data dictionary: A descriptive list of data elements to be collected in an information system or database

Data element domain: A specification (list or range) of the valid, allowable values that can be assigned for each data element in a data set

Data Elements for Emergency Department Systems (DEEDS): A collection of data elements designed to provide uniform specifications for information that emergency departments may use in their record systems

Data set: A list of recommended data elements with uniform definitions

Dental codes: Codes used for billing for dental procedures, classified in the Current Procedural Terminology (CPT)

Department of Health and Human Services (HHS): A cabinet-level agency that oversees all the health and human services-related activities of the federal government

Derived classification: One based on a reference classification such as ICD or ICF by adopting the reference classification structure and categories and providing additional detail or through rearrangement or aggregation of items from one or more reference classifications

Description: In a controlled medical vocabulary, the combination of a concept and a term

Descriptive text: One component of the DSM, text that describes mental disorders under the following headings: Diagnostic Features; Subtypes and/or Specifiers; Recording Procedures; Associated Features and Disorders; Specific Culture, Age, and Gender Features; Prevalence, Course, Familial Pattern, and Differential Diagnosis

Descriptor: Wording that represents the official definition of an item or service that can be billed using a particular code

Designated standards maintenance organization (DSMO): A category of organization established by the Health Insurance Portability and Accountability Act to maintain the electronic transaction standards mandated by HIPAA

***Diagnostic and Statistical Manual of Mental Disorders* (DSM):** A nomenclature to standardize the diagnostic process for patients with psychiatric disorders, which includes codes that correspond to ICD-9-CM codes; most recent version is fourth edition (text revision), or DSM-IV-TR, published in 2000

Diagnostic classification: A listing of all the disorders, diagnostic codes, subtypes, specifiers, and notes that are unique to a system such as DSM-IV

Diagnostic criteria: Extensive diagnostic criteria that indicate what symptoms must be present and not present for a patient to meet the qualifications for a particular mental diagnosis

Differentiation: The degree to which a tumor resembles the normal tissue from which it arose

Digital Imaging and Communications in Medicine (DICOM): A standard for the interchange of computerized biomedical images and image-related information within and between healthcare providers

Documentation paradigm: A disease-specific format developed by the individual provider for the purpose of establishing standard clinical documentation forms

Domain: A sphere or field of activity and influence

Dose form: The form in which a drug is administered to a patient as opposed to the form in which the manufacturer supplied it

Drug Component: The elements that together constitute the clinical drug

Drug knowledge base: Similar to a drug terminology but enables clinical screening and provides integrated and referential knowledge

Drug Listing Act 1972: The act that amended the Food, Drug, and Cosmetic Act so that drug estab-lishments engaged in the manufacture, preparation, propagation, compounding, or processing of a drug are required to register their establishments and list all their commercially marketed drug products with the Food and Drug Administration

DSM-IV-TR: *See Diagnostic and Statistical Manual of Mental Disorders* (DSM)

Durable medical equipment (DME): Medical equipment designed for long-term use in the home, including eyeglasses, hearing aids, surgical appliances and supplies, orthotics and prostheses, and bulk and cylinder oxygen

ECRI: An independent, nonprofit, health services research agency established to promote safety, quality, and cost-effectiveness in healthcare to benefit patient care through research, publishing, education, and consultation; formerly called the Emergency Care Research Institute

EHR system (EHR-S): A system that ensures the longitudinal collection of electronic health information for and about persons; enables immediate electronic access to person- and population-level information by authorized users; provides knowledge and decision support that enhance the quality, safety, and efficiency of patient care; and supports efficient processes for healthcare delivery

Electronic data interchange (EDI): A standard transmission format using strings of data for business information communicated among the computer systems of independent organizations

Electronic health record (EHR): A health record in an information system designed to provide access to complete and accurate clinical data, practitioner alerts and reminders, clinical decision support systems, and links to medical knowledge

Electronic prescribing (e-Rx): When a prescription is written from the personal digital assistant and an electronic fax or when an actual electronic data interchange transaction is generated that transmits the prescription directly to the retail pharmacy's information system

Essential Medical Data Set (EMDS): A standardized medical history data set containing the data elements for demographics, problem lists, medications, allergies, and previous critical encounters

Etiology axis: The cause of the disease or injury

Evaluation and management (E/M) codes: CPT codes that describe patient encounters with healthcare professionals for assessment counseling and other routine healthcare services

Fiscal intermediary (FI): An organization that contracts with CMS to serve as the financial agent between providers and the federal government in the local administration of Medicare Part A claims. See also Medicare Administrative Contractors

Food and Drug Administration (FDA): Federal agency responsible for protecting the public health by ensuring the safety, efficacy, and security of human and veterinary drugs, biological products, medical devices, the nation's food supply, cosmetics, and products that emit radiation

Food, Drug, and Cosmetic Act (FDCA): The basic authority intended to ensure that foods are pure and wholesome, safe to eat, and produced under sanitary conditions; that drugs and devices are safe and effective for their intended uses; that cosmetics are safe and made from appropriate ingredients; and that all labeling and packaging is truthful, informative, and not deceptive

Formulary: A listing of drugs classified by therapeutic category or disease class

Fully specified name: In SNOMED CT, the unique text assigned to a concept that completely describes it

Generic device group: The actual nomenclature or naming level by which a product or a group of similar products can be classified in the Global Medical Dictionary Nomenclature using a selected generic descriptor and its unique code

Global Assessment of Functioning (GAF) Scale: A 100-point tool rating overall psychological, social, and occupational functioning of individuals, excluding physical and environmental impairment

Global Medical Device Nomenclature (GMDN): A collection of internationally-recognized terms used to describe and catalog medical devices, in particular, the products used in the diagnosis, prevention, monitoring, treatment, or alleviation of disease or injury in humans

Granularity: Level of detail

HCPCS level I: Current Procedural Terminology, developed by the American Medical Association

HCPCS level II: Codes not covered by CPT and modifiers that can be used with all levels of codes, developed by the Centers for Medicare and Medicaid Services

HCPCS level III: Codes, often called local codes, developed by local Medicare and/or Medicaid carriers for use in their particular geographic locations; eliminated on December 31, 2003

Health Insurance Portability and Accountability Act (HIPAA): The federal legislation enacted to provide continuity of health coverage, control fraud and abuse in healthcare, reduce healthcare costs, and guarantee the security and privacy of health information

Health Level Seven (HL7): An organization, accredited by the American National Standards Institute, that develops standards regarding clinical and administrative data

Healthcare Common Procedure Coding System (HCPCS): A two-level classification system introduced in 1983 to standardize the coding systems used to process Medicare and Medicaid claims

Healthcare Information Technology Standards Panel (HITSP): An organization developed under the auspices of the American National Standards Institute (ANSI) to address interoperability in healthcare by harmonizing health information technology standards.

Histology: The study of the microscopic structure of tissue

ICD-9-CM Coordination and Maintenance Committee: Committee composed of representatives from the National Center for Health Statistics

(NCHS) and the Centers for Medicare and Medicaid Services (CMS) that is responsible for maintaining the United States' clinical modification version of the International Classification of Diseases, 9th revision (ICD-9-CM) code sets; holds open meetings that serve as a public forum for discussing (but not making decisions about) proposed revisions to ICD-9-CM

ICD-10-CM/PCS Coordination and Maintenance Committee: A body to be formed to follow the same procedures currently used by the ICD-9-CM Coordination and Maintenance Committee to consider new codes and revisions to existing codes

ICNP Catalogues: A set of precoordinated statements being developed by the International Council of Nurses that will consist of subsets of nursing diagnoses, interventions, and outcomes for a specific area of practice

Informaticians: Individuals in a field of study (informatics) that focuses on the use of technology to improve access to, and utilization of, information

Information model: A model that combines the elements necessary to fully represent the meaning of clinical information and that supports semantic interoperability among the heterogeneous computer-based systems that form an integrated information system

Institute of Electrical and Electronics Engineers Standards Association (IEEE-SA): An activity of the IEEE that develops standards in a broad range of industries including healthcare

Intelligent prompting®: A means in tables and forms for displaying only clinically relevant items

International Classification for Nursing Practice® (ICNP®): A "unified nursing language system into which nursing terminologies can be cross-mapped for designated purposes" (Coenen 2003)

International Classification of Diseases—Oncology (ICD-O): A classification system used for reporting incidences of malignant disease

International Classification of Diseases, Ninth Revision, Clinical Modification (ICD-9-CM): A classification system used in the United States to report morbidity information

International Classification of Diseases, Tenth Revision (ICD-10): The most recent revision of the disease classification system developed and used by the World Health Organization to track morbidity and mortality information worldwide

International Classification of External Causes of Injury (ICECI): One of the WHO Family of International Classifications (WHO-FIC), this classification includes external causes but not injuries and is related to ICD-10 chapter XX, External causes of morbidity and mortality

International Classification of Function, Disability, and Health (ICF): A classification system released by the World Health Organization in 2001 that describes how people live with their health conditions

International Classification of Impairments, Disabilities, and Handicaps (ICIDH): Published by the World Health Organization to measure the consequences of disease and divided into three classifications: impairments, disabilities, and handicaps; the precursor to ICF

International Classification of Primary Care (ICPC): A classification system for patient data related to general and family practice and primary care

International Conference on Harmonization of Technical Requirements for Registration of Pharmaceuticals for Human Use (ICH): A joint project established in 1990 that brought together the drug regulatory authorities of the European Union, Japan, and the United States, as well as representative associations of the pharmaceutical research-based industry in the three regions

International Council of Nurses (ICN): A federation of national nurses' associations representing millions of nurses worldwide that was instrumental in developing the International Classification for Nursing Practice

International Health Terminology Standards Development Organisation (IHTSDO): A nonprofit organization based in Denmark to which the responsibility for the ownership, maintenance, and distribution of SNOMED CT was transferred from the College of American Pathologists in April 2007

International Organization for Standardization (ISO): The world's largest developer of standards whose principal activity is the development of technical standards, which often have important economic and social repercussions

Interface terminology: A systemic collection of healthcare-related phrases or terms that supports clinicians' entry of patient-related information into computer programs

Interoperability: The ability of information technology systems, software applications, and networks to exchange and use information

IS-A relationships: Relationships that link concepts within a hierarchy

Labeler: Any firm that manufactures, repacks, or distributes a drug product

Lexicon: A collection of words or terms and their meanings for a particular domain, such as drug terms

Likert scale: A rating scale that presents a set of attitude statements with which subjects are asked to express agreement or disagreement on a five-point scale

Local codes: *See* HCPCS Level III

Logical Observation Identifiers, Names, and Codes® (LOINC®): A database protocol developed by the Regenstrief Institute for Health Care aimed at standardizing laboratory and clinical codes for use in clinical care, outcomes management, and research

LOINC committee: A voluntary group of interested experts organized by the Regenstrief Institute in 1994 to initiate the development of LOINC

Major drug class: A general therapeutic or pharmacological classification scheme for prescription drug products reported to the Food and Drug Administration under the provisions of the Drug Listing Act

Mapping: Creation of a cross-map that links the content from one classification or terminology scheme to another

MEDCIN®: A proprietary clinical terminology developed as a point-of-care tool for electronic medical record documentation at the time and place of patient care

Medical Dictionary for Regulatory Activities (MedDRA): A vocabulary developed within the regulatory environment as a pragmatic, clinically validated medical terminology with an emphasis on ease-of-use data entry, retrieval, analysis, and display, with a suitable balance between sensitivity and specificity

Medical Subjects Headings (MeSH): The National Library of Medicine's controlled vocabulary for indexing journal articles

Medicare Administrative Contractors (MACs): Medicare contract entities replacing Medicare Part A and Part B Fee-for-Service (FFS) claims payment contractors as a result of Medicare contract reform

MetamorphoSys: The installation wizard and customization program included in each release of the Unified Medical Language System

Metathesaurus®: The very large, multipurpose, and multilingual vocabulary database that is the central vocabulary component of the Unified Medical Language System

Minimum Data Set for Long-term Care (MDS): A core set of screening, clinical, and functional status elements, including common definitions and coding categories that Medicare- and/or Medicaid-certified nursing facilities must collect on nursing home residents

Miscellaneous codes: National codes that are used when a supplier is submitting a bill for an item or service that no existing national code describes

Modifier: A two-digit designation listed after a procedure code to indicate that a service was altered in some way from the stated CPT or HCPCS descriptor without changing the definition

Morbidity: The state of being diseased (including illness, injury, or deviation from normal health); the number of sick persons or cases of disease in relationship to a specific population

Morphology: The science of structure and form of organisms without regard to function

Morphology axis: Structural change in tissue

Mortality: The incidence of death in a specific population; also, the loss of subjects during the course of a clinical research study, which is also called attrition

Mortality Reference Group (MRG): A body established by WHO to make recommendations on mortality issues relating to ICD-10 to the WHO Updating and Revision Committee (URC)

Multiaxial: The ability of a nomenclature to express the meaning of a concept across several axes

Multiaxial system: An evaluation that involves a five-level assessment, with each level or axis evaluating a different domain of clinical information that can be used in prognosis and treatment planning

National Center for Health Statistics (NCHS): The federal agency responsible for collecting and disseminating information on health services utilization and the health status of the population in the United States; developed the clinical modification to the International Classification of Diseases, Ninth Revision (ICD-9) and is responsible for updating the diagnosis portion of the ICD-9-CM

National Committee on Vital and Health Statistics (NCVHS): A public policy advisory board that recommends policy to the National Center for Health Statistics and other health-related federal programs

National Council for Prescription Drug Programs (NCPDP): A not-for-profit ANSI-accredited SDO founded in 1977 that produces standards, implementation guides, and a data dictionary for data interchange and processing standards for pharmacy transactions

National Drug Code (NDC): A code set used for medical codes maintained and approved by the FDA; the code set designated by the Department of Health and Human Services for reporting drugs and biologics on standard retail pharmacy transactions

National Drug Code (NDC) Directory: The directory of the NDC system

National Drug File Reference Terminology (NDF-RT): A nonproprietary drug reference terminology that includes drug knowledge and classifies drugs, most notably, by mechanism of action and physiologic effect

Nomenclature: A systematic listing of proper names

Normalized: Conversion of various representational forms to standard expressions so that those that have the same meaning will be recognized by computer software as synonymous in a data search

Notice of Proposed Rulemaking (NPRM): A publication in which the federal government calls for public comments on policy, which the government then analyzes and uses to make any necessary changes published as a final rule in the *Federal Register*

Nursing informatics: The part of informatics designed for, and relevant to, nurses

Nursing Information and Data Set Evaluation Center (NIDSEC): An organization established by the American Nurses Association to review, evaluate against defined criteria, and recognize information systems from developers and manufacturers that support the documentation of nursing care within automated nursing information systems or computer-based patient record systems

Nursing Management Minimum Data Set (NMMDS): A data set that supports the description, analysis, and comparison of nursing care and nursing care resources with greater precision regarding the effects of context on complex healthcare outcomes

Nursing Minimum Data Set (NMDS): A minimum set of elements with uniform definitions and categories concerning the specific dimensions of nursing

Ontololgy: In information science, a common vocabulary organized by meaning, allowing for an understanding of the structure of descriptive information that facilitates interoperability

Outcomes and Assessment Information Set (OASIS): A core group of data elements that represent items of a comprehensive assessment for an adult home care patient

Package Code: The part of the National Drug Code that identifies package size

Patient Care Data Set (PCDS): A nursing vocabulary intended to provide standard terms for representing and capturing clinical data for patient care information systems

Patient medical record information (PMRI): Information about a single patient generated by healthcare professionals as a direct result of interaction with the patient, or with individuals who have personal knowledge of the patient, or both

Perioperative Nursing Dataset (PNDS): A data set developed by the Association of Perioperative Registered Nurses to identify the perioperative experience of the patient from preadmission to discharge

Permanent national codes: HCPCS level II codes that provide a standard coding system managed by private and public insurers

Physiologic effects: Cellular, tissue, or organ processes or functions altered by drugs

Post-coordination: Post-coordination describes representation of a clinical meaning using a combination of two or more codes. SNOMED CT allows many concepts to be represented in a post-coordinated form. One form of post-coordination involves creating a single expression consisting of several concepts related by attributes (IHTSDO 2008)

Pre-coordination: When a single concept identifier is used to represent a clinical idea. SNOMED CT also allows the use of post-coordinated expressions (see post-coordination) to represent a meaning using a combination of two or more concept identifiers. Including commonly used concepts in a pre-coordinated form makes the terminology easier to use (IHTSDO 2008)

Preferred term: In SNOMED CT, the description or name assigned to a concept that is used most commonly; in the UMNDS classification system, a representation of the generic product category, which is a list of preferred concepts that name devices

Product Code: The part of the National Drug Code that identifies a specific strength, dosage form, and formulation for a particular drug

Product trade name: Name (also referred to as catalog name) assigned or supplied by the labelers (firms) as required under the Food, Drug, and Cosmetic Act

Prospective payment system (PPS): A type of reimbursement system based on preset payment levels rather than actual charges billed after a service has been provided; specifically, one of several Medicare reimbursement systems based on predetermined payment rates or periods and linked to the anticipated intensity of services delivered as well as the beneficiary's condition

Read Codes: A comprehensive list of terms developed in the United Kingdom by the National Health Service Centre for Coding and Classification, which is used by healthcare professionals to describe and report the care and treatment of their patients; *See* Clinical Terms Version 3

Reasons for encounter (RFE): In the ICPC system, the reasons a patient sees a provider from the patient's viewpoint

Reference terminology: A set of concepts and relationships that provide a common reference point for comparisons and the aggregation of data about the entire healthcare process, recorded by multiple different individuals, systems, or institutions

Regenstrief Institute, Inc.: An internationally-respected, nonprofit, medical research organization associated with Indiana University, which initiated the development of LOINC

Regenstrief LOINC Mapping Assistant (RELMA): A free Microsoft Windows software download that provides LOINC users help in working with LOINC database files

Regenstrief Medical Records System (RMRS): One of the nation's first electronic medical record systems and the keystone of Regenstrief Institute activities

Related classification: Partially refers to a reference classification or is associated with the reference classification at specific levels of structure only and describes important aspects of health or the health system not covered by reference or derived classifications

Relationship: A type of connection between two terms

Relative value unit (RVU): A measurement that represents the value of the work involved in providing a specific professional medical service in relation to the value of the work involved in providing other medical services

Root concept: A single special concept that represents the root of the entire content in SNOMED CT

Routed generic: The combination of an active ingredient(s) or generic name, plus a route; useful in decision support functions for drug interactions to distinguish a topical drug, which may not interact with another drug, from its oral formulation, which may interact

Rubric: A category; in ICPC, the two digits following the first character of an ICPC code and representing the second axis, components

RxNorm: A nonproprietary terminology that represents drugs at the level of granularity needed to support clinical practice

RxNorm concept unique identifier (RXCUI): A numeric identifier in RxNorm that designates the same concept, regardless of the form of the name or the table in which it is located; also represents an opaque identifier found in the UMLS Metathesaurus

Semantic: Referring to the meaning of a word or term

Semantic branded drug: In RxNorm, the semantic clinical drug (SCD) with the brand name, i.e., <SCD> [Brand name]. For example, Amoxicillin 250 MG Oral Capsule [Amoxil]. Amoxil is the brand name.

Semantic data model (SDM): A natural application modeling mechanism that can capture and express the structure of an application environment

Semantic interoperability: Mutual understanding of the meaning of data exchanged between information systems

Semantic Network: The network that represents a consistent categorization of all concepts represented in the UMLS Metathesaurus

Semantic normal form (SNF): The preferred term for clinical drugs in RxNorm

Semicolon: A punctuation mark [;] placed after a procedure description within a CPT code set to avoid repeating common information

Separate procedure: A procedure that is commonly part of another, more complex procedure, but that may be performed independently or otherwise unrelated to the other procedure (CPT)

SNF clinical formulation or semantic clinical drug (SCD): One of the two types of semantic normal forms created in RxNorm for every clinical drug; consists of components and a dose form

SNF drug component or semantic clinical drug component (SCDC): One of the two types of semantic normal forms created in RxNorm for every clinical drug; consists of an active ingredient and strength

SOAP: An acronym for a component of the problem-oriented medical record, which refers to how each progress note contains documentation relative to **s**ubjective observations, **o**bjective observations, **a**ssessments, and **p**lans

SPECIALIST Lexicon: A tool that supplies the lexical information needed for the SPECIALIST natural language processing system

Standards development organization (SDO): A private or governmental organization involved in the development of healthcare informatics standards at a national or international level

Surgical package: A global package for surgical procedures that refers to the payment policy of bundling payment for the various services associated with a surgery into a single payment covering professional services for preoperative care, the surgery itself, and postoperative care

Systematized Nomenclature of Dentistry (SNODENT): A comprehensive taxonomy that contains codes for identifying not only diseases and diagnoses, but also anatomy, conditions, morphology, and social factors that may affect health or treatment

Systematized Nomenclature of Medicine Clinical Terms® (SNOMED CT®): A systematized, multiaxial, and hierarchically organized controlled terminology developed by the College of American Pathologists and currently owned by the International Health Terminology Standards Development Organisation

Taxonomy: The study of the general principles of scientific classification

Temporary national codes: Codes that give insurers the flexibility to establish codes that are needed before the next January 1 annual update for permanent national codes

Term type (TTY): Each element of the normalized term in RxNorm

Terminology: A set of terms representing the system of concepts of a particular subject field

Topography: Description of a part of the body

Transmission standards: Standards that support the uniform format and sequence of data during transmission from one healthcare entity to another; also referred to as communication, messaging, and transaction standards

UMLS Knowledge Source Server (UMLSKS): The tool that provides Internet access to the Knowledge Sources and other related resources made available by developers using the Unified Medical Language System

Unified Medical Language System® (UMLS®): A program initiated by the National Library of Medicine to build an intelligent, automated system that can understand biomedical concepts, words, and expressions and their interrelationships; includes concepts and terms from many different source vocabularies

Unified Medical Language System (UMLS) Metathesaurus: A list containing information on biomedical concepts and terms from more than 100 healthcare vocabularies and classifications, administrative health data, bibliographic and full-text databases, and expert systems

Uniform Ambulatory Care Data Set (UACDS): A core set of data elements for reporting ambulatory data elements in a standardized manner; created through the work of the National Committee on Vital and Health Statistics

Uniform Hospital Discharge Data Set (UHDDS): A core set of data elements collected by acute care short-term stay (usually less than thirty days) hospitals to report inpatient data elements in a standardized manner

Universal Medical Device Nomenclature System (UMDNS): A standard international nomenclature and computer coding system for medical devices; developed by ECRI

Updating and Revision Committee (URC): A body established by WHO in 2000 to recommend mortality and morbidity changes to ICD-10, manage the ICD-10 update process, and recommend changes to the Heads of WHO Collaborating Centres each year

URU principle: The guiding principle for modeling concepts in SNOMED CT that states that all concepts must be understandable, reproducible, and useful

Vocabulary: A list or collection of clinical words or phrases with their meanings; also, the set of words used by an individual or group within a particular subject field

WHO Family of International Classifications (WHO-FIC): The group of classifications promoted by the World Health Organization as being appropriate for use in health settings throughout the world

Wonca International Classification Committee (WICC): The current name of the Wonca Classification Committee, the group that designed the International Classification of Primary Care

World Health Organization (WHO): The United Nations specialized agency created to ensure the attainment by all peoples of the highest possible level of health; the international organization responsible for a number of international classifications, including *The International Statistical Classification of Diseases and Related Health Problems* (ICD-10) and *The International Classification of Functioning, Disability and Health* (ICF)

World Organization of Family Doctors (Wonca): The organization instrumental in the development of the International Classification of Primary Care; formerly called the World Organization of National Colleges, Academics, and Academic Associations of General Practitioners/Family Physicians (Wonca)

References

American Medical Association. 2009. *Current Procedural Terminology (CPT),* fourth edition. Chicago: American Medical Association.

Coenen, A. 2003. The International Classification for Nursing Practice (ICNP) Programme: Advancing a unifying framework for nursing. *Online Journal of Issues in Nursing.*

Goltra, Peter S. 1997. *MEDCIN: A New Nomenclature for Clinical Medicine.* New York City: Springer Verlag.

Hardiker, N.R., Hoy, D., Casey, A. Standards for nursing terminology. *Journal of the American Medical Informatics Association,* 7:6,523–528.

International Health Terminology Standards Development Organisation. 2008. SNOMED Clinical Terms User Guide. http://www.ihtsdo.org/fileadmin/user_upload/Docs_01/SNOMED_CT_Publications/SNOMED_CT_User_Guide_20080731.pdf.

National Center for Complementary and Alternative Medicine 2009. http://nccam.nih.gov/health/whatiscam/.

Index